BRITISH HERBAL PHARMACOPOEIA

1996

BRITISH HERBAL PHARMACOPOEIA 1996

Published by the
BRITISH HERBAL MEDICINE ASSOCIATION

and completely revised by its
SCIENTIFIC COMMITTEE

Copyright © 1996 British Herbal Medicine Association

ISBN 0 903032 10 4

1st edition, Section One 1971
1st edition, Section Two 1972
1st edition, Section Three 1974
1st consolidated edition (comprising Sections One, Two and Three) 1974

2nd edition, Part 1 1976
2nd edition Part, 2 1979
Part 1 Reprinted 1980
2nd edition Part 3, 1981
2nd consolidated edition (comprising Parts 1, 2 and 3) 1983
Reprinted 1987, 1989, 1991, 1995

3rd edition (abridged) 1990

4th edition 1996

British Library Cataloguing-in-Publication Data
A Catalogue Record for this Book is available from the British Library

Compiled and typeset by
Martin J. Willoughby and Simon Y. Mills
University of Exeter, Exeter.
Printed and bound in Great Britain by
Biddles Ltd, Guildford and King's Lynn

CONTENTS

Lucerne

Marigold
Marshmallow Leaf
Marshmallow Root
Maté
Matricaria Flower
Meadowsweet
Melilot
Milk Thistle Fruit
Mistletoe Herb
Motherwort
Mugwort
Mullein Leaf
Myrrh

Nettle Herb
Nettle Root

Oak Bark

Parsley Herb
Parsley Root
Passiflora
Peppermint Leaf

Pilewort Herb
Poke Root
Prickly Ash Bark
Psyllium Seed
Pulsatilla
Pumpkin Seed

Quassia
Queen's Delight

Raspberry Leaf
Red Clover Flower
Rhatany Root
Rhubarb
Roman Chamomile Flower
Rosemary Leaf

Sage Leaf
Sarsaparilla
Saw Palmetto Fruit
Senega Root
Senna Fruit, Alexandrian
Senna Fruit, Tinnevelly
Senna Leaf
Shepherd's Purse

Skullcap
Slippery Elm Bark
Squill
Squill, Indian
St. John's Wort
Stramonium Leaf

Thyme

Valerian Root
Vervain
Violet Leaf

White Deadnettle
White Horehound
Wild Carrot
Wild Cherry Bark
Wild Lettuce
Wild Thyme
Wild Yam
Willow Bark
Wormwood

Yarrow

PREFACE

The British Herbal Pharmacopoeia 1996 provides monographs of quality standards for 169 herbs commonly used in the United Kingdom for the preparation of botanical drugs.

Following the success of the British Herbal Pharmacopoeia 1990 and after numerous requests for inclusion of additional plants, the British Herbal Medicine Association took the decision to review the current 84 monographs and add a further 85 to produce a fully revised and updated 1996 volume.

As time advances, more herbal materials have been included in official pharmacopoeias and to avoid duplication of work, some of the monographs in this volume have been abbreviated, making reference to the official monograph where appropriate.

Particular attention has been paid to developing thin layer chromatographic techniques for comparative identification of the new botanical drugs. TLC identities developed for the BHP 1990 have proved very successful and these methods have been improved and updated wherever possible. All of the TLC methods have been designed to be within the scope of the average wet chemical laboratory; complex procedures and the need for a wide range of chemical markers were deliberately avoided.

Physical specifications for the new herbs were determined by extensive consultation with the industry, medical herbalists and academics to arrive at what is a realistic control specification which assures quality without excluding perfectly satisfactory material of commerce.

Quantitative analysis for active principles has not been included in the monographs because in most cases it is not possible to determine individually active components within a herb. Herbs are composed of a complex and synergistic mixture of active compounds which rarely have the same potency when isolated.

The monograph format employed for the BHP 1990 has been retained along with descriptions of powdered material and material of commerce and a brief reference to the action of the herb.

The task of producing this revised and updated volume was entrusted to the Scientific Committee of the British Herbal Medicine Association, a group of dedicated and enthusiastic volunteers, who have given much time and effort in the production of this work. Thanks are due to their employers who, in many cases, have allowed the time for meetings and research work.

As with previous editions of the BHP, consultant pharmacognocists have been employed to produce the macroscopical and microscopical descriptions for each full monograph, and chromatography specialists have been used to develop the TLC methods.

It is hoped that this revised and updated volume will be used to enhance further the quality of plant material used in the manufacture of herbal medicines by ensuring specificity and purity whilst being realistic in its requirements.

P. Wetton
Chairman, BHMA Scientific Committee

THE BRITISH HERBAL MEDICINE ASSOCIATION

The BHMA was founded in 1964 to advance the science and practice of herbal medicine in the United Kingdom and to ensure its continued statutory recognition at a time when all medicines were becoming subject to greater regulatory control.

Following the Medicines Act 1968 the legislative detail applicable to herbal medicines increased substantially. During the 1980s, as part of the EC Review of Medicines, all UK manufacturers were required to complete a thorough technical appraisal of their products and to provide evidence on quality, safety and efficacy to the Department of Health.

Throughout these years the BHMA has supported the interests of its members with advice and comment on legislation and by providing essential scientific information - of which the British Herbal Pharmacopoeia and British Herbal Compendium are notable examples.

Members of the BHMA include companies involved in the manufacture of herbal medicines or supply of botanical drugs, herbal practitioners, academics, pharmacists, students of phytotherapy and many others. The BHMA Board is representative of these interests and includes four Members with over 30 years of outstanding service to the Association.

In 1989 the BHMA became a founder-member of ESCOP, the European Scientific Co-operative for Phytotherapy, together with comparable organisations from Belgium, France, Germany the Netherlands and Switzerland. The aims of ESCOP are to advance the status of herbal medicines throughout Europe and to assist with harmonisation of their regulatory status at the European level. To date, ESCOP represents a total of 11 countries.

THE BHMA SCIENTIFIC COMMITTEE

From its inception, the BHMA recognised a need for the improved specification of botanical drugs, particularly those not described in official pharmacopoeias.

The Scientific Committee was formed in 1965 and its work led to publication of the first monographs of the British Herbal Pharmacopoeia, as Section One, in 1971. Section Two followed in 1972 and Section Three in 1974.

With this foundation the Scientific Committee embarked on an enlarged edition. Updated monographs from 1974 were published as Part 1 in 1976, additional monographs were introduced as Part 2 in 1979 and Part 3 in 1981 - a total of 232 monographs and the culmination of 16 years of study, involving many distinguished contributors, under the Chairmanship of Mr. F. Fletcher-Hyde. With minor amendments the monographs were published in a unified edition as the British Herbal Pharmacopoeia 1983, under the Chairmanship of Mr. H. W. Mitchell.

After preparatory work during the mid-1980s, the Scientific Committee convened in December 1987, with Mr. P. R. Bradley as Chairman, to proceed with a fully revised edition of the Pharmacopoeia. The culmination of this work was the publication of the BHP 1990 which included 84 monographs in an updated format. As with other pharmacopoeia, quality standards were of prime importance with less emphasis placed on therapeutics. Therapeutic data was presented in a separate volume, The British Herbal Compendium, edited by Mr. P. R. Bradley and published in 1992.

The present Committee chaired by Mr. P. Wetton, is fortunate to include past Chairmen, representatives from industry, academia and the herbal professions. Dr. Betty Jackson, who served on the Committee from 1976 to 1983, has also contributed to the volume.

6

MEMBERS OF THE SCIENTIFIC COMMITTEE

Peter Wetton BSc CChem FRSC FIQA   Chairman

Technical Manager,
G. R. Lane Health Products Limited.

Peter R. Bradley MSc CChem FRSC

Development Manager,
Whitehall International.

Sheila E. Drew BPharm PhD MRPharmS

Quality Assurance Manager,
William Ransom & Son plc.

Simon Y. Mills MA MCPP FNIMH

Director, Centre for Complementary Health Studies,
University of Exeter.

Hugh W. Mitchell HonMNIMH

President, British Herbal Medicine Association
Managing Director,
Mitchfield Botanics Limited.

Arnold R. Webster CChem MRSC

Technical Manager,
Peter Black Healthcare Limited.

Martin J. Willoughby BSc PhD

Research Fellow, Centre for Complementary Health Studies,
University of Exeter.

Hein H. Zeylstra MCPP

Principal, The School of Phytotherapy,
Bucksteep Manor, Bodle Street Green, Hailsham.

ACKNOWLEDGEMENTS

Many individuals and organisations have contributed to the production of the British Herbal Pharmacopoeia 1996 and grateful thanks are extended to the following:

The consultant pharmacognosists Dr Betty P. Jackson, Mr Derek W. Snowdon and Ms Janet Peck for the time and effort spent preparing and checking macroscopical and microscopical descriptions.

Member of the Scientific Committee Dr Martin J. Willoughby for his work in producing and testing the TLC methods, for the mammoth task of compiling the draft monographs and preparing the publication for press.

Mention should be made of those companies who made laboratory facilities and staff available, providing ongoing technical and administrative support to the project:

> University of Exeter, G. R. Lane Health Products Limited,
> Mitchfield Botanics Limited, Peter Black Healthcare Limited,
> Whitehall International, and William Ransom & Son plc.

Invaluable assistance was also provided by the following organisations and the BHMA Scientific Committee would like to record their gratitude to all who unfailingly responded to requests for samples and quantitative data:

> H. Ambrosius GmbH., Dixa AG., Flachsmann GmbH.,
> Mitchfield Botanics Ltd., Paul Muggenburg GmbH & Co.,
> Potters Herbal Supplies Ltd., William Ransom & Son plc,
> Slater & Frith Ltd., and Whyte Chemicals Ltd.

Grateful thanks are extended to Mrs Hillary Judd of the British Pharmacopoeia Commission for her help and advice, and the European Pharmacopoeia Commission, and the Controller of Her Majesty's Stationery Office for permission to reproduce extracts from official texts.

The BHMA Scientific Committee would like to thank Paul Shelton for his help with the preparation and evaluation of thin-layer chromatograms, Penelope Jackson for her untiring work in word processing the monographs, and all the staff of Biological Sciences (Hatherly Laboratories), University of Exeter, for their support, particularly Anna Davey and Neville Barratt.

Also, thanks are extended to the laboratory staff of G.R. Lane Health Products Ltd.,especially Paul Henly, for testing some of the TLC methods.

FOREWORD

This new edition of the British Herbal Pharmacopoeia (BHP) will be welcomed by everyone who is concerned about the quality of medicinal herbs and will be particularly of interest to manufacturers of herbal products and medical herbalists. There is a continuing and ever increasing demand for herbal remedies by the public despite the many pharmaceutical preparations which are available for the treatment of disease. Consumer groups, regulatory agencies and academics have continued to demand that herbs used for medicinal purposes should be of high standard, free from contaminants and of reliable batch-to-batch quality.

The new expanded edition of the BHP contains monographs on 169 medicinal herbs and herbal materials. 85 of these monographs have been added since the previous edition. Over recent years, the European Pharmacopoeia has produced monographs on some medicinal herbs and where these or monographs in the British Pharmacopoeia exist the BHP provides only an abbreviated monograph. However, for the majority of herbs included in this volume of the BHP there are no published European Pharmacopoeia or British Pharmacopoeia monographs. The Scientific Committee of the BHMA are to be congratulated on providing modern monographs for many of the medicinal herbs which are currently available to the general public in the UK.

What is included in these monographs? Each herb is clearly identified by its pharmaceutical name, binomial Latin name and family in addition to its common name and synonyms. The plant part used is indicated and in some instances harvesting details and geographical sources are given because these may well affect the yield and nature of the therapeutic constituents. Detailed macroscopical and microscopical descriptions are provided, in many cases by new examination of currently available commercial samples. Microscopical descriptions are particularly important for assessing the identification and quality of medicinal herbs which may occur either in broken fragments or in powdered form. Each herb is characterised by a simple thin-layer chromatographic (TLC) identification test. The exact conditions for carrying out such tests are described. The TLC provides a "fingerprint" of defining constituents and occasionally highlights characteristic compounds. In general, there are no specified quantitative assessments for active ingredients although these are available for those herbs which are the subject of either European Pharmacopoeia or British Pharmacopoeia monographs.

Quantitative standards have been set for the majority of herbs in terms of acceptable limits for foreign matter, total ash, ash insoluble in hydrochloric acid and water, or alcohol extractable material. A brief statement of therapeutic action is given in each monograph, but further detailed information is provided by the British Herbal Compendium which is the sister volume to the BHP.

Other standards utilised for quality assurance of medicinal herbs such as permitted levels of microbial contamination, toxic elements, pesticides, mycotoxins, fumigants or radioactive residues are not defined in the individual monographs. The section on General Notices discusses such requirements and references are supplied to official EC and UK guidelines for Quality of Herbal Remedies.

Adequate quality assurance is the cornerstone by which the public may be guaranteed that the medicinal herbs which they demand do not contain ingredients which may be toxic or have different therapeutic action. The new edition of the BHP goes a long way to provide adequate standards for the quality of a substantial number of the medicinal herbs which are used in the UK.

Professor J. D. Phillipson MSc, PhD, DSc, FRPharmS, FLS
Emeritus Professor of Pharmacognosy
The School of Pharmacy, University of London

INTRODUCTION

25 years have passed since the first monographs of the British Herbal Pharmacopoeia (BHP) were published in 1971. The foresight of the BHMA Board in initiating a pharmacopoeia devoted entirely to plant drugs and the enterprise and meticulous work of the BHMA Scientific Committee in producing the first and second editions continue to provide inspiration to others who follow in their footsteps. The unified second edition published in 1983 is now a classic, still in print and in demand around the world for the wide range of materials it includes and its unique and concise therapeutic information.

In 1990 significant changes in format were introduced, which will by now be familiar to users of the BHP. The monographs were fully revised as specifications for commercially available and widely used plant drugs, with a distinctive style but broadly in line with the format used in many national pharmacopoeias. Apart from a brief pharmacological Action stated at the end of each monograph, therapeutic information is no longer included in the BHP itself. However, as a separate work but designed to be a companion to the BHP, the British Herbal Compendium was introduced in 1992. Monographs of the Compendium, covering exactly the same range of plant drugs as the Pharmacopoeia, include sections on constituents and therapeutics together with regulatory information and extensive literature references. Separation of the pharmacopoeial specifications from other scientific data proved a success, enabling the Compendium to be developed flexibly with information which would be inappropriate in a pharmacopoeia.

This concept has been continued in the 1996 edition of the BHP, which comprises the monographs of the 1990 volume (amended where necessary) together with many fully revised monographs, bringing the total to 169. Volume 1 of the Compendium covered the 84 plant drugs included in the BHP 1990 and a further volume in preparation will cover the 85 new monographs in the BHP 1996.

A primary reason for production of the original BHP was that monographs on plant drugs were being progressively deleted from official pharmacopoeias. It is encouraging to note a substantial reverse of this trend in Europe. Numerous additional monographs on plant drugs are planned for publication in the European Pharmacopoeia and in due course they will be reproduced in the national pharmacopoeias of countries party to the European Pharmacopoeia Convention. It is not the purpose or intention of the BHP to compete with pharmacopoeias official in the UK but rather to provide specifications for plant drugs for which official monographs are not available in English. Since a herbal pharmacopoeia would be incomplete without mention of the official drugs, abbreviated texts making reference to official monographs have been included where relevant. This compromise also facilitates coverage of the official plant drugs in the Compendium. Inevitably some full monographs in this edition of the BHP will be superseded over the next few years by new monographs of the European Pharmacopoeia and/or British Pharmacopoeia; in such cases the BHP monographs will be reduced to abbreviated versions at the next opportunity.

Monographs appearing for the first time in the British Herbal Pharmacopoeia are:

Agnus Castus	Ginkgo Leaf
Artichoke	Hawthorn Flowering Top
Ascophyllum	Horse-chestnut Seed
Birch Leaf	Java Tea
Clove	Melilot
Coriander	Milk Thistle Fruit
Eucalyptus Leaf	Nettle Root
Fennel, Bitter	Pumpkin Seed
Fennel, Sweet	White Deadnettle

The general format and style of the 1990 monographs has been retained, the only change being the addition of botanical family names to the headings. Plant families are quoted in accordance with *Vascular Plant Families and Genera* compiled by R.K. Brummitt. Abbreviations for authors of species are quoted in accordance with a related book, *Authors of Plant Names* edited by R.K. Brummitt and C.E. Powell. Both books were published by the Royal Botanic Gardens, Kew, in 1992.

Macroscopical and microscopical descriptions in the monographs have been prepared by leading pharmacognosists and refer to material in the whole or large fragment form. When materials are commercially supplied in powder form a less comprehensive examination for diagnostic structures is appropriate. In most cases therefore, a submonograph on the powdered drug, with a description of the characteristic features, has been included.

Identification of plant drugs by thin-layer chromatography is now a basic requirement and suitable systems have been devised for the monographs. This technique offers a simple yet sensitive analytical tool using equipment which should be available in every quality control laboratory. Major bands relative to marker substances or the solvent front are described with no attempt to name the constituents forming individual bands. As stated under General Notices and worthy of re-emphasis here, a chromatogram of an authenticated sample of the plant drug in question, prepared on the same plate as the sample under test for comparison purposes, always enhances the reliability of identification. The use of certain solvent systems and spray reagents described in the English version of *Plant Drug Analysis* by H. Wagner, S. Bladt and E.M. Zgainski (Springer-Verlag, 1984) is acknowledged; since its publication this extensively illustrated book has become a standard reference in many laboratories analysing plant drugs.

The quantitative criteria of earlier editions of the Pharmacopoeia have been reappraised and extended, based on assessment of copious laboratory data kindly provided by companies in the herbal industry. Where available, information from textbooks and foreign pharmacopoeias has also been used in the evaluation. The standards set are intended as practical criteria for commercially supplied plant drugs, to distinguish those of pharmacopoeial quality from substandard material.

Although it is beyond the BHMA Scientific Committee's resources to validate for inclusion in the BHP suitable procedures for the determination of chemical constituents of plant drugs, references to published methods, where available in the literature, will continue to be included in the British Herbal Compendium,

An essential feature of this edition, as in 1990, is the inclusion of Appendices describing methods of analysis and reagents pertaining to the monographs. With the kind permission of the respective authorities, the majority of methods and reagents described are those of the European Pharmacopoeia or the British Pharmacopoeia. Texts of the European Pharmacopoeia or corresponding texts in national pharmacopoeias of various European countries are, of course, available in a number of languages, which may prove helpful to some overseas users of this Pharmacopoeia.

It should be borne in mind that the criteria included in the monographs will not indicate the presence or absence of certain possible contaminants, either chemical or biological. For this purpose more specialised techniques may be required and the nature or frequency of testing will depend on various factors, both historical and batch-related. A summary of guidance on this subject is included in the General Notices.

Considerable effort has been made to ensure that the analytical criteria and procedures defined in this volume are appropriate for the botanical drugs in question. However, the practical experience of many users of the British Herbal Pharmacopoeia can provide useful validation towards subsequent editions. In due course the Scientific Committee would welcome data or comments based upon extensive use of the monographs.

GENERAL NOTICES

The following information is intended to supplement statements made elsewhere in this edition of the British Herbal Pharmacopoeia, primarily in the monographs and appendices. It is also intended to offer guidance, or to indicate other useful publications, pertaining to certain general quality requirements for plant drugs which are not otherwise mentioned in this volume.

In the text of the British Herbal Pharmacopoeia the unqualified word "Pharmacopoeia" means the British Herbal Pharmacopoeia. The correct abbreviation for British Herbal Pharmacopoeia is BHP. A herbal material is not of BHP quality unless it complies with all the requirements of the relevant monograph. However, statements under the heading Characteristics are not to be interpreted in a strict sense and are not to be regarded as analytical requirements.

USE OF THE MONOGRAPHS

Temperatures
All temperatures are expressed on the Celsius thermometric scale.

Reference Samples
For comparison purposes in the laboratory evaluation of a plant drug it is advantageous to maintain a reference sample of the drug which has been authenticated by an experienced pharmacognosist or other authority and has previously been found to conform with the requirements of the Pharmacopoeia.

Characteristics
The botanical evaluation of samples of crude drugs requires an ability to interpret morphological and anatomical descriptions of plants and a knowledge of the terms used, gained either from formal training or by the study of suitably illustrated text books. The methodology used for macroscopical and microscopical examination of plant material is adequately described in the following books:

Evans WC. *Trease and Evans' Pharmacognosy, 13th Edition*. London: Bailliére Tindall, 1989. ISBN 0-7020-1357-9.

Jackson BP and Snowdon DW. *Atlas of Microscopy of Medicinal Plants, Culinary Herbs and Spices*. London: Belhaven Press (now Chichester: John Wiley), 1990. ISBN 1-85293-081-0.

Another useful book, with many photographs and photomicrographs of plant drugs, is:

Bisset NG, editor (translated from Wichtl M.), *Herbal Drugs and Phytopharmaceuticals: A handbook for practice on a scientific basis*. Boca Raton-London: CRC Press, Stuttgart: Medpharm Scientific, 1994. ISBN 0-8493-7192-9.

Macroscopical descriptions in the monographs refer to features which can be seen by the unaided eye or with the aid of a hand lens. The characteristic structures described for powdered material should be read in conjunction with the microscopical description of the whole drug.

Identification

Thin-layer Chromatography has been employed as the principal means of positive identification of plant materials defined in the monographs. In a few cases where isolated constituents of plant drugs are commercially available, chromatographically-separated constituents are related to known constituents used as markers. In other cases a fingerprint of the separated constituents is obtained and the positions of major bands in the chromatogram are described relative to a non-constituent marker or to the solvent front.

In describing certain chromatograms the term 'doublet' refers to two bands close together - visibly separate but with approximately the same Rf value. The term 'fine detail' refers to multiple, closely spaced, faint bands over a range of Rf values.

Description in words of the colours, intensities and positions of an often complex array of bands on a chromatogram presents obvious difficulties and only the major bands can be described in detail. Furthermore the positions and appearance of individual bands may vary slightly depending on experimental conditions. Although not specifically required in the monographs, it cannot be over-emphasized that in order to enhance the reliability of identification **a chromatogram of an authentic sample of the plant drug in question should be developed on the same plate, in parallel with the sample under test**. This enables full comparison of all the separated bands and should be adopted as standard practice whenever possible.

Natural variations in the levels of constituents in different samples of a plant drug may also lead to minor deviations from one chromatogram to another. The extent of deviation allowed before samples are considered incorrect or contaminated with foreign material depends on experience and careful judgement. Further investigations should be carried out in all cases of suspect material.

Where standardised Solvent Systems or Spray Reagents are indicated by letter suffixes, these are described in Appendix 1. "Freshly prepared", with respect to Spray Reagents or other items, means prepared within 24 hours of use. "Water-bath" means a bath of boiling water unless otherwise specified.

Quantitative Standards

"%" means "% w/w" with respect to the limits specified for Loss on Drying, Foreign Matter, Total Ash, Ash Insoluble in Hydrochloric Acid, Ethanol-soluble Extractive, Ethanol-insoluble Residue and Water-soluble Extractive, but "% v/w" with respect to the limits specified for Volatile Oil.

In Loss on Drying tests where no time duration is prescribed the material is dried to constant weight; this is implicit in the text of Appendix 2. All quantitative determinations prescribed in the monographs are carried out on material which has not been specially dried and calculations are made accordingly except where otherwise stated. When "calculated with reference to the oven-dried material" is stated, the result of the Loss on Drying test should be applied to the calculation.

Material of Commerce

This section is for information only and does not constitute a standard. Authentic material in other physical forms or from other geographical sources is not excluded.

Storage

The statements, where included, are advisory only.

Action

The pharmacological actions stated do not imply any regulatory acceptance in the United Kingdom for the purpose of Product Licences for medicines.

GENERAL QUALITY CRITERIA FOR PLANT DRUGS

Monographs of the British Herbal Pharmacopoeia define specific criteria of quality applicable to individual plant drugs. However, such materials and preparations derived from them should also meet adequate general standards of quality, particularly with regard to possible contaminants.

Ideally, the exact geographical source of a herbal material and the conditions under which it has been grown, harvested, dried and stored should be known, as well as any chemical treatments, such as pesticides or fumigants, to which it may have been subjected. In many cases this is not possible, since plant drugs are obtained from varied geographical and commercial sources. The appropriate level of testing additional to the monograph criteria must therefore be carefully assessed, based on various factors including the nature of the material, knowledge of its batch history and test results from previous batches.

Regulatory Guidance on the Quality of Herbal Medicines
A Note for Guidance on 'Quality of Herbal Remedies' is included in:
The Rules Governing Medicinal Products in the European Community, Volume III: Guidelines on the quality, safety and efficacy of medicinal products for human use. ISBN 92-825-9619-2 (English language edition).Catalogue Number: CB-55-89-843-EN-C. Published by the Office for Official Publications of the European Communities, 1989. Available from Her Majesty's Stationery Office.

Contaminants
The above Note for Guidance does not specify limits for contaminants in herbal medicines, nor are statutory limits specified in UK legislation under the Medicines Act. General guidelines do, however, require that contaminants be controlled. Specific limits may be included in the quality criteria defined for raw materials or finished products in the documentation pertaining to individual UK Product Licences.

The European Pharmacopoeia defines criteria with respect to microbial quality of herbal medicines and pesticide residues in plant drugs. Where limits for contaminants are not otherwise specified, plant drugs should at least meet the standards defined in food legislation.

Microbial Contamination
The total viable counts of raw botanical drugs may vary widely and, to an extent, the acceptable level should be based on historical data for the material in question.

The European Pharmacopoeia defines limits for microbial contamination in various categories of pharmaceutical preparations under Part 1, VIII.15 *Microbial Quality of Pharmaceutical Preparations* (1995), in which the following criteria are given:

CATEGORY 4   *Herbal remedies*

A. *Herbal remedies to which boiling water is added before use*
  – Total viable aerobic count. Not more than 10^7 aerobic bacteria and not more than 10^5 fungi per gram or per millilitre.
  – Not more than 10^2 *Escherichia coli* per gram or per millilitre.

B. *Other herbal remedies*
  – Total viable aerobic count. Not more than 10^5 aerobic bacteria and not more than 10^4 fungi per gram or per millilitre.
  – Not more than 10^3 enterobacteria and certain other gram-negative bacteria per gram or per millilitre.
  – Absence of *Escherichia coli* (1.0 g or 1.0 ml).
  – Absence of *Salmonella* (10.0 g or 10.0 ml).

Of particular importance in the microbiological quality control of herbal products are:

- Routine screening of plant drugs and preparations derived from them.
- Assessment in relation to trends in historical data.
- Validation to confirm that products have been manufactured in accordance with the principles of Good Pharmaceutical Manufacturing Practice and do not favour the multiplication of micro-organisms.

Potentially Toxic Elements

The term 'heavy metals' has traditionally been used to describe those elements which should be restricted in ingested materials because of their toxic effects. This term includes not only lead but other metals such as chromium, iron, copper, zinc, nickel and tungsten, some of which are essential nutrients in trace amounts (e.g. copper, iron, zinc) and some of which have relatively low toxicity (e.g. nickel, chromium). Mercury, which has been classed as a noble metal, and the 'metalloid' arsenic are also elements which should be controlled in foods and medicines because of their toxic natures. 'Potentially toxic elements' therefore seems a more satisfactory term than 'heavy metals' in this context.

There are no specific UK legal criteria for maximum levels of toxic elements in medicines, although many conventional drug substances will contain levels up to perhaps 10 ppm, which is acceptable having due regard to the nature and source of the material and the relatively low amounts which will be ingested. UK statutory limits and guideline limits for various elements in foods are summarised below.

The Arsenic in Food Regulations 1959 (SI 1959 No. 831 as amended) define a general limit of 1 part per million (ppm) for arsenic in food: higher limits apply to certain specified foodstuffs, pertinent examples being 2 ppm for liquorice (dried extract) and for dried hops other than those intended for use in commercial brewing, and 5 ppm for spices and dried herbs.

The Lead in Food Regulations 1979 (SI 1979 No. 1254 as amended) define a general limit of 1 mg/kg for lead in food: higher limits applicable to certain specified foodstuffs include 2 mg/kg in cocoa powder and in dried or dehydrated fruit or vegetables, 5 mg/kg in dandelion coffee and in tea, and 10 mg/kg in dried herbs, spices and mustard and in hops.

The Tin in Food Regulations 1992 (SI 1992 No. 496) define a general limit of 200 mg/kg for tin in foodstuffs.

Guideline limits on copper and zinc have been set for food and, although not statutory, they may be invoked as evidence that the Food Safety Act 1990 has been contravened. The general guideline limit for copper in foods other than beverages sold ready-to-drink is 20 mg/kg; exceptions include chicory dried or roasted, flavourings and coffee beans 30 mg/kg, cocoa powder 70 mg/kg (on the fat-free substance) and tea 150 mg/kg. There are no guideline limits for cadmium and mercury, but the recommendation is that food should only be admitted into the UK if the levels of cadmium or mercury are acceptable in its country of origin.

With regard to medicinal plants, the toxic elements which may be present in sufficient quantity to cause concern vary from plant to plant as their physiological uptake of these elements varies: amounts present also depend on the location, varying according to the quality of the soil or aerial pollution. A general screen on plant materials will give a guide as to what specific elements in which plants may be of concern. Lead is probably not a problem in most plants, for example, but arsenic and mercury might be found at higher levels.

Seaweeds are unique in that they may contain relatively high quantities of toxic elements, and the Medicines Control Agency have laid down a provisional maximum daily limit of 75 µg of total 'heavy metals' from seaweed-containing preparations, arsenic and lead being of primary concern (although levels of cadmium, chromium and mercury may also be monitored).

Testing for heavy metals and other potentially toxic elements by traditional methods can be problematical. Atomic Absorption Spectrophotometry is a more precise technique, enabling individual elements to be assayed, although the instrumentation is expensive. Considerable technical expertise and experience are required to obtain reproducible results.

Pesticides
The European Pharmacopoeia defines limits for plant drugs with respect to 34 specific pesticides under Part 1, V.4.6 *Pesticide Residues* (1995) and offers methods of analysis under Part 1, VIII.17 *Tests for Pesticides* (1995). Limits applying to other pesticides not specified in the V.4.6 text, and whose presence is suspected for any reason, are in accordance with European Community Directives 76/895 and 90/642: in UK legislation the latter limits are given in *The Pesticides (Maximum Residue Levels in Crops, Food and Feeding Stuffs) Regulations 1994* (SI 1994 No. 1985).

The appropriate frequency of testing for pesticide residues in plant drugs should be determined on the basis of historical data for particular materials and the level of knowledge on their sources and pesticide treatments (if any). Determinations for pesticide residues will be beyond the scope of most routine quality control laboratories but analytical screening for a wide range of pesticides may be contracted to specialised laboratories in the UK.

Other Contaminants
The possibility of mycotoxins, fumigant residues or radioactive residues should also be assessed and testing arranged if deemed necessary.

MONOGRAPHS

AGNUS CASTUS
Verbenaceae

Agni casti fructus

Synonym: Chaste Tree fruits.

Agnus Castus consists of the dried, ripe fruits of *Vitex agnus-castus* L.

CHARACTERISTICS

Macroscopical Description
Almost spherical or slightly ovoid fruits, up to 4 mm diameter, usually shortly pedicellate, with a few smaller, immature fruits in close groups of up to six; each fruit more than three-quarters ensheathed in the closely-attached, enlarged, persistent calyx, bearing five, often indistinct, short teeth; externally the calyx is dull greyish-green and minutely felted; fruit wall only slightly rough, very dark reddish-brown to almost black; apex with a slight depression and, more obvious on larger fruits, four faint grooves at right-angles to one another; the fruits are extremely hard.

Microscopical Description
Calyx Outer epidermis of small, isodiametric polygonal cells, densely covered by short, bent or undulate, uni- or bicellular covering trichomes of fairly uniform length; inner epidermal cells a little larger, walls slightly wavy, some thickened, trichomes absent.

Fruit A narrow pericarp, four loculi, each filled with a single ovoid seed. Epicarp largely of cells having a thick outer wall with conspicuous pitted thickening on the inside; in surface view the cells are subrectangular or slightly elongated polygonal, and show large, simple pits; among the thickened cells are short-stalked glandular trichomes with uni- or multicellular heads; few short, covering trichomes; outer mesocarp, a few layers of brown pigmented parenchymatous cells; inner mesocarp extending into septa, finely pitted sclerenchymatous cells, some only moderately thick-walled, most are typical, isodiametric stone cells with small lumen; endocarp a layer of small brown cells. Seeds, cotyledons large, of thin-walled, oil-containing parenchyma; endosperm of three or four layers of similar, slightly larger cells. Inner and outer coats of testa, single layers of small, brown-pigmented cells, enclosing a region, two to four cells thick, of fairly large, thin-walled, lignified cells, having numerous, fine, reticulate bands of thickening.

Odour and Taste
Odour faintly aromatic; taste unpleasant, bitter, reminiscent of sage.

IDENTIFICATION

Carry out the method for Thin-layer Chromatography as described in Appendix 1, using Solvent System A.

Apply 20 µl of each of the following solutions separately to the plate: (1) extract 1 g powdered Agnus Castus with 10 ml methanol by warming on a water-bath for 10-15 minutes, cool and filter; (2) 0.025% rutin in methanol.

Spray the plate with Spray Reagent A and examine in ultraviolet light 366 nm.

Major bands relative to rutin are approximately as follows: turquoise 2.15, yellow 1.8, yellow 1.55*, yellow 1.28*, yellow 0.6.

*These are the prominent bands of the chromatogram.

QUANTITATIVE STANDARDS

Foreign Matter
Not more than 2%   Appendix 3

Total Ash
Not more than 8%   Appendix 4

Ash Insoluble in Hydrochloric Acid
Not more than 2%   Appendix 5

Water-soluble Extractive
Not less than 8%   Appendix 7

MATERIAL OF COMMERCE Agnus Castus is harvested from the wild and supplied as whole fruits. It is obtained mainly from Mediterranean countries, especially Albania and Morocco.

19

Powdered Agnus Castus

Complies with the requirements for Identification and Quantitative Standards stated for Agnus Castus.

Characteristic Features
A greyish powder with a musty, slightly aromatic odour and rather unpleasant, bitter taste, reminiscent of sage; abundant, more or less isodiametric stone cells of varying wall thickness and degree of pitting; ovoid lignified cells with thin bands of reticulate thickening; calyx epidermis with closely-spaced, short covering trichomes; epicarp cells with large pits in the outer wall; thin-walled parenchymatous cells and globules of fixed oil; small glandular trichomes.

ACTION Hormonal modulator.

AGRIMONY   Rosaceae

Agrimoniae herba

Synonyms: Common Agrimony (*A. eupatoria*); Fragrant Agrimony (*A. procera*).

Agrimony consists of the dried aerial parts of *Agrimonia eupatoria* L. or *Agrimonia procera* Wallr., harvested during the flowering period.

CHARACTERISTICS

Macroscopical Description
Stems Simple or infrequently branched, up to 60-90 cm long, cylindrical or slightly angular, finely striated, green or with reddish patches, abundant long, tangled hairs.

Leaves Compound imparipinnate, up to 15 cm long, alternate on stem; four to six almost opposite pairs of leaflets and a terminal leaflet, distal leaflets largest; between each pair of large leaflets one or more pairs of much smaller, often unequal, stipule-like leaflets; large leaflets rugose, up to 7 cm long, 3.5 cm wide, narrowly elliptic, sessile, margin deeply serrate to serrate-dentate, finely ciliate; venation pinnate, veins prominent below, lighter coloured, depressed above; upper surface dark green, shiny, slightly rough due to small excrescences, few hairs; lower surface lighter greyish-green with numerous shaggy hairs.

Flowers Numerous, spirally arranged in a terminal spike, pentamerous, hermaphrodite, perigynous; very shortly pedicellate, borne in axil of a deeply divided hairy bract with three or five unequal narrow linear lobes; sepals shorter than petals, pointed ovate, dark green, few short hairs; calyx closely surrounded by numerous terminally-hooked spines on rim of the very hairy receptacle; petals free, yellow or slightly orange yellow, obconic, apex blunt or slightly emarginate, surfaces glabrous, margins sparingly ciliate; stamens ten to twenty, short, inwardly curled, anthers brown; carpels two, styles short, separate.

Fruit Turbinate, pendulous, up to 4-6 mm long, 3 mm wide, greenish-brown, deeply grooved from pointed base to receptacle rim bearing spiny, hooked bristles; two achenes enclosed.

Microscopical Description
Stem Section almost circular, epidermal cells small, slightly convex, cuticle ridged; occasional dome-shaped elevation of pigmented cells forming base of long, unicellular, lignified covering trichome; glandular trichomes up to five-celled stalk, head almost spherical; outer cortex orange-brown, small round to ovoid cells, moderately thickened; inner cortex colourless, larger, thin-walled parenchyma; pericycle continuous wide band, slender, thin-walled, lignified fibres; phloem narrow; xylem rows of vessels of uniform size, inconspicuous medullary rays; pith extensive, large, thin-walled parenchymatous cells; scattered cluster crystals in cortex and pith; epidermis in surface view thin-walled, elongated cells, at intervals rows of wider, shorter cells with few stomata; vessels bordered-pitted and relatively large spirally thickened.

Leaf Dorsiventral, enclosed in the palisade layer isolated rhomboidal crystals 40-50 μm, spongy mesophyll cells and intercellular spaces small, with cluster crystals, singly or in short files; upper epidermal cells isodiametric or slightly elongated-rectangular, anticlinal walls thin, straight to slightly wavy, stomata absent or very infrequent, palisade uniform, closely packed; lower epidermis cells similar in shape, slightly smaller, more angularly sinuous, faintly beaded, stomata very numerous, most anomocytic, a few anisocytic; trichomes on both surfaces, very numerous on lower; covering all unicellular, lignified, varying greatly in length, longer straight or bent, shorter straight, erect; lumen wide at base with brown contents, narrowing considerably, almost occluded in upper part; surface with small, scattered nodules, longer trichomes with faint spiral markings; glandular trichomes less numerous, small, variable, most numerous with up to four-celled stalk, erect or bent, fewer with very short stalk; head pale brown, almost spherical, up to four-celled, thin-walled.

Bract Inner and outer epidermal cells similar, a little elongated, straight or slightly sinuous, stomata very numerous in outer, absent from inner; trichomes of both types on both surfaces; many of the covering type very long, enlarged at base; mesophyll with very numerous clusters and prisms.

Flower Sepals fringed with short, bent or twisted, unicellular covering trichomes and small glandular trichomes; epidermal cells straight to sinuous walled; stomata in outer epidermis; both types of trichomes numerous on outer surface, infrequent on inner; mesophyll densely packed with clusters and prisms. Petals, few widely spaced, covering trichomes along margins; epidermal cells thin-walled, elongated, straight to sinuous, cuticle finely striated; infrequent stomata in outer epidermis near apex; irregularly-occurring grouped prisms and cluster crystals in inner tissues. Stamens, fibrous layer of anther small polygonal cells, thickenings well-marked; pollen ovoid to sub-spherical, up to 60 μm long, 35 μm wide, exine thin, smooth, three pores.

Odour and Taste
Virtually odourless; taste very slightly bitter and astringent.

IDENTIFICATION

Carry out the method for Thin-layer Chromatography as described in Appendix 1, using Solvent System A.

Apply 20μl of each of the following solutions separately to the plate: (1) extract 1g powdered Agrimony with 10ml methanol by warming on a water-bath for 10-15 minutes, cool and filter; (2) 0.025% rutin in methanol.

Spray the plate with Spray Reagent A and examine in ultraviolet light 366 nm.

Major bands relative to rutin are approximately as follows: yellow 2.2, yellow 1.8, yellow 1.5*, yellow 1.4*, yellow 1.2, yellow 1.0.

* Bands may coalesce in high concentration.

QUANTITATIVE STANDARDS

Foreign Matter
Not more than 2%   Appendix 3

Total Ash
Not more than 10%   Appendix 4

Ash Insoluble in Hydrochloric Acid
Not more than 2%   Appendix 5

Water-soluble Extractive
Not less than 12%   Appendix 7

MATERIAL OF COMMERCE Agrimony is supplied in the cut or crushed condition. It is obtained from European countries including the UK, and particularly Bulgaria and Hungary.

Powdered Agrimony

Complies with the requirements for Identification and Quantitative Standards stated for Agrimony.

Characteristic Features
Brownish-green, odourless, slightly astringent; numerous lignified, unicellular, warted trichomes, some spirally marked; leaf lamina with rhomboidal crystals in palisade layer, anomocytic stomata; bract and calyx tissue, densely packed clusters and prisms; fragments of small glandular trichomes; deeply pigmented portions of tapering, hooked spines of fruit; bordered-pitted and spirally-thickened vessels; multiple layers of slender, sinuous, lignified, fibrous cells from fruit; groups of thick-walled, partially lignified, polyhedral cells, almost filled with a large crystal, from inner wall of receptacle; large, thin-walled parenchyma of stem; ovoid pollen grains with smooth, thin exine.

ACTION Astringent.

ALOES, BARBADOS
Aloaceae

Aloe barbadensis

Synonym: Curaçao Aloes.

Barbados Aloes consists of the concentrated and dried juice of the leaves of *Aloe barbadensis* Miller.

This material complies with the requirements of the European Pharmacopoeia for Barbados Aloes.

MATERIAL OF COMMERCE Barbados Aloes is supplied as large, opaque blocks or in the broken or crushed condition. It is obtained from the Netherlands Antilles.

ACTION Stimulant laxative.

ALOES, CAPE
Aloaceae

Aloe capensis

Cape Aloes consists of the concentrated and dried juice of the leaves of various species of Aloe, mainly *Aloe ferox* Miller and its hybrids.

This material complies with the requirements of the European Pharmacopoeia for Cape Aloes.

MATERIAL OF COMMERCE Cape Aloes is supplied as large, translucent blocks or in the broken or crushed condition. It is obtained principally from South Africa.

ACTION Stimulant laxative.

AMMONIACUM
Umbelliferae

Ammoniaci gummiresina

Synonym: Gum Ammoniacum.

Ammoniacum consists of the gum-resin exuded from the flowering and fruiting stems of *Dorema ammoniacum* Don and possibly other species of *Dorema*.

CHARACTERISTICS

Macroscopical Description
Ammoniacum occurs in two forms, tears and lumps, which are often mixed in commercial samples.

Tear Ammoniacum Composed of separate, small, rounded to ovoid or irregular masses varying from about 0.5-3 cm in diameter, hard and brittle, but softening when warmed; surface dull, pale yellow, darkening to pale brown on ageing; fractured surface milky-white to pale brownish-yellow, opaque with a waxy lustre.

Lump Ammoniacum Composed of tears and larger pieces of the gum-resin agglutinated together with a bluish, resinous substance and frequently mixed with varying amounts of extraneous materials such as stones, fragments of the fruit and stem, and other debris; structure of the pieces of gum resin similar to that of the tears.

Odour and Taste
Odour resinous, characteristic but not strong; taste unpleasant, bitter and acrid.

IDENTIFICATION

Carry out the method for Thin-layer Chromatography as described in Appendix 1, using Solvent System C.

Apply 40 µl of each of the following solutions separately to the plate; (1) extract 1 g powdered Ammoniacum, shaking with 10 ml ethanol (96%) for 5 minutes; (2) 0.1% cineole in toluene.

Spray the plate with Spray Reagent D, heat at 105°C for 10-15 minutes, then examine in daylight.

Major bands relative to cineole are ap-

proximately as follows: red/brown 0.85, brown 0.4, purple 0.2-0.

There are many faint bands from 2.0-1.0, but all prominent bands are in the region 1.0-0. This latter region exhibits much fine detail with purple, brown and low banding.

QUANTITATIVE STANDARDS

Total Ash
Not more than 7%   Appendix 4

Ethanol-soluble Extractive
Not less than 60%   Appendix 6A

MATERIAL OF COMMERCE Ammoniacum is supplied in tears or nodular masses. It is obtained from the Middle East, especially Iran.

ACTION Expectorant.

ANGELICA ROOT   Umbelliferae

Angelicae radix

Synonyms: European Angelica root, Garden Angelica root.

Angelica Root consists of the dried rhizome and roots of *Angelica archangelica* L. [*Archangelica officinalis* Hoffm.], harvested in Autumn.

CHARACTERISTICS

Macroscopical Description
Rhizome Vertical, up to 5 cm diameter and 10 cm long, more or less cylindrical; dark brownish-grey to reddish-brown; at apex short remains of leaves, stem scars, buds; lower part bearing numerous, closely-spaced, often entwined, adventitious roots.
Roots Up to 1 cm thick at point of origin, tapering, 25-30 cm long; greyish-brown, rough surfaced with longitudinal furrows and irregular, sometimes incompletely en-

circling, transverse ridges; few, small wiry rootlets; fracture short, uneven; medullary rays well-marked, bark greyish-white with irregular splits, darker tissue showing radially arranged secretion ducts; wood greyish-yellow, medullary rays wide.

Microscopical Description
Root Section irregularly circular; radial and tangential lacunae in outer bark; xylem about one third of total diameter; cork several layers, weakly lignified; cortical parenchyma tangentially elongated, thin-walled cells, occasional secretion canals; frequent small starch granules, 2-4 µm, very rarely small prismatic crystals; phloem, medullary rays multiseriate, cells elongated and thin-walled; blocks of sieve tissue wide, enclosing well-separated secretion canals, increasing in diameter from cambium to cortex, about 50 µm to 250 µm, circular or tangentially orientated ovoid; secretory epithelium

thin-walled, pale yellow-brown, lumen of canal sometimes with amorphous, pale greyish contents; sieve tissue largely uniform polygonal to rounded cells; cambiform tissue a layer of several cells; xylem rays with reticulately thickened, lignified vessels, up to about 70 µm diameter, in small, closely-spaced groups of up to about five, embedded in small, round-celled, sometimes, adjacent to medullary rays, collenchymatously thickened, unlignified xylem parenchyma; medullary rays, unlignified, almost as wide as xylem rays. Roots sectioned near point of origin have a small parenchymatous pith.

Rhizome Structure similar to root; extensive pith containing secretion ducts.

Odour and Taste

Penetrating aromatic odour; taste aromatic, strong, slightly pungent and numbing; rather lingering.

IDENTIFICATION

Carry out the method for Thin-layer Chromatography as described in Appendix 1, using Solvent System D with non-saturated conditions.

Apply 40 µl of each of the following solutions separately to the plate: (1) extract 1 g powdered Angelica Root with 10 ml methanol by warming on a water-bath for 30 minutes, cool, filter and concentrate to approximately 2 ml; (2) 1% coumarin in methanol.

Examine the plate under ultraviolet light 366 nm.

The chromatogram is characterised by multiple white bands throughout the Rf range

0.85-0.

If the plate is then sprayed with 1.8M ethanolic potassium hydroxide solution and re-examined in ultraviolet light 366 nm, major bands of the above spectrum relative to coumarin are approximately as follows: white 0.7, white 0.45.

No appreciable amount of coumarin is visible in the chromatogram.

QUANTITATIVE STANDARDS

Foreign Matter
Not more than 5%   Appendix 3

Total Ash
Not more than 10%   Appendix 4

Ash insoluble in Hydrochloric Acid
Not more than 2%   Appendix 5

Water-soluble Extractive
Not less than 30%   Appendix 7

MATERIAL OF COMMERCE Angelica Root is supplied as entire or longitudinally sliced rhizome and roots. It is obtained from plants cultivated in Northern Europe including the UK.

Powdered Angelica Root

Complies with the requirements for Identification and Quantitative Standards stated for Angelica Root.

ACTION Aromatic bitter, spasmolytic.

ANISEED

Umbelliferae

Anisi fructus

Synonym: Anise.

Aniseed consists of the whole dry cremocarp of *Pimpinella anisum* L.

This material complies with the requirements of the European Pharmacopoeia for Aniseed.

MATERIAL OF COMMERCE Aniseed is supplied as whole dried fruits. Indigenous to the Near East, it is cultivated in many countries and obtained principally from Egypt, Turkey and Spain.

ACTION Expectorant; carminative.

ARNICA FLOWER

Compositae

Arnicae flos

Synonym: European Arnica.

Arnica Flower consists of the dried flower-heads of *Arnica montana* L.

CHARACTERISTICS

Macroscopical Description

Flowers Capitulum, more or less obconical, about 2 cm diameter and 1.5 cm in height, involucre of twenty to twenty-five somewhat leathery, linear-lanceolate bracts in two rows, outer surface dark, brownish-green, dull and rough, pubescent, inner surface lighter, greyish-green, slightly shiny, longitudinally grooved, less-markedly pubescent, margins with numerous, longish, white hairs; receptacle 3-8 mm diameter, flat or slightly convex, numerous closely spaced, almost circular depressions, giving a honeycomb appearance, each depression surrounded by extremely short bristles; florets brownish-yellow, disc florets numerous, hermaphrodite, pappus of white silky filaments, nearly equalling the length of the corolla tube, corolla pentamerous, sympetalous, actinomorphic, up to 7-8 mm long, slightly expanded at apex into five toothed lobes, five epipetalous stamens, anthers syngenesious, ovary inferior, monocarpellary, up to 7 mm long, five very fine longitudinal ridges, surface with short, upwardly directed, appressed white hairs, style filiform, with spreading, bifid stigma; ray florets female, sixteen to twenty in a single row, up to 2-3.5 cm long, 3-5 mm wide, three, four or five acute apical teeth, seven to nine veins, anastomosing near the apex, pappus 7-8 mm, gynoecium as in disc florets.

Fruits Slender achenes, 5-7 mm long, mid-brown, finely ribbed, pappus filaments approximately same length as the achene.

Pedicels 2-3 cm long, 1-1.5 mm thick, dark brown surface wrinkled and rough, very numerous short, deeply pigmented hairs, fewer, long white hairs.

Microscopical Description

Bract Inner epidermal cells near apex isodiametric or a little elongated, anticlinal walls slightly sinuous; in mid-region cells more elongated, more markedly sinuous, beaded; towards the base, cells markedly elongated, varying from sinuous to straight-walled; glandular trichomes, uni- or biseriate stalk of short component cells, and multicellular globose head; covering trichomes, up to eight cells long, uniseriate; stomata absent. Outer epidermis, cells near apex subrectangular, anticlinal walls markedly sinuous, beaded; mid-region cells more elongated, walls quite angularly-sinuous, beaded; towards the base, cells elongated rectangular, walls sinuous; numerous, quite large, deeply pigmented glandular trichomes with broad multicellular base tapering to multicellular, uni- or biseriate stalk, having shorter cells, with slightly thickened walls, near the base, bearing a multicellular, pyriform head; cell contents impart a brownish-red colour to choral hydrate solution; smaller, non-pigmented, glandular trichomes with uni- or biseriate stalk and globose multicellular head; non-glandular trichomes with up to six to eight thin-walled cells; abundant anomocytic stomata.

Ray floret Inner epidermal cells of corolla, near apex subrectangular to polygonal, periclinal wall weakly papillose, anticlinal walls slightly wavy; mid-region and towards base, cells more elongated, sinuous in outline, papillae more well-marked; stomata absent; covering trichomes, most numerous in the lower region, six to eight cells, the basal cell short, slightly swollen, progressively longer distal cells; glandular trichomes, short, uni- or biseriate stalk, globose multicellular head; outer epidermal cells subrectangular or slightly elongated, walls slightly wavy, papillae absent; anomocytic stomata, more numerous near corolla lobes; glandular and covering trichomes similar to those of inner epidermis, covering rather more numerous.

Disc floret Epidermal cells subrectangular to somewhat elongated, anticlinal walls almost straight to fairly wavy; inner epidermal cells of corolla lobes with well-marked, finger-like papillae; trichomes similar to those of ray florets, especially numerous on outer basal epidermis. Pappus long, five to six cells thick at base, finely tapering to one, surface barbed due to exserted, slightly reflexed, terminal portion of the cells. Style, stigmas reflexed, upper surface densely covered with uniform, tubular papillae. Pollen spherical, 40-50 μm, exine very finely granular with numerous spines up to about 8 μm; three pores and three furrows.

Achene Epidermal cells slightly elongated, rectangular, straight-walled; numerous upwardly-directed, twin trichomes with constituent cells of slightly unequal length, diverging at their apices, pits present in the contiguous walls; quite short glandular trichomes, uni- or biseriate stalk, multicellular head.

Receptacle Surface bearing short trichomes of one, two or three cells, acutely pointed, conspicuously thickened at point of insertion.

Pedicel Pigmented glandular trichomes as on bracts, many very large; long covering trichomes with up to ten to twelve cells, others, more numerous, short, bluntly conical, with one to three cells.

Odour and Taste
Odour sweet, pleasant aromatic; taste bitter and acrid.

IDENTIFICATION

Carry out the method for Thin-layer Chromatography as described in Appendix 1, using Solvent System A.

Apply 20 μl of each of the following solutions separately to the plate: (1) extract 1g powdered Arnica Flower with 10 ml methanol by warming on a water-bath for 10-15 minutes, cool and filter; (2) 0.025% rutin in methanol.

Spray the plate with Spray Reagent A and examine in ultraviolet light 366 nm.

Major bands relative to rutin are approximately as follows: turquoise doublet 1.95, yellow doublet 1.4, white 1.2.

Note: *Arnica montana* does not exhibit a yellow band corresponding to rutin in the chromatogram.

QUANTITATIVE STANDARDS

Foreign Matter
Not more than 2%   Appendix 3

Total Ash
Not more than 8%   Appendix 4

MATERIAL OF COMMERCE Arnica Flower is supplied as whole, dried flowerheads. Material harvested from the wild is obtained principally from Spain.

Arnica montana grows in mountainous regions of central and southern Europe and in the plains of northern Europe to southern Scandinavia and Russia. In many countries it is a protected species in the wild and cultivation has proved difficult.

Powdered Arnica Flower

Complies with the requirements for Identification and Quantitative Standards stated for Arnica Flower.

ACTION Topical healing.

ARTICHOKE   Compositae

Cynarae folium

Synonyms: Globe Artichoke Leaf, Cynara.

Artichoke consists of the dried radical leaves of *Cynara scolymus* L.

CHARACTERISTICS

Macroscopical Description
Leaves very large, up to about 50 cm long and 25 cm broad with a long petiole about 1 cm thick; lamina deeply pinnatifid forming flat, lanceolate segments with coarsely-toothed margins; upper surface brownish-green, lower surface greyish-white and densely covered with hairs; segments with pinnate venation, the side veins terminating in a short point on each marginal tooth; midrib and petiole deeply grooved on the upper surface, the lower surface prominently

raised, with several longitudinal ridges and covered with long, whitish hairs.

Microscopical Description

Lamina Dorsiventral, the cells of the palisade layer fairly large and loosely packed; cells of the upper epidermis with straight to slightly sinuous anticlinal walls, those of the lower epidermis more wavy-walled; anomocytic stomata on both surfaces, more numerous on the lower; covering trichomes scattered on the upper epidermis, especially over the veins, very abundant on the lower epidermis; individual trichomes mostly of the whip-lash type with several small cells forming the uniseriate bases and very long, narrow and sinuous terminal cells intertwining to form a felted mass covering the surface; other, less numerous, uniseriate covering trichomes composed of four to six cells, tapering to a blunt apex with the cells sometimes more or less globular to ovoid; fairly large glandular trichomes also abundant on both surfaces, with a short, one or two-celled stalk and a spherical head filled with brownish secretion.

Midrib and Petiole Epidermal cells in surface view rectangular and longitudinally elongated, with scattered glandular and covering trichomes similar to those on the lamina; cut transversely shows bands of collenchyma below both epidermises and a large vascular bundle in each ridge on the lower surface with a number of smaller bundles arranged in an arc surrounding the groove on the upper surface; vascular bundles composed of a dense group of pericyclic fibres with thick, lignified walls, a wide area of thin-walled sieve tissue and a lignified xylem containing small vessels, tracheids and xylem parenchyma; below each xylem group a mass of lignified fibres which, in the larger bundles, extends as a narrow layer on either side of the vascular tissue to join with the fibres of the pericycle; ground tissue composed of large-celled, rounded parenchyma, some with lignified walls.

Odour and Taste

Odour faint, slightly sour; taste salty at first, then bitter.

IDENTIFICATION

Carry out the method for Thin-layer Chro-matography as described in Appendix 1, using Solvent System A.

Apply 20 µl of each of the following solutions separately to the plate: (1) extract 1 g powdered Artichoke with 10 ml methanol by warming on a water-bath for 10-15 minutes, cool and filter; (2) 0.025% rutin in methanol.

Spray the plate with Spray Reagent A and examine in ultraviolet light 366 nm.

Major bands relative to rutin are approximately as follows: yellow 2.3, turquoise (doublet) 2.1*, yellow 1.5, turquoise 1.2, yellow 1.0.

* The turquoise doublet may appear as a single band.

QUANTITATIVE STANDARDS

Foreign Matter
Not more than 2%   Appendix 3

Total Ash
Not more than 15%   Appendix 4

Ash Insoluble in Hydrochloric Acid
Not more than 4%   Appendix 5

Water-soluble Extractive
Not less than 25%   Appendix 7

MATERIAL OF COMMERCE Artichoke is supplied as whole or cut leaves. It is obtained from Southern Europe and North Africa.

Powdered Artichoke

Complies with the requirements for Identification and Quantitative Standards stated for Artichoke.

Characteristic Features

Greyish-green to brown powder with a faint odour and a taste, at first, salty, then rather bitter; fragments of the lamina with more or less sinuous walls and anomocytic stomata; covering trichomes, scattered, or in felted masses, and large, glandular trichomes with brown contents; groups of lignified fibres and vessels from the midrib and petiole, the larger vessels with reticulate thickening.

ACTION Hepatic.

ASAFOETIDA

Ferulae gummiresina

Synonyms: Asafetida, Asant.

Asafoetida is the oleo-gum resin obtained by incising the living rhizomes and roots of *Ferula assa-foetida* L., *F. rubricaulis* Boiss., *F. foetida* Regel and other species of *Ferula*.

CHARACTERISTICS

Description
Irregular masses of agglutinated tears up to 4 cm long or rounded to ovoid tears up to 3 cm in diameter, greyish-white, dull yellow or reddish-brown in colour; freshly exposed surface white becoming pink or red.

Odour and Taste
Strong, persistent, alliaceous odour; bitter, acrid and alliaceous taste.

IDENTIFICATION

A. Boil 0.1 g Asafoetida with 5 ml ethanol (90%) for l or 2 minutes, cool and filter into 5 ml ethanol (90%) made strongly alkaline with 18M ammonia, no blue fluorescence is produced.
B. Boil 0.1 g Asafoetida with 2 ml 4M hydrochloric acid, cool and filter into 5 ml 4M ammonia; a blue fluorescence is produced.
C. Carry out the method for Thin-layer Chromatography as described in Appendix 1, using Solvent System A.
 Apply 20 µl of each of the following solutions separately to the plate: (1) extract 1 g crushed Asafoetida with 10 ml methanol on a water-bath for 5 minutes, cool and filter; (2) 0.025% rutin in methanol.
 Spray the plate with Spray Reagent A and examine in ultraviolet light 366 nm.
 Major bands relative to rutin are approximately as follows: whitish-blue 2.6, blue 2.6.

QUANTITATIVE STANDARDS

Foreign Matter
Not more than 10%   Appendix 3

Total Ash
Not more than 15%   Appendix 4

Ethanol (60%)-soluble Extractive
Not less than 25%   Appendix 6A

MATERIAL OF COMMERCE Asafoetida is supplied as agglutinated masses frequently mixed with fruits, fragments of root and earth, or as rounded or flattened tears. It is obtained principally from Afghanistan and Iran.

ACTION Spasmolytic.

ASCOPHYLLUM

Ascophylli thallus

Synonym: Knotted Wrack.

Ascophyllum consists of the entire thallus of *Ascophyllum nodosum* Le Jol., dried as soon as possible after collection.

CHARACTERISTICS

Macroscopical Description
The thallus, which grows to a length of 2 m or more, consists of dichotomously branched, strap-shaped axes, bearing numerous, short, lateral branches and dilated at intervals by single, conspicuous, ovoid vesicles; tips of the lateral branches swell and constitute the receptacles containing the reproductive organs.
 On drying, the thallus becomes hard and brittle and usually occurs in commerce as dark, greyish-black, flattened pieces, smooth, up to about 5 mm wide and 1-2 mm thick, the vesicles shrunken and frequently broken, margin entire; interior surface lighter greyish-brown; fragments from the receptacles closely covered on both sides

with numerous small, rounded protuber-ances.

Microscopical Description
Outer layer (meristoderm) covered by a thick, mucilaginous cuticle, and composed of dark brown, palisade-like cells, thick-walled and irregularly polygonal in surface view; cortex of relatively large cells with irregularly thick-ened walls, closely arranged and becoming more longitudinally elongated towards the inside and grading to the central medulla, where the cells are distinctly elongated; lon-gitudinal walls often gelatinised in the cells of the cortex, and especially the medulla, but transverse walls remain intact; occa-sional hyphae develop from the medulla cells, which are elongated longitudinally and in-tertwine to form loose masses.

Fertile conceptacles occur in the recep-tacles and contain either oogonia or antheridia; mature oogonia sub-spherical to ovoid, up to about 16 mm long and contain-ing four ova; antheridia smaller, more elon-gated, about 25 mm long and containing nu-merous, minute spermatozoids.

Odour and Taste
Odour characteristic of seaweed; taste salty, mucilaginous and unpleasant.

IDENTIFICATION

Thin-layer Chromatographic analysis is in-appropriate for this material, macroscopic and microscopic identification should be relied upon for this purpose.

QUANTITATIVE STANDARDS

Foreign Matter
Not more than 2%   Appendix 3

Total Ash
Not more than 22%   Appendix 4

Ash Insoluble in Hydrochloric Acid
Not more than 3%   Appendix 5

Water-soluble extractive
Not less than 20%   Appendix 7

MATERIAL OF COMMERCE Ascophyllum is supplied in crushed, cut or powdered form. It is obtained mainly from the Atlantic coasts of northern Europe, particularly from Norway.

Commercial material often contains a proportion (perhaps 10%) of *Fucus* species, which are inextricably harvested with the Ascophyllum.

Powdered Ascophyllum

Complies with the requirements for Identifi-cation and Quantitative Standards stated for Ascophyllum.

Characteristic Features
A greenish powder with a seaweed-like odour and an unpleasantly salty and mucilaginous taste; fragments of thick-walled, polygonal cells of the epidermis with dense brown contents; groups of larger, elongated cells, some with partly gelatinised walls; very oc-casionally masses of thin-walled hyphae from the medulla.

ACTION Thyroactive.

BALM LEAF   Labiatae

Melissae folium

Synonyms: Lemon Balm, Melissa Leaf.

Balm Leaf consists of the dried leaves and flowering tops of *Melissa officinalis* L.

CHARACTERISTICS

Macroscopical Description
Stems Quadrangular, much branched,

bearing numerous pairs of opposite leaves; up to about 4 mm wide, surface pale green or brownish with scattered hairs and longitu-dinal ridges.

Leaves Petiolate, broadly ovate, up to about 5 cm long; margin deeply dentate, apex acute; upper surface dark green, lower surface paler with conspicuous raised vena-tion; scattered hairs on both surfaces.

Flowers Small, in whorls in the axils of

the upper leaves; calyx bilobed, pale green, conical, with long spreading hairs; corolla white or pinkish, two-lipped, the upper lip notched, the lower lip three-lobed, spreading.

Microscopical Description

Stem Epidermal cells thin-walled and axially elongated with occasional stomata; covering and glandular trichomes similar to those on the leaf or, more usually, cicatrices showing their position; cortex narrow, parenchymatous with collenchyma in the ridges; groups of pericyclic fibres with moderately thickened and lignified walls; phloem and xylem forming a complete ring surrounding a parenchymatous pith; xylem completely lignified, composed of fibres and parenchyma together with small spirally or annularly thickened vessels interspersed with larger, bordered-pitted vessels.

Leaf Dorsiventral; epidermal cells markedly wavy-walled with diacytic stomata on the lower surface only; very short, conical, unicellular covering trichomes with a finely striated cuticle occur abundantly, especially over the veins on the lower surface; multicellular uniseriate covering trichomes also occur composed of from two to five cells, wide at the base and narrowing rapidly towards the tip, with slightly thickened, warty walls; glandular trichomes also very abundant, some small with a unicellular stalk and a unicellular or bicellular head, others large, of the typical Labiate type, with a unicellular stalk and a spherical to ovoid head composed of eight cells.

Flower Epidermis of the calyx wavy-walled with numerous covering and glandular trichomes similar to those on the leaf, the multicellular covering type particularly abundant on the outer surface; epidermal cells of the corolla distinctly papillose; pollen grains spherical, about 40 μm in diameter, with six pores and furrows and a finely warty exine.

Odour and Taste
Faintly aromatic and lemon-like.

IDENTIFICATION

Carry out the method for Thin-layer Chromatography as described in Appendix 1, using Solvent System A.

Apply 20 μl of each of the following solutions separately to the plate: (1) extract 1 g powdered Balm Leaf with 10 ml methanol by warming on a water-bath for 10-15 minutes, cool and filter; (2) 0.025% rutin in methanol.

Spray the plate with Spray Reagent A and examine in ultraviolet light 366 nm.

Major bands relative to rutin are approximately as follows: turquoise 2.2, yellow 1.6, turquoise 1.4 , purple 1.2

There is an area of diffuse turquoise fine detail between 2.1-1.8.

QUANTITATIVE STANDARDS

Foreign Matter
Not more than 2%   Appendix 3

Total Ash
Not more than 14%   Appendix 4

Ash Insoluble in Hydrochloric Acid
Not more than 3%   Appendix 5

Water-soluble Extractive
Not less than 15%   Appendix 7

MATERIAL OF COMMERCE Balm Leaf is supplied in the cut or crushed condition. It is cultivated in many European countries and obtained particularly from Bulgaria, Romania and Spain.

Powdered Balm Leaf

Complies with the requirements for Identification and Quantitative Standards stated for Balm Leaf.

Characteristic Features
Greyish-green with a slightly aromatic odour and taste reminiscent of lemon; abundant fragments of vascular tissue from the stems composed of lignified fibres, vessels and parenchyma; epidermis of the leaf and stem, that of the leaf wavy-walled with numerous short, conical, covering trichomes and glandular trichomes of the Labiate type; scattered glandular trichomes and fragments of multicellular covering trichomes; lower epidermis of the leaf with diacytic stomata; large-celled rectangular parenchyma from the pith; very infrequent pollen grains, spherical, with six pores and furrows and a finely warty exine.

ACTION Sedative; topical antiviral.

BALM OF GILEAD BUD   **Salicaceae**

Populi gemma

Synonym: Poplar Buds.

Balm of Gilead Bud consists of the air-dried winter leaf buds and flower buds of *Populus nigra* L. or certain other species of Populus including *P. candicans* Ait. [*P. gileadensis* Rouleau] and *P. tacamahaca* Mill. [*P. balsamifera* Du Roi].

CHARACTERISTICS

Macroscopical Description
Leaf Buds Pyramidal or conical, straight or slightly curved, up to 2.5 cm long, 7-8 mm wide, reddish-brown to dark brown with a variable covering of brown to nearly black, shiny, sticky, resinous secretion; at the bud centre a small number of embryonic leaves enclosed by ten to twelve full-length, imbricated, elliptical, concave, innermost scales; two or three outer scales, short, ovoid, markedly concave, similar in size but less closely appressed to the inner part of the bud; scales stiff and woody in texture, smooth with a dull lustre, larger scales finely striated longitudinally.
Flower Buds More uniformly conical, straight or somewhat arcuate, up to 2 cm long, 3 mm wide; central embryonic catkin tightly enclosed by three full-length scales, imbricated; two or sometimes three outer scales, shorter and of unequal length, not fully encircling and less firmly bound to the bud.
Leaf and flower buds of *P. candicans* and *P. tacamahaca* are somewhat larger.

Microscopical Description
Epidermal cells small, ovoid to roughly quadrangular and more rectangular at the apex, anticlinal walls thin-walled except towards the base where the cells, singly or in groups of two to fifty, have moderately thickened walls with numerous pits and rounded lumen; trichomes absent; mesophyll of small cells with dark-brown contents except for a narrow strip of less pigmented cells along the margins, numerous cluster crystals of calcium oxalate, 5-25 μm in diameter, often in short, longitudinal files, more abundant towards the base; elongated groups of large, irregular, thick-walled sclereids with small lumens and associated with some prismatic crystals of calcium oxalate; xylem vessels with spiral and annular thickening.
P. candicans and *P. tacamahaca* have unicellular trichomes, 250-450 μm long, 15 μm wide, thick-walled and bent towards the apex.

Odour and Taste
Fragrant and balsamic odour; aromatic, bitter and acrid taste, somewhat lingering.

IDENTIFICATION

Carry out the method for Thin-layer Chromatography as described in Appendix 1 using Solvent System A.
Apply 20 μl of each of the following solutions separately to the plate: (1) extract 1 g chopped Balm of Gilead Bud with 10 ml methanol by refluxing on a water-bath for 10-15 minutes, cool, filter and concentrate to about 2 ml; (2) 0.025% rutin in methanol.
Spray the plate with Spray Reagent A and examine in ultraviolet light 366 nm.
Major bands relative to rutin are approximately as follows: reddish-brown 2.8, greenish-blue 2.6, yellow 1.65, whitish-blue 1 .4.

QUANTITATIVE STANDARDS

Foreign Matter
Not more than 2%   Appendix 3

Total Ash
Not more than 4%   Appendix 4

Ash Insoluble in Hydrochloric Acid
Not more than 1%   Appendix 5

Ethanol-soluble Extractive
Not less than 40%   Appendix 6

MATERIAL OF COMMERCE Balm of Gilead Bud is supplied in the whole or crushed condition. It is obtained from European countries and the USA.

ACTION Expectorant.

BARBERRY BARK
Berberidaceae

Berberidis cortex

Barberry Bark consists of the dried stem-bark of *Berberis vulgaris* L.

CHARACTERISTICS

Macroscopical Description
Small, irregular, flat pieces up to 2 mm thick or longer, curved pieces up to 0.5 mm thick; outer surface dark yellowish-grey with shallow, longitudinal furrows or, on the thicker pieces, with deeper cracks and fissures; occasional black apothecia of lichens; inner surface dark yellow to brown, distinctly longitudinally striated and glistening, frequently with patches of paler yellow wood attached; fracture short in the outer part, which readily separates, fibrous in the inner part.

Microscopical Description
Outer rhytidome consisting of successive areas of thin-walled, lignified cork cells alternating with dark yellowish-brown areas of dead cortex and secondary phloem; secondary phloem with tangential bands of fibres, usually one or two cells wide, alternating with wider bands of sieve tissue and separated by medullary rays two to four cells wide; phloem fibres small, yellow, thick-walled and lignified with very numerous, conspicuous pits; sieve tissue consisting of narrow sieve tubes and small-celled parenchyma; many of the medullary ray cells containing large prism crystals of calcium oxalate, one or occasionally two in each cell, others containing starch granules; some medullary ray cells, especially where adjacent to the phloem fibres, developed as stone cells with moderately thickened walls.

Odour and Taste
Odour faintly aromatic; taste bitter, imparting a yellow colour to the saliva.

IDENTIFICATION

Carry out the method for Thin-layer Chromatography as described in Appendix 1, using toluene:ethyl acetate:diethylamine (70:20:10) as the solvent system.

Apply 60 µl of the following solutions to the plate: (1) moisten 1 g powdered Barberry Bark with 1 ml 1.8M ammonia solution and then extract with 10 ml methanol by warming on a water-bath for 10 minutes, cool and filter; (2) 0.2% berberine chloride in methanol.

Examine in ultraviolet light 366 nm.

The major bands relative to the solvent front are approximately as follows: thin blue 0.6, lemon yellow 0.5-0. The yellow band will correspond to the band produced by berberine chloride. In the case of Golden Seal Root, a major blue band is observed above the thin blue band in the chromatogram of Barberry Bark. This serves as a method of differentiation between the two extracts.

QUANTITATIVE STANDARDS

Foreign Matter
Not more than 2%   Appendix 3

Total Ash
Not more than 10%   Appendix 4

Ash Insoluble in Hydrochloric Acid
Not more than 2.5%   Appendix 5

Water-soluble Extractive
Not less than 12%   Appendix 7

MATERIAL OF COMMERCE   Barberry Bark is supplied as broken quills. It is obtained from Europe, North Africa and Western Asia.

Powdered Barberry Bark

Complies with the requirements for Identification and Quantitative Standards stated for Barberry Bark.

Characteristic Features
Yellowish-brown, odour faintly aromatic, taste bitter; fragments of thin-walled, lignified, polygonal cork cells; abundant short, yellow fibres occurring singly or in small groups, with thick, lignified walls and very numerous pits; thin-walled sieve tubes and associated parenchyma; prism crystals of calcium oxalate in medullary ray cells

and scattered, individual crystals, occasionally twinned; small, simple starch granules, rounded to ovoid; groups of rectangular stone cells with moderately thickened walls and numerous pits; abundant groups of yellowish-brown crushed parenchyma; occasional lignified fibres and vessels from the adherent xylem, the vessels with numerous closely-packed bordered pits or reticulately thickened.

ACTION Cholagogue.

BAYBERRY BARK Myricaceae

Myricae radicis cortex

Synonyms: Myrica, Wax Myrtle Bark, Candle Berry Bark.

Bayberry Bark consists of the dried root-bark of *Myrica cerifera* L.

CHARACTERISTICS

Macroscopical Description
Quills or curved pieces up to about 8 cm long, 1.5 cm broad and 1-2 mm thick; outer surface smooth, whitish or silvery-grey when cork present, but this usually removed or exfoliating giving a reddish-brown, smooth or slightly reticulated surface; inner surface dark brown and finely striated longitudinally; fracture granular in the outer part, fibrous in the inner part; fractured surface reddish-brown.

Microscopical Description
Outer layers of thin-walled cork cells; phelloderm parenchymatous with some of the innermost layers converted to stone cells with moderately thickened and pitted walls; remainder of cortex parenchymatous with scattered groups of stone cells and, in the inner part, occasional small groups of lignified, thick-walled fibres; individual stone cells varying in size and shape but usually large, rectangular to polygonal with strongly thickened walls and numerous slit-shaped pits; secondary phloem with small groups of lignified fibres in more or less tangential rows alternating with wider areas of sieve tissue and large-celled parenchyma and separated by medullary rays two or three cells wide; all the fibre groups surrounded by sheaths of parenchymatous cells containing prism crystals of calcium oxalate; occasional parenchymatous cells throughout the cortex and secondary phloem filled with small, irregularly prismatic crystals of calcium oxalate, the remainder containing starch; starch granules simple or two or three compound, individual granules up to 12 µm in diameter.

Odour and Taste
Odour aromatic; taste slightly bitter and astringent, becoming pungent and unpleasant.

IDENTIFICATION

Carry out the method for Thin-layer Chromatography as described in Appendix 1, using Solvent System C.

Apply 60 µl of each of the following solutions separately to the plate: (1) extract 1 g powdered Bayberry Bark by shaking with 20 ml dichloromethane for 20 minutes. Filter, evaporate the filtrate to dryness and dissolve the residue in 2 ml toluene; (2) 0.1% cineole in toluene.

Spray the plate with Spray Reagent D, heat at 105°C for 10-15 minutes, then examine in daylight.

Major bands relative to cineole are approximately as follows: purple 0.7, dark purple 0.3, brown 0.15.

QUANTITATIVE STANDARDS

Foreign Matter
Not more than 3%   Appendix 3

Total Ash
Not more than 10%   Appendix 4

Ash Insoluble in Hydrochloric Acid
Not more than 3%   Appendix 5

Water-soluble Extractive
Not less than 10%   Appendix 7

MATERIAL OF COMMERCE Bayberry Bark is supplied as small broken pieces. It is obtained from south-eastern states of the USA.

Powdered Bayberry Bark

Complies with the requirements for Identification and Quantitative Standards stated for Bayberry Bark.

Characteristic Features
Light to reddish brown and sternutatory; odour aromatic, taste bitter and pungent; abundant starch granules, simple and rounded or two or three compound; calcium oxalate prism crystals scattered and in crystal sheaths associated with groups of thick-walled, lignified fibres; stone cells occurring singly or in groups, with moderately thickened walls and showing considerable variation in size and shape; fragments of polygonal, reddish-brown cork cells; thick-walled parenchyma with dense yellowish to reddish-brown contents.

ACTION Astringent.

BEARBERRY LEAF   Ericaceae

Uvae ursi folium

Synonyms: Arctostaphylos, Uva Ursi.

Bearberry Leaf consists of the dried leaves of *Arctostaphylos uva-ursi* (L.) Spreng.

This material complies with the requirements of the European Pharmacopoeia for *Bearberry Leaf*.

MATERIAL OF COMMERCE Bearberry Leaf is usually supplied as whole or slightly broken leaves. It is collected from the wild and obtained from many countries in Europe.

ACTION Urinary antiseptic.

BELLADONNA HERB   Solanaceae

Belladonnae herba

Synonyms: Atropa, Deadly Nightshade.

Belladonna Herb consists of the dried leaf or the dried leaf, flowering tops and occasionally fruits of *Atropa belladonna* L.

This material complies with the requirements of the European Pharmacopoeia for *Belladonna Leaf* and the British Pharmacopoeia for Belladonna Herb or, when the material is in powder, Powdered Belladonna Herb.

MATERIAL OF COMMERCE Belladonna Herb is supplied in the broken or crushed condition. It is usually obtained from plants cultivated in northern Europe or the USA; it is also collected from the wild in south-eastern Europe.

ACTION Antispasmodic.

BIRCH LEAF

Betulae folium

Synonyms: Silver Birch Leaf *(Betula pendula)*; Downy Birch Leaf *(Betula pubescens)*. The names *B. alba* and European White Birch have been used for both species.

Birch Leaf consists of the dried leaves of *Betula pendula* Roth [*Betula verrucosa* Ehrh.] or *Betula pubescens* Ehrh.

CHARACTERISTICS

Macroscopical Description
Betula pendula Upper surface green, lower surface light green, both glabrous; 2.5-6 cm long, up to 3.5 cm wide; rhomboid, less often triangular or ovoid, variable; margin conspicuously biserrate; apex sharply pointed; base, devoid of serrations, broadly tapering, cuneate; venation fine, pinnate, more obvious on lower surface, lateral veins terminating in larger, marginal teeth, smaller veinlets forming a fine network.
Betula pubescens Somewhat smaller; shapes similar, more variable; margin serrate, the single teeth smaller and less obviously apically directed; venation more well marked; surface sometimes finely pubescent all over, or hairs only associated with veins on lower surface, occasionally few along margin.
Leaves of both species thin; petiole less than half the length of lamina.

Microscopical Description
The anatomy of both species very similar. Dorsiventral, palisade usually of two layers, the upper closely-packed typical cells, somewhat the longer in *B. pendula*, the second layer of less typical cells, rather short, indistinctly obconical, more loosely spaced; spongy mesophyll cells with spreading arms, in *B. pubescens* well-marked, more elongated parallel to leaf surface, in *B. pendula* the cells more or less spherical, the projections less distinct. Upper epidermal cells with almost flat outer wall, slightly thickened, cuticle smooth; inner periclinal wall distinctly inwardly curved, pushing into palisade layer; lower epidermal cells smaller,

not so deep, inner and outer periclinal walls flat; stomata present, slightly raised; occasional cluster crystals in the spongy mesophyll. Midrib with upper xylem of narrow, lignified elements, small areas of sieve tissue below; above and below the vascular tissue moderately thick-walled, lignified fibres, the upper in a narrow, almost continuous band, the lower of narrowly separated, irregular groups; immediately adjacent to the outer limits of the fibre bands, infrequent single prism crystals; numerous cluster crystals in the parenchymatous ground tissue; epidermal cells above and below midrib small, outer wall convex; subjacent to both, several layers of collenchymatous parenchyma. In surface view, upper epidermal cells almost straight-walled, uniform, isodiametric, polygonal; stomata absent; palisade cells small, uniform, closely packed; lower epidermal cells isodiametric, straight-walled, polygonal, considerably smaller; numerous stomata with four to eight subsidiary cells; cluster crystals in the spongy mesophyll, scattered and, more usually, in short rows near veins; associated with the underside of some larger veins, as well as midrib, short, discontinuous, isolated files of parenchymatous cells containing single prism crystals; glands, sessile or very shortly-stalked, on both surfaces, most numerous in association with veins; pale brown or almost colourless, usually with conspicuous, thin, swollen bladder and made up of a few layers of small, more or less rectangular cells in radial rows, the innermost cells more thickened and darker brown; in some, more mature glands, the central cell structure less well-defined; glands in sectional view wide, shallow and gently convex above, seated in small depressions close to the epidermis. In *B. pubescens* only, of variable frequency, unicellular covering trichomes, thick-walled, lumen very narrow except near base where there are brown contents; conical and usually straight; length variable, some longer trichomes bent or undulate; walls unlignified and smooth; occasional larger trichomes with faintly warted surface.

Odour and Taste
Odourless or faintly aromatic; tasteless or very slightly bitter.

IDENTIFICATION

Carry out the method for Thin-layer Chromatography as described in Appendix 1 using Solvent System A.

Apply 20 µl of each of the following solutions separately to the plate: (1) extract 1 g powdered Birch Leaf with 10 ml methanol by warming on a water-bath for 10-15 minutes, cool and filter; (2) 0.025% rutin in methanol.

Spray the plate with Spray Reagent A and examine in ultraviolet light 366nm.

Major bands relative to rutin are approximately as follows: turquoise 2.1, yellow 2.0, yellow 1.8, yellow1.7, yellow 1.5. There is an area of fine detail from 1.5-1.2.

QUANTITATIVE STANDARDS

Foreign Matter
Not more than 3%   Appendix 3

Total Ash
Not more than 6%   Appendix 4

Ash Insoluble in Hydrochloric Acid
Not more than 4%   Appendix 5

Water-soluble Extractive
Not less than 10%   Appendix 7

MATERIAL OF COMMERCE Birch Leaf is supplied in the whole or broken condition. It is harvested from the wild and obtained mainly from eastern European countries, the former USSR and China.

Powdered Birch Leaf

Complies with the requirements for Identification and Quantitative Standards stated for Birch Leaf.

ACTION Diuretic; antirheumatic.

BLACK COHOSH   Ranunculaceae

Cimicifugae rhizoma

Synonyms: Cimicifuga, Black Snakeroot, Actaeae racemosae radix.

Black Cohosh consists of the dried rhizome and roots of *Cimicifuga racemosa* (L.) Nutt.

CHARACTERISTICS

Macroscopical Description
  Rhizomes Dark-brown, hard, sub-cylindrical and somewhat knotted, 1-2 cm in diameter and 5-15 cm long, with numerous, closely-arranged, upright or curved branches each terminating in the remains of a bud or in a circular, cup-shaped scar; branches about 1 cm thick and up to 3 cm long and marked with distinct, encircling leaf scars; fracture, horny; transverse surface showing a thin outer bark surrounding a ring of numerous pale, narrow wedges of vascular tissue alternating with dark medullary rays; a large central pith. Roots attached to the under surface of the rhizome or more usu-

ally broken off leaving circular scars.
  Roots Dark brown, 1-3 mm in diameter, brittle, nearly cylindrical or obtusely quadrangular, longitudinally wrinkled; fracture short; transverse surface showing a distinct cambium line separating a wide outer bark from a central region composed of three to six wedges of lignified xylem tissue united by their apices and separated by broad, nonlignified medullary rays.

Microscopical Description
  Rhizome Suberised epidermal cells tabular in surface view with moderately thickened walls, parenchymatous cortex filled with starch; xylem wedges lignified and composed of numerous, small vessels with bordered pits or reticulately-thickened walls, thin-walled fibres and xylem parenchyma, unlignified parenchyma of pith and medullary rays filled with starch granules, spherical or polygonal, simple or two to three or even up to six-compound, individual

granules 3-15 µm in diameter with central slit-shaped hilum.

Root Tissues similar.

Odour and Taste
No odour; slightly bitter taste.

IDENTIFICATION

Carry out the method for Thin-layer Chromatography as described in Appendix 1, using Solvent System A.

Apply 20 µl of each of the following solutions separately to the plate: (1) extract 1 g powdered Black Cohosh with 10 ml methanol by refluxing on a water-bath for 15-20 minutes, cool and filter; (2) 0.025% rutin in methanol.

Spray the plate with Spray Reagent A and examine in ultraviolet light 366 nm.

Major bands relative to rutin are approximately as follows: whitish-blue 2.2, pale blue 1.9, whitish-blue 1.65.

QUANTITATIVE STANDARDS

Stem Bases
Not more than 5%

Foreign Matter
Not more than 2%   Appendix 3

Total Ash
Not more than 10%   Appendix 4

Ash Insoluble In Hydrochloric Acid
Not more than 4%   Appendix 5

Water-soluble Extractive
Not less than 10%   Appendix 7

MATERIAL OF COMMERCE Black Cohosh is supplied in the whole or broken condition. It is obtained from Canada and northern USA.

Powdered Black Cohosh

Complies with the requirements for Identification and Quantitative Standards stated for Black Cohosh.

Characteristic Features
Light brown powder, odourless with a bitter taste; abundant starch granules, often occurring in masses in numerous fragments of thin-walled parenchyma; groups of small, lignified vessels with closely-arranged bordered pits or, less frequently, with reticulate thickening; lignified thin-walled fibres and xylem parenchyma; fragments of brown suberised cells with thickened walls.

ACTION Anti-inflammatory.

BLACK HAW BARK   Caprifoliaceae

Viburni prunifolii cortex

Synonyms: Stagbush Bark, American Sloe Bark.

Black Haw Bark consists of the dried root-bark and/or stem-bark of *Viburnum prunifolium* L.

CHARACTERISTICS

Macroscopical Description
Dull grey-brown, channelled or curved pieces, rarely quilled, up to 10 cm in length and 1-4 mm wide. Outer surface irregularly fissured and scaly; inner surface, yellow or orange-brown, longitudinally striated, cream adherent xylem fragments sometimes present. Fracture short and granular.

Microscopical Description
Root bark Exfoliating, stratified cork comprising several layers of tabular cells with brown cell content alternating with several rows of lignified cells; outer cortical cells collenchymatous, inner parenchymatous; phloem, interspersed with narrow med-

ullary rays, consisting of sieve tissue, parenchyma and small groups of lignified, striated, pitted sclereids. Many parenchymatous cells contain cluster crystals of calcium oxalate, 10-25 μm in diameter, and/or oil globules; isolated oval starch granules, 5-20 μm in length, may occur.

Stem bark Additionally, occasional small groups of non or lightly lignified, thick walled pericyclic fibres.

Odour and Taste
Odour slight and resembling Valerian; taste bitter and astringent.

IDENTIFICATION

Carry out the method for Thin-layer Chromatography as described in Appendix 1, using chloroform: acetone: formic acid (75:16.5:8.5) as the solvent system.

Prepare two separate plates (Plates 1 and 2), applying 40 μl of the following solution to each plate: defat 2 g powdered Black Haw Bark by heating under reflux with 50 ml light petroleum for 15 minutes, filter and extract the residue with 20 ml methanol by warming on a water bath for 20 minutes, then cool and filter; evaporate the filtrate to approximately 1 ml.

Spray Plate 1 with Spray Reagent A and examine in ultraviolet light 366 nm.

Major bands relative to the solvent front are approximately as follows: white 0.7, white 0.6, white 0.55, yellow 0.4*, white 0.05.

* The presence of the yellow band at Rf 0.4 distinguishes Black Haw Bark from Cramp Bark (from *Viburnum opulus* L.); this band is absent in a chromatogram of the latter.

As a further test for substitution or adulteration with Cramp Bark, spray Plate 2 with Spray Reagent F and examine the plate in daylight. No brown-red band at Rf 0.1-0.2 is observed in the chromatogram of Black Haw Bark, but this band is characteristic for Cramp Bark.

QUANTITATIVE STANDARDS

Foreign Matter
Not more than 3%   Appendix 3

Total Ash
Not more than 12%   Appendix 4

Ash Insoluble in Hydrochloric Acid
Not more than 4%   Appendix 5

Water-insoluble Extractive
Not less than 10%   Appendix 7

MATERIAL OF COMMERCE
Black Haw Bark is supplied as small pieces of root-bark and/or stem-bark of irregular shape. It is obtained from central and eastern USA.

Powdered Black Haw Bark

Complies with the requirements for Identification and Quantitative Standards stated for Black Haw Bark.

Characteristic Features
Light reddish-fawn powder with a slight but characteristic odour and bitter, astringent taste; fragments of yellowish-brown cork some lignified; abundant collenchyma, some beaded, and parenchyma cells containing calcium oxalate cluster crystals or oil globules; groups of elongated, oval or irregularly shaped, occasionally isodiametric or cube-shaped, lignified sclereids with thick, pitted, striated walls; infrequent oval starch granules and prismatic crystals of calcium oxalate; rare fragments of lignified xylem vessels. Fragments of epiphyte and lightly lignified, thick-walled fibres from stem bark.

ACTION Spasmolytic.

BLACK HOREHOUND Labiatae

Ballotae nigrae herba

Synonyms: Ballota, *Marrubium nigrum* Crantz.

Black Horehound consists of the dried aerial parts of *Ballota nigra* L. [*Ballota foetida* Lam.] collected during the flowering period.

CHARACTERISTICS

Macroscopical Description
Stems Branched, erect, main axis up to 90 cm, four-angled, longitudinally striated, corners accentuated; upper dark green, lower reddish-brown; variably hairy, most short, bent and downwardly directed.

Leaves Opposite, petiolate, ovate to orbicular, lamina 2-5 cm, base more or less cuneate; margin irregularly crenate; soft-textured, hairy, somewhat rugose; venation pinnate, veins slightly depressed on upper, prominent on lower surface.

Flowers Several whorls of many flowers in axils of paired upper leaf-like bracts; flowers shortly pedicellate with three subulate hairy bracteoles; calyx funnel-shaped, hairy, 5-7 mm long, ten-ribbed, opening to five broadly ovate teeth with acutely pointed apices, 1-2 mm; teeth spreading or recurved in fruit; corolla purple, 1-2 cm, tube shorter than calyx, upper lobe very hairy, lower lip less hairy or glabrous, tube paler in colour, hairy on upper outer surface; within tube, less than half way above base, a complete ring of hairs.

Fruits Four small slightly elongated-ovoid, three-sided achenes, shiny, dark brown to almost black.

Microscopical Description
Stem Section square, rounded, extensions at corners, small irregularities along sides; epidermal cells small, outer wall convex, occasional stomata; covering trichomes, weakly lignified, up to three cells, on slightly raised multicellular base, cell junctions thickened and swollen; infrequent small glandular trichomes, stalk very short, one to three-celled, head almost spherical; areas of collenchymatous cells in corners; endodermis well-marked; continuous band of sclerenchymatous tissue including rows of larger vessels at the corners, smaller groups at intervals along sides; vessels strongly lignified, spirally thickened and bordered-pitted; pith, with central hollow, thin-walled parenchymatous cells.

Leaf Dorsiventral; upper epidermal cells thin-walled, more or less rectangular, deeply and widely sinuous, stomata absent or very infrequent; lower epidermal cells slightly smaller, more sinuous; numerous stomata, anomocytic, three or four subsidiary cells, fewer with two subsidiary cells, diacytic. Both epidermises with one to three-celled swollen-jointed trichomes, slender pointed, terminal cell longest; few glandular trichomes, up to four-celled globose heads, short stalk of two cells unequal in length; very few almost sessile glands, eight-celled head and conspicuous cuticular bladder.

Flower Calyx epidermal cells thin-walled, loosely sinuous, stomata in outer epidermis; both epidermises with numerous unicellular, narrowly conical trichomes, apically directed, shorter on inner surface; ribs of outer surface bear longer two to three-celled, curved, swollen-jointed trichomes, basal cell short and wide, thicker walled; few glandular trichomes, stalks up to five cells long. Corolla inner epidermal cells of upper lobe small polygonal, papillose, outer epidermal cells rectangular, sinuous; margins of lobe with one to three-celled, almost straight trichomes with swollen joints; central upper area of lobe densely covered with cluster trichomes having an erect, two or three-celled central component; the short, wide basal cell constricting abruptly into the second, much narrower cell, is surrounded by a spreading rosette of five to seven much shorter, unicellular components, conical, many undulate; lower lip glabrous or with few hairs; tube, upper outer epidermis with long thin-walled trichomes, the majority unicellular, few bicellular, the basal cell short, wide; tube inner, ring of long, very closely-spaced, oblong-lanceolate, thin-walled straight trichomes up to 650 μm long, 30 μm wide; above ring to near throat of corolla, two rows of much shorter, slightly wider, lanceolate unicellular trichomes, bases slightly constricted. Pollen grains 25-30 μm, spherical to slightly oval, three pores, exine smooth.

Odour and Taste
Disagreeable.

IDENTIFICATION

Carry out the method for Thin-layer Chromatography as described in Appendix 1, using Solvent System A.

Apply 20 μl of each of the following solutions separately to the plate: (1) extract 1 g powdered Black Horehound with 10 ml methanol by warming on a water-bath for 10-15 minutes, cool and filter; (2) 0.025% rutin in methanol.

Spray the plate with Spray Reagent A and examine in ultraviolet light 366 nm.

Major bands relative to rutin are approximately as follows: turquoise 2.0, turquoise 1.8, turquoise 1.6, yellow 1.3, turquoise 1.0, turquoise 0.8, yellow 0.7, turquoise 0.6.

QUANTITATIVE STANDARDS

Foreign Matter
Not more than 2%   Appendix 3

Total Ash
Not more than 11%   Appendix 4

Ash Insoluble in Hydrochloric Acid
Not more than 1%   Appendix 5

Water-soluble Extractive
Not less than 10%   Appendix 7

MATERIAL OF COMMERCE Black Horehound is supplied in the cut or broken condition. It is a Mediterranean herb, harvested from wild or cultivated plants in southern Europe.

Powdered Black Horehound

Complies with the requirements for Identification and Quantitative Standards stated for Black Horehound.

ACTION Anti-emetic.

BLADDERWRACK   Fucaceae

Fuci thallus

Synonyms: Fucus, Seawrack, Kelpware.

Bladderwrack consists of the entire thallus of *Fucus vesiculosus* L., dried as soon as possible after collection.

CHARACTERISTICS

Macroscopical Description
Grey to black, thin, flattened pieces of thallus; hard and brittle when dry, becoming softer and mucilaginous when wet; occasional air vesicles present.

Microscopical Description
Outer epidermis of thin-walled cells, polygonal in surface view and rectangular, often palisade-like, in side view; cortex of several layers of parenchymatous cells; central medulla tissue of loosely interwoven strands of elongated cells which are cross-connected and have a branched appearance, oval antheridia borne terminally on branches near the base of much branched short hairs having swollen elongated cells; long, unbranched paraphyses occasionally associated with spherical oogonia which are sessile or borne on a short unicellular stalk.

Odour and Taste
Typical sea-weed odour; bland and mucilaginous taste.

IDENTIFICATION

Carry out the method for Thin-layer Chromatography as described in Appendix 1, using a mixture of butan-1-ol: propan-1-ol:

glacial acetic acid: water (3:1:1:1) as the Solvent System.

Apply 20 µl of each of the following solutions separately to the plate: (1) extract 2 g powdered Bladderwrack with 10 ml 30% methanol by refluxing on a water-bath for 30 minutes, cool and filter; (2) 0.025% L-methionine in methanol.

Spray the plate with Ninhydrin Reagent, heat at 105°C for 20-30 minutes and examine in daylight.

Major bands relative to L-methionine are approximately as follows: pink 0.54, pinkish-yellow 0.38.

QUANTITATIVE STANDARDS

Foreign Matter
Not more than 2%   Appendix 3

Total Ash
Not more than 22%   Appendix 4

Ash Insoluble in Hydrochloric Acid
Not more than 4%   Appendix 5

Water-soluble Extractive
Not less than 15%   Appendix 7

MATERIAL OF COMMERCE Bladderwrack is usually supplied in the cut condition and is obtained from West European coastal regions, particularly of Ireland and France.

Powdered Bladderwrack

Complies with the requirements for Identification and Quantitative Standards stated for Bladderwrack.

Characteristic Features
Reddish-brown powder with an odour of sea-weed and a mucilaginous taste; numerous fragments of epidermis with polygonal cells; elongated hypodermal cells and irregular fragments of pseudoparenchyma with thick, mucilaginous walls.

ACTION Thyroactive.

BLUE FLAG   Iridaceae

Iridis versicoloris rhizoma

Blue Flag consists of the dried rhizome of *Iris versicolor* L. or *Iris caroliniana* Watson.

CHARACTERISTICS

Macroscopical Description
Rhizomes often branched, up to 20 cm long and 3 cm wide at the nodes, usually flattened dorsiventrally and divided by slight constrictions 3-5 cm apart; outer surface greyish-brown to purplish-brown, wrinkled longitudinally and bearing annular scars; lower surface showing numerous root scars or occasional transversely wrinkled roots; upper surface bearing remains of leaf bases; fracture short, the broken surface varying in colour from cream to purplish-brown and exhibiting whitish fibro-vascular bundles scattered throughout the stele.

Microscopical Description
Narrow zone of greyish-brown to purplish-brown cork; hypodermis of several layers with occasional groups of sclereids with uniformly thickened walls, often associated with epidermal cells with brownish walls; ground tissue composed of rounded parenchymatous cells with non-lignified beaded walls and conspicuous pits, the large intercellular spaces containing prismatic crystals of calcium oxalate, 200-350 µm and sometimes up to 600 µm long, with oblique or chisel-shaped ends; some parenchymatous cells containing amylodextrin granules, spherical or elliptical in shape and up to 25 µm in diameter, which stain red with iodine solution; occasional starch granules; many rounded resin cells containing reddish-brown amorphous substance; endodermis with U-shaped lignified thickening; vascular

41

bundles with a central group of sieve tissue surrounded by lignified xylem with groups of vessels having annular, spiral and pitted thickening, sometimes associated with fibres.

Odour and Taste
Slightly aromatic odour; sweet and slightly acrid taste.

IDENTIFICATION

Carry out the method for Thin-layer Chromatography as described in Appendix 1 using Solvent System A.

Apply 20 µl of each of the following solutions separately to the plate: (1) extract 1 g powdered Blue Flag with 10 ml methanol on a water-bath for 10-15 minutes, cool, filter and concentrate the filtrate to about 5 ml; (2) 0.025%, rutin in methanol.

Spray the plate with Spray Reagent A and examine in ultraviolet light 366 nm.

Major bands relative to rutin are approximately as follows: green 1.3, green 1.2 and green 1.0.

QUANTITATIVE STANDARDS

Leaf Bases
Not more than 5%

Foreign Matter
Not more than 2%   Appendix 3

Total Ash
Not more than 8%   Appendix 4

Ash Insoluble in Hydrochloric Acid
Not more than 2%   Appendix 5

Ethanol (60 %) Soluble Extractive
Not less than 25%   Appendix 6A

MATERIAL OF COMMERCE Blue Flag is supplied as broken pieces. It is obtained from eastern and central North America and from southern Europe.

Powdered Blue Flag

Complies with the requirements for Identification and Quantitative Standards stated for Blue Flag.

Characteristic Features
Reddish-brown powder with a slight, aromatic odour and a sweet and slightly acrid taste; numerous fragments of parenchyma associated with resin cells, large prismatic crystals of calcium oxalate; parenchymatous cells containing granules of amylodextrin; vessels with spiral or annular thickening.

ACTION Laxative.

BOGBEAN   Menyanthaceae

Menyanthidis folium

Synonyms: Menyanthes, Buckbean.

Bogbean consists of the dried leaves of *Menyanthes trifoliata* L. collected after flowering.

CHARACTERISTICS

Macroscopical Description
Long stalked, trifoliate leaves with sheathing base; leaflets dull green or yellowish-green, 3.5-7 cm long and 1-4 cm wide; lamina glabrous, ovate or elliptical with an entire, occasionally sinuous margin and a spathulate, almost sessile base; apex subacute and venation pinnate; petiole yellowish-green, 7-15 cm long, finely striated and often twisted.

Microscopical Description
Epidermal cells straight or slightly sinuous on upper surface, more sinuous on lower surface; anomocytic stomata more numerous on lower surface with adjacent cells showing radiate, cuticular striations; elongated epidermal cells over veins and at margins, usually papillose with a striated cuti-

cle; two to four layers of palisade cells; midrib showing an arc of collateral bundles; petiole with a ring of collateral bundles embedded in aerenchyma; narrow lignified vessels with spiral or annular thickening.

Odour and Taste
Slight but distinctive odour; very bitter taste.

IDENTIFICATION

Carry out the method for Thin-layer Chromatography as described in Appendix 1, using Solvent System A.

Apply 20 µl of each of the following solutions separately to the plate: (1) extract 1 g powdered Bogbean with 10 ml methanol on a water-bath for 10-15 minutes, cool, filter and concentrate to about 2 ml; (2) 0.025% rutin in methanol.

Spray the plate with Spray Reagent A and examine in ultraviolet light 366 nm.

Major bands relative to rutin are approximately as follows: pale blue 1.5, orange 1.3, yellowish-white 1.2, orange 1.0, pale blue 0.85.

QUANTITATIVE STANDARDS

Foreign Matter
Not more than 2%   Appendix 3

Total Ash
Not more than 10%   Appendix 4

Ash Insoluble in Hydrochloric Acid
Not more than 2%   Appendix 5

Water-soluble Extractive
Not less than 23%   Appendix 7

MATERIAL OF COMMERCE Bogbean is usually supplied as the crushed leaf. It is obtained from eastern Europe.

Powdered Bogbean

Complies with the requirements for Identification and Quantitative Standards stated for Bogbean.

Characteristic Features
Yellowish-green powder with a slight odour and a bitter taste; fragments of leaf lamina with straight or sinuous anticlinal walls; some fragments with anomocytic stomata and adjacent cells with radiate striations; papillose epidermal cells with longitudinally striated cuticle.

ACTION Bitter.

BOLDO   Monimiaceae

Boldo folium

Boldo consists of the dried leaves of *Peumus boldus* Molina.

CHARACTERISTICS

Macroscopical Description
Greyish-green, somewhat glossy, coriaceous and brittle; up to 6 cm long and 2.5-3 cm wide, oblong-ovate to broadly ovate, apex obtuse, often slightly emarginate, base equal, rounded; margin entire, smooth or somewhat undulate, thickened and more or less revolute; venation pinnate, veins prominent on lower surface, fawnish, finely pubescent; upper surface with numerous prominent, warty excrescences, lower surface with less well-marked warts; petioles 2-3 mm, woody.

Microscopical Description
Dorsiventral, palisade of two layers composed of cells of nearly equal length; upper epidermal cells polygonal, thick-walled, indistinctly beaded, straight or slightly sinuous anticlinal walls, stomata absent; lower epidermal cells somewhat larger, straight or sinuous-walled, very numerous slightly raised anomocytic stomata with two or three of the subsidiary cells smaller than the oth-

ers; stellate trichomes with up to sixteen thick-walled, unicellular components, lignified, present on both epidermises; inconspicuous scars of fallen trichomes; hypodermis, usually of one layer but may be up to three or more layers in places, beneath the upper epidermis, cells resembling those of the epidermis, thick-walled, pitted in both the anticlinal and periclinal walls; vascular strand with narrow xylem elements, thick-walled sclerenchymatous fibres and lignified pitted parenchymatous cells; numerous almost-spherical oil cells in the spongy mesophyll; aggregations of small, blunt-ended prismatic crystals in many cells of the mesophyll.

Odour and Taste
Odour faintly aromatic and pungent; taste aromatic, somewhat unpleasant, reminiscent of thymol, bitter and slightly astringent.

IDENTIFICATION

Carry out the method for Thin-layer Chromatography as described in Appendix 1 using Solvent System C.

Apply 60 μl of each of the following solutions to the plate: (1) extract 2 g of powdered Boldo by shaking with 20 ml of dichloromethane for 20 minutes. Filter, evaporate the filtrate just to dryness and dissolve the residue in 2 ml of toluene; (2) 0.1% cineole in toluene.

Spray the plate with Spray Reagent D, heat at 105°C for 10-15 minutes and examine in daylight.

Major bands relative to cineole are approximately as follows: purple 2.15, brown 1.1, blue 1.0, green 0.8, brown 0.45.

QUANTITATIVE STANDARDS

Foreign Matter
Not more than 2%   Appendix 3

Total Ash
Not more than 15%   Appendix 4

Ash Insoluble in Hydrochloric Acid
Not more than 9%   Appendix 5

Water-soluble Extractive
Not less than 15%   Appendix 7

MATERIAL OF COMMERCE Boldo is supplied in the whole or broken form. It is obtained from Chile and Peru.

Powdered Boldo

Complies with the requirements for Identification and Quantitative Standards stated for Boldo.

Characteristic Features
Greyish-green powder with an aromatic and slightly pungent odour and taste; numerous whole and fragmented stellate trichomes, unicellular components, some of which may show a slender, superficial, widely-spaced, spiral band; abundant oil cells; upper epidermis, usually associated with hypodermis; lower epidermis with frequent anomocytic stomata; infrequent parenchyma with small crystals, thick-walled fibres, and lignified pitted parenchyma.

ACTION Cholagogue.

BROOM TOP

Leguminosae-Papilionoideae

Cytisi scoparii herba

Synonyms: Scoparium, Scotch Broom.

Broom Top consists of the dried flowering tops of *Cytisus scoparius* (L.) Link [*Sarothamnus scoparius* (L.) Wimm. ex Koch].

CHARACTERISTICS

Macroscopical Description

Stems Dark green, glabrous with five prominent, longitudinal ridges; 2-4 mm in diameter.

Leaves Alternate, ternate with short petiole on lower stem, simple and sessile on upper; dark green, distinctly pubescent when young; leaves lanceolate, 4-7 mm long, margin entire, apex acute, base even; leaflets more ovate.

Flowers Axillary, 20 mm long; calyx, short two-lipped tube with five minute teeth; five yellow, papilionate petals enclosing ten stamens and a long spirally coiled style. Elongated, unilocular ovary with marginal placentation and several ovules.

Microscopical Description

Stem Polygonal epidermal cells with straight, thickened anticlinal walls; cuticle, thick and smooth; stomata anomocytic, very numerous; several rows of cortical parenchyma, outer layers with chloroplasts, groups of fibres occur in tip and central area of ridges; stele with secondary growth consisting of compacted ring of phloem with groups of pericyclic fibres; wide ring of lignified xylem containing thin-walled fibres with acute apices and narrow diameter vessels and tracheids with annular or reticulate thickening; central parenchymatous pith, completely lignified in older stems.

Leaf Epidermal cells of both surfaces, polygonal with straight anticlinal walls; cuticle smooth but striated on leaf margins; frequent anomocytic stomata and thick-walled covering trichomes 200-400 µm long, some finely warty, unicellular, rarely bicellular with additional short basal cell. Isobilateral, two layers of palisade below each surface, upper continuous over midrib. Midrib vascular bundle, collateral, containing small areas of phloem and xylem only.

Flower Calyx, polygonal cells with straight anticlinal walls; outer epidermis with slightly beaded walls; inner epidermis, non-beaded with infrequent anomocytic stomata. Corolla, polygonal cells; inner surface of upper petals, wavy-walled with internal projections in apical areas, sinuous and beaded nearer base, cuticle faintly striated; inner surface of keel petals papillose with striated cuticle; outer epidermis, wavy, slightly thickened anticlinal walls; narrow, elongated cells occur on all margins. Stamen, lignified fibrous layer of anther wall; spherical pollen grains, 20-25 µm in diameter, with three pores and a smooth or very finely pitted exine.

Odour and Taste

Odour slight; taste bitter and unpleasant.

IDENTIFICATION

Carry out the method for Thin-layer Chromatography as described in Appendix 1, using Solvent System A.

Apply 20 µl of each of the following solutions separately to the plate: (1) extract 1 g powdered Broom Top with 10 ml methanol by warming on a water-bath for 10-15 minutes, cool and filter; (2) 0.025% rutin in methanol.

Spray the plate with Spray Reagent A and examine in ultraviolet light 366 nm.

Major bands relative to rutin are approximately as follows: turquoise 2.1, yellow 1.8, yellow 1.6, yellow 1.5, turquoise 0.82.

QUANTITATIVE STANDARDS

Foreign Matter
Not more than 2%   Appendix 3

Total Ash
Not more than 3%   Appendix 4

Acid Insoluble in Hydrochloric Acid
Not more than 2%   Appendix 5

Water-soluble Extractive
Not less than 9%   Appendix 7

MATERIAL OF COMMERCE Broom Top is supplied in the cut condition. It is mainly harvested from the wild and obtained from southern and central Europe.

Powdered Broom Top

Complies with the requirements for Identification and Quantitative Standards stated for Broom Top.

Characteristic Features
Dark green powder with a slight odour and a bitter, unpleasant taste; leaf and stem fragments with polygonal epidermal cells and anomocytic stomata, often numerous; unicellular, rarely bicellular, thick-walled, sometimes warty, covering trichomes, free and accompanied by epidermal cells; narrow, lignified xylem conducting elements with annular or reticulate thickening, sometimes accompanied by thin-walled fibres; polygonal epidermal cells of corolla, papillose or beaded with striated cuticle, or wavy-walled and evenly thickened, or having internal projections; straight-walled, beaded epidermal cells of the calyx; lignified fibrous anther wall; pollen grains with smooth or very finely pitted exine; occasional groups of lignified, pitted parenchyma.

ACTION Anti-arrhythmic, diuretic.

BUCHU   Rutaceae

Barosmae folium

Synonyms: Agathosma, Round or Short Buchu.

Buchu consists of the dried leaves of *Barosma betulina* Bartl. et Wendl. [*Agathosma betulina* (Berg.) Pillans] collected at the fruiting stage.

CHARACTERISTICS

Macroscopical Description
Wrinkled, simple leaves, 10-20 mm long and 6-10 mm wide with some smaller leaves present; bright green to yellowish green, darker on the upper surface; obovate, coriaceous and brittle; upper surface almost glabrous with small scattered prominences; lower surface finely wrinkled; margin dentate in the apical half and serrate in the lower half with an oil gland at the base of each dentation; apex blunt and recurved, base equal and acute.

Microscopical Description
Cells of the upper epidermis fairly large and polygonal with moderately thickened walls, frequently pitted or beaded; cells of the lower epidermis thin-walled and smaller; abundant anomocytic stomata in the lower epidermis only; mucilage which stains pink with Ruthenium Red Solution and yellow, feathery or sphaero crystals of diosmin which stain bright yellow with Potassium Hydroxide Solution are present in the epidermal cells; occasional unicellular covering trichomes with thick, slightly warty walls; mesophyll of moderately thickened parenchyma cells containing cluster crystals of calcium oxalate and surrounding large spherical oil glands; the mid-rib and larger veins contain abundant fibres, usually with thickened, lignified walls.

Odour and Taste
Strong aromatic odour reminiscent of blackcurrants; strong aromatic taste, becoming bitter.

IDENTIFICATION

Carry out the method for Thin-layer Chromatography as described in Appendix 1, using Solvent System A.

Apply 20 µl of each of the following solutions separately to the plate: (1) extract 1 g powdered Buchu with 10 ml methanol on a water-bath for 5 minutes, cool, filter and concentrate to about 5 ml; (2) 0.025% rutin in methanol.

Spray the plate with Spray Reagent A and examine in ultraviolet light 366 nm.

Major bands relative to rutin are approximately as follows: blue 2.4, blue 2.3, blue 1.3, orange 1.0.

QUANTITATIVE STANDARDS

Stems
Not more than 5%

Foreign Matter
Not more than 1%   Appendix 3

Total Ash
Not more than 5%   Appendix 4

Ash Insoluble in Hydrochloric Acid
Not more than 1.5%   Appendix 5

Water-soluble Extractive
Not less than 14%   Appendix 7

Volatile Oil
Not less than 1.3%   Appendix 9

MATERIAL OF COMMERCE Buchu is supplied as whole or coarsely broken leaves. It is obtained from South Africa.

Powdered Buchu

Complies with the requirements for Identification and Quantitative Standards stated for Buchu.

Characteristic Features
Greenish-yellow powder with a characteristic aromatic odour and taste; fragments of upper epidermis showing mucilage and crystals of diosmin, fragments of the lower epidermis with abundant stomata; abundant crystals of diosmin; cluster crystals of calcium oxalate; large, spherical oil glands; abundant fibres.

ACTION Urinary antiseptic.

BURDOCK LEAF   Compositae

Bardanae folium

Synonym: Lappa Leaf.

Burdock Leaf consists of the dried leaves of *Arctium lappa* L. [*Arctium majus* Bernh.] or *Arctium minus* Bernh. collected during the first year of growth.

CHARACTERISTICS

Macroscopical Description
Leaves petiolate, ovate-cordate, up to 40 cm long, with an undulating margin and acute apex; upper surface pale yellowish-green with scattered white hairs and pale, small, rounded, projecting glands; lower surface densely covered with a thick, greyish-white down composed of long felted hairs; petiole solid and furrowed (*A. iappa*) or hollow and finely longitudinally striated (*A. minus*).

Microscopical Description
Upper epidermal cells with sinuous to wavy anticlinal walls, with occasional covering trichomes of the whip-lash type with a uniseriate stalk composed of two to six cells and a terminal cell which is narrow, much elongated and curled, forming the lash, up to 500 μm long and 90 μm wide at the base frequently collapsed; scattered large, glandular trichomes with a short bi-cellular stalk and a head formed of two rows of cells enclosed in a bladder-like membrane; stomata absent, lower epidermal cells with wavy anticlinal walls with numerous anomocytic stomata, but the entire epidermis obscured

by a very abundant covering of trichomes similar to those on the upper epidermis; small prismatic crystals of calcium oxalate in the mesophyll.

Odour and Taste
Slight odour; bitter taste.

IDENTIFICATION

Carry out the method for Thin-layer Chromatography as described in Appendix 1 using Solvent System A.

Apply 20 µl of each of the following solutions separately to the plate: (1) extract 1 g powdered Burdock Leaf with 10 ml methanol on a water-bath for 10-15 minutes, cool and filter; (2) 0.025% rutin in methanol.

Spray the plate with Spray Reagent A and examine in ultraviolet light 366 nm.

Major bands relative to rutin are approximately as follows: pale bluish-green 2.2, orange 1.55, yellowish orange 1.45, blue 1.2.

QUANTITATIVE STANDARDS

Foreign Matter
Not more than 2%   Appendix 3

Total Ash
Not more than 15%   Appendix 4

Ash Insoluble in Hydrochloric Acid
Not more than 3%   Appendix 5

Water-soluble Extractive
Not less than 20%   Appendix 7

MATERIAL OF COMMERCE Burdock Leaf is usually supplied as large felted masses of leaves. It is obtained chiefly from Bulgaria, Hungary, Poland and the former Yugoslavia.

Powdered Burdock Leaf

Complies with the requirements for Identification and Quantitative Standards stated for Burdock Leaf.

Characteristic Features
Greyish-green powder with a slight, leafy odour and a bitter taste; abundant covering trichomes forming a felted mass, frequently with terminal cells detached and stalk cells still attached to fragments of lower epidermis; fragments of upper epidermis showing rounded glandular trichomes; portions of vascular tissue from the petioles with thin-walled lignified fibres and groups of reticulately-thickened vessels.

ACTION Dermatological agent.

BURDOCK ROOT   Compositae

Bardanae radix

Synonym: Lappa Root.

Burdock Root consists of the air-dried roots of *Arctium lappa* L. [*A. majus* Bernh.] or *Arctium minus* Bernh.

CHARACTERISTICS

Macroscopical Description
Cylindrical or flattened pieces of varying length and up to 1.5 cm in diameter; outer surface yellowish-brown to dark brown, longitudinally wrinkled with occasional scars of secondary roots; fracture short and horny, internal surface pale brownish-buff;

smoothed transverse surface showing an outer region occupying about one quarter of the radius separated by a dark cambium from the indistinctly radiate xylem; the central region in older roots usually much shrunken.

Microscopical Description
Cork composed of a number of layers of rather indistinct, rectangular, thin-walled cells; underlying phelloderm cells with brown contents; phloem fairly wide and composed mainly of large, thin-walled parenchymatous cells with narrow, radial strands of sieve tissue; resin canals arranged in an interrupted ring, often present in the outer

part of the phloem in young roots; in older roots small groups of fibres with moderately thickened, slightly lignified walls; xylem very parenchymatous and largely unlignified with small groups of lignified vessels and fibres arranged in narrow, radiating strands separated by wide medullary rays; vessels up to about150 μm in diameter with bordered pits or reticulately thickened walls; parenchymatous cells throughout the root containing angular masses of inulin and only occasional starch grains.

Odour and Taste
Odourless; mucilaginous, sweetish then slightly bitter taste.

IDENTIFICATION

Carry out the method for Thin-layer Chromatography as described in Appendix 1, using Solvent System A and allowing the solvent front to ascend a distance of 10 cm above the line of application.

Apply 20 μl of each of the following solutions separately to the plate: (1) extract 1 g powdered Burdock Root with 10 ml ethanol by shaking gently for 15 minutes, filter and evaporate to about 1 ml; (2) 0.025% rutin in methanol.

Spray the plate with Spray Reagent A and examine in ultraviolet light 366 nm.

Major bands relative to rutin are approximately as follows: narrow intense blue 2.35, whitish blue 2.1, pale blue 1.75, pale blue 1.4.

QUANTITATIVE STANDARDS

Loss on Drying
Not more than 15% when dried in an oven at 100-105°C. Use 2-3 g   Appendix 2

Foreign Matter
Not more than 2%   Appendix 3

Total Ash
Not more than 12% calculated with reference to the oven-dried material   Appendix 4

Ash Insoluble in Hydrochloric Acid
Not more than 3% calculated with reference to the oven-dried material   Appendix 5

Water-soluble Extractive
Not less than 24% calculated with reference to the oven-dried material   Appendix 7

MATERIAL OF COMMERCE Burdock Root is supplied as cylindrical or flattened pieces, often longitudinally split, showing inner tissue much shrunken, or as chopped pieces. It is obtained chiefly from Bulgaria, Hungary, Poland and the former Yugoslavia.

Powdered Burdock Root

Complies with the requirements for Identification and Quantitative Standards stated for Burdock Root.

Characteristic Features
Buff-coloured powder with little odour and a slightly bitter, mucilaginous taste; parenchymatous cells, many containing birefringent masses of inulin; some brown resin-like cell contents; xylem vessels with reticulately thickened walls or with bordered pits.

STORAGE Store in a cool, dry place in well closed containers.

ACTION Dermatological agent.

CALAMUS

Calami rhizoma

Synonyms: Acorus, Calamus Rhizome, Sweet Flag Root.

Calamus consists of the dried rhizomes of *Acorus calamus* L. var. *americanus* Wulff or *A. calamus* L. var. *vulgaris* L., free from roots and leaf bases, peeled or unpeeled.

CHARACTERISTICS

Macroscopical Description
Rhizome subcylindrical, almost straight or slightly curved, 5-15 cm long, up to 2 cm wide and 1.5 cm thick; infrequent lateral branching. Unpeeled: well-marked, irregular wrinkles, earthy to dark brown; upper surface with conspicuous, quite closely approximated, narrowly triangular leaf scars, continuing some way to lower surface, edges raised, short projecting fibres; underside rows of up to twelve closely -spaced, raised, root scars with central stele and narrow cortex, alternate rows inclined at an angle to one another, producing an irregular zig-zag pattern of scars; larger rhizomes sometimes split longitudinally. Peeled; similar shape and length, but more slender, almost always split, the interior shrunken, forming an ill-defined groove; external surface irregularly prismatic, with variably sized angular facets; surface pinkish-white or pale fawn, somewhat rough, scurfy; some remains of root scars, only infrequent traces of leaf scars; rarely, small patches of brown epidermal remains in regions of original deeper wrinkles; fracture short, mealy, somewhat spongy, pale fawn to faint pinkish-white.

Microscopical Description
Epidermal cells small, upright rectangular in transverse section, outer wall slightly thickened, smooth; in surface view, short, rectangular, anticlinal walls only slightly irregular; in regions of leaf scars, areas of larger, variable sub-epidermal corky cells; outer layers of cortex small-celled collenchymatous parenchyma without intercellular spaces, occasional pigmented tannin cells and larger, almost colourless, volatile oil cells; remaining parenchyma of ground tissue filled with starch grains, 3-6 µm, most simple, more or less ovoid, few up to eight-compound; progressively towards endodermis, intercellular spaces occur developing to well-marked lacunae; in longitudinal section the lacunae are axially elongated; contiguous walls of the lacunae cells with numerous, small, simple pits; oil cells abundant; cortex traversed by small number of oblique leaf-trace vascular bundles. Endodermis cells thin-walled, slightly tangentially elongated, starch-free. Fibro-vascular bundles collateral, phloem small-celled, lignified vessels, variable in size, thin-walled, angular outline, thickening spiral, annular, reticulate and scalariform, some with associated small pigmented cell; sheath of lignified fibres, up to four cells wide, encloses most bundles of cortex and stele, bundles immediately adjacent to endodermis without sheath, or only partially sheathed, fibres of narrow diameter, moderately thickened; in longitudinal section show few scattered small pits, outer fibres of sheaths accompanied by sub-rectangular thin-walled parenchyma cells, some containing quite small prismatic crystals; ground tissue of stele almost entirely lacunose, volatile oil cells numerous, occasional tannin cells and the starch-filled parenchyma.

Odour and Taste
Pleasant aromatic odour; taste bitter and pungent.

IDENTIFICATION

Carry out the method for Thin-layer Chromatography as described in Appendix 1, using Solvent System C.

Apply 60 µl of each of the following solutions separately to the plate: (1) extract 2 g powdered Calamus by shaking with 20 ml dichloromethane for 20 minutes. Filter, evaporate the filtrate just to dryness and dissolve the residue in 1 ml toluene; (2) 0.1% cineole in toluene.

Spray the plate with Spray Reagent D, heat at 105°C for 10-15 minutes, then examine in daylight.

The chromatogram of Calamus is characterised by a series of violet, brown-violet and purple bands throughout the entire Rf range corresponding to approximately 30 components of its essential oil.

Samples of Calamus display wide variability but major bands relative to cineole are approximately as follows: purple 1.85, purple 1.5, pink 0.95, purple 0.4.

QUANTITATIVE STANDARDS

Foreign Matter
Not more than 2%   Appendix 3

Total Ash
Not more than 6%   Appendix 4

Ash Insoluble in Hydrochloric Acid
Not more than 1.5%   Appendix 5

MATERIAL OF COMMERCE Calamus is supplied as sliced rhizomes. It is obtained mainly from Eastern Europe (var. *vulgaris*) or North America (var. *americanus*). Material from Asian sources, primarily the Indian subcontinent, is often unsuitable for me-

dicinal use due to its high content (4-8%) of β-asarone.

Powdered Calamus

Powdered Calamus complies with the requirements for Identification and Quantitative Standards stated for Calamus.

Characteristic Features
Pale, pink-tinged, fawn powder with spicy, aromatic odour and pungent, bitter taste; abundant, small, mainly simple, starch grains; thin-walled, ovoid, simple-pitted parenchyma; slightly larger, unpitted oil cells; irregular, small fragments of brown amorphous matter; narrow lignified vessels; slender, thin-walled fibres associated with short files of small prism crystals.

ACTION Carminative.

CALUMBA ROOT   Menispermaceae

Calumbae radix

Synonyms: Jateorhiza, Colombo Root.

Calumba Root consists of the dried, transverse or oblique slices of the roots and occasionally the rhizomes of *Jateorhiza palmata* (Lam.) Miers.

CHARACTERISTICS

Macroscopical Description
Roots Irregularly circular or oval slices of root depressed in the centre, 2-8 cm in diameter and 3-12 mm thick; yellow to yellowish-brown; cork thin, reddish-brown to greyish-brown and longitudinally wrinkled; transverse surface shows a dark cambium line separating a broad, outer greenish-yellow zone from a greyish inner wood.
Rhizomes Slices usually 2-3 cm in diameter and not depressed (sometimes raised) in the centre, which consists of lignified tissue.

Microscopical Description
Root Up to fifty radial rows of dark-brown polygonal cork cells with yellow or

yellow-green contents; cortex parenchymatous with isolated, irregular or rectangular, lignified sclereids near the cork; sclereids unevenly thickened with greenish-yellow walls and several prismatic crystals of calcium oxalate up to 30 µm long in the lumen; vascular region mainly parenchymatous, some lignified vessels with reticulate thickening or with bordered pits near to the cambium and in the centre of root; the walls of the sclereids and vessels turn green when mounted in 12M sulphuric acid; parenchymatous cells containing simple, occasionally two or three compound, spherical to oval, starch granulex 20-85 µm long with an eccentric, distinct, radiate or cleft hilum.
Rhizome Very similar to root but with a lignified, parenchymatous pith.

Odour and Taste
Slight odour; bitter, but not astringent taste.

IDENTIFICATION
Carry out the method for Thin-layer Chromatography as described in Appendix 1, using Solvent System A.

Apply 20 µl of each of the following solutions separately to the plate: (1) extract 1 g powdered Calumba Root with 10 ml methanol by refluxing on a water-bath for 10-15 minutes, cool and filter; (2) 0.025% rutin in methanol.

Spray the plate with Spray Reagent A and examine in ultraviolet light 366 nm.

Major bands relative to rutin are approximately as follows: green 1.3, whitish 1.2.

QUANTITATIVE STANDARDS

Foreign Matter
Not more than 2%   Appendix 3

Total Ash
Not more than 10%   Appendix 4

Ash Insoluble in Hydrochloric Acid
Not more than 2.5%   Appendix 5

Water-soluble Extractive
Not less than 15%   Appendix 7

MATERIAL OF COMMERCE Calumba Root is supplied as slices of root and rhizome and only occasionally in the broken condition. It is obtained mainly from South East Africa and Madagascar.

Powdered Calumba Root

Complies with the requirements for Identification and Quantitative Standards stated for Calumba Root.

Characteristic Features
Yellowish-brown powder with a greenish tinge, with a slight odour and a bitter but not astringent taste; fragments of cork cells with sinuous walls and yellow or yellowish-green contents; rectangular sclereids containing prismatic crystals of calcium oxalate; greenish-yellow vessels with reticulate or bordered-pitted thickening, abundant parenchyma and abundant starch; vessels and sclereids become green when mounted in 12M sulphuric acid.

ACTION Appetite stimulant.

CARAWAY   Umbelliferae

Carvi fructus

Synonyms: Caraway Seed, Caraway Fruit.

Caraway consists of the dried ripe fruits of *Carum carvi* L.

This material complies with the requirements of the British Pharmacopoeia for Caraway or, when the material is in powder, Powdered Caraway.

MATERIAL OF COMMERCE Caraway is supplied as whole fruits. It is cultivated in many countries and obtained mainly from Europe, North Africa and Turkey.

ACTION Carminative.

CARDAMOM FRUIT   Zingiberaceae

Cardamomi fructus

Synonym: Cardamon Fruit.

Cardamom Fruit consists of the dried, nearly ripe, fruits of *Elettaria cardamomum* Maton var. *minuscula* Burkill.

This material complies with the requirements of the British Pharmacopoeia for Cardamom Fruit.

MATERIAL OF COMMERCE Cardamom Fruit is supplied as whole fruits or as the seeds sealed in tins to prevent loss of volatile oil. It is harvested from cultivated plants and obtained mainly from Sri Lanka, southern India and Guatemala.

ACTION Carminative.

CASCARA

Rhamnaceae

Rhamni purshiani cortex

Synonym: Cascara Sagrada.

Cascara consists of the dried bark of *Rhamnus purshianus* DC. [*Frangula purshiana* (DC.) A. Gray ex J.C. Cooper].

This material complies with the requirements of the European Pharmacopoeia for Cascara and the British Pharmacopoeia for Cascara or, when the material is in powder, Powdered Cascara.

MATERIAL OF COMMERCE Cascara is supplied as quills, channelled or nearly flat pieces or in the broken condition. It is obtained mainly from western North America, particularly Oregon, Washington and British Columbia.

ACTION Stimulant laxative.

CASSIA BARK

Lauraceae

Cinnamomi cassiae cortex

Synonyms: Chinese Cinnamon, Cassia lignea.

Cassia Bark consists of the dried bark of stems or branches of *Cinnamomum cassia* Blume [*Cinnamomum aromaticum* Nees] from which the outer tissues may have been wholly or partly removed.

CHARACTERISTICS

Macroscopical Description
Channelled or slightly curved pieces, 2-3 mm thick, up to 2-3 cm wide, varying considerably in length, up to 30 or 40 cm; outer surface dark greyish-brown, slightly uneven, with dull lustre, numerous more or less round to elliptical lenticels, only occasionally lighter than surrounding surface; few, faint and uneven, longitudinal ridges; inner surface dull cinnamon brown, smooth or finely striated, occasional lighter, greyish-brown areas; larger pieces with few, irregular, longitudinal splits; fracture short, granular, inconspicuous fibres in inner region. Some samples may have had much of the outer tissues removed.

Microscopical Description
Section of unscraped bark, occasional areas with small epidermal cells, outer walls slightly thickened; cork, a variable number of alternating layers of more or less uniformly thickened, thin-walled and thicker-walled cells; a single innermost layer with the outer and side walls more markedly thickened, lignified; cortex of thin-walled parenchyma, with scattered larger cells containing mucilage or volatile oil, single or small groups of uniformly thickened sclereids; pericycle a continuous band, two or three cells thick, of sclereids, the inner and radial walls thickened, small groups of thick-walled fibres associated with outer pericycle; phloem with multiseriate medullary rays, irregular tangential bands of obliterated sieve tissue, infrequent single, thick-walled fibres, scattered secretion cells; small acicular crystals of calcium oxalate in cells of medullary rays; abundant simple or up to four-compound starch granules.

Odour and Taste
Odour strongly resembling that of cinnamon bark, less delicate; taste cinnamon-like, mucilaginous and astringent.

IDENTIFICATION

Carry out the method for Thin-layer Chromatography as described in Appendix 1, using Solvent System C.
    Apply 60 µl of each of the following solutions to the plate: (1) extract 1 g of pow-

dered Cassia Bark by shaking with 10 ml of dichloromethane for 20 minutes. Filter, evaporate the filtrate just to dryness and dissolve the residue in 1 ml of toluene; (2) 0.1% cineole in toluene.

Spray the plate with Spray Reagent D, heat at 105°C for 10-15 minutes and examine in daylight.

Major bands relative to cineole are approximately as follows: purple 2.2, brown 1.7, brown 1.15, pink 0.9, purple 0.4.

Cassia Bark may be distinguished from Cinnamon, using the same system, in the following manner: Cinnamon exhibits a chromatogram similar to Cassia Bark but with the addition of a purple band just above the brown band at 1.15.

QUANTITATIVE STANDARDS

Foreign Matter
Not more than 2%   Appendix 3

Total Ash
Not more than 5%   Appendix 4

Ash Insoluble in Hydrochloric Acid
Not more than 2%   Appendix 5

MATERIAL OF COMMERCE Cassia Bark is supplied in the whole or powdered condition and is obtained from southern China and south-east Asia.

Powdered Cassia Bark

Complies with the requirements for Identification and Quantitative Standards stated for Cassia Bark.

Characteristic Features
Dark reddish-brown, odour and taste cinnamon-like, somewhat less pleasant. rather astringent and mucilaginous; abundant sclereids, lumen usually quite large, walls either uniform in thickness or one markedly thinner, striated and simple-pitted; abundant starch granules, single grains often 10-20 µm; thick-walled fibres, up to 40 µm diameter, usually singly, sparsely pitted; small cork cells; acicular crystals up to 8 µm, in small-celled parenchyma; larger, ovoid secretion-cells.

ACTION Carminative.

CATECHU   Rubiaceae

Uncariae extractum siccum

Synonyms: Pale Catechu, Gambir, Gambier.

Catechu is a dried aqueous extract prepared from the leaves and young shoots of *Uncaria gambier* (Hunter) Roxb.

This material complies with the requirements of the British Pharmacopoeia 1988 for Cat-echu or, when the material is in powder, Powdered Catechu.

MATERIAL OF COMMERCE Catechu is supplied as cubes or broken pieces. It is obtained from Indonesia and Malaysia.

ACTION Astringent.

CAYENNE PEPPER Solanaceae

Capsici fructus acer

Synonyms: Capsicum, Chillies, Tabasco Pepper.

Cayenne Pepper consists of the dried ripe fruits, usually devoid of the calyx, of *Capsicum frutescens* L. sensu latiore.

CHARACTERISTICS

Macroscopical Description
Ovoid-conical pods about 15-25 mm long and 5-8 mm wide, apex obtuse, abruptly tapering at the base where the calyx and pedicel may be attached; pericarp orange-red, translucent, glabrous, leathery and somewhat shrivelled; fruit divided into two loculi by a membranous, longitudinal dissepiment, each loculus containing five to ten seeds, loose or attached to the dissepiment; seeds flattened, subreniform, about 3-4 mm long, 2.5-3 mm wide and 0.5-1 mm thick, with a smooth, hard, yellowish-brown testa. Calyx greenish-brown, hard, about 4 mm long, cup-shaped with five inconspicuous teeth; pedicel slender, smooth, about 1-2 cm long.

Microscopical Description
Epicarp a single layer of sub-rectangular cells, often arranged in rows of five to seven, with thickened outer walls and a striated cuticle; mesocarp thin-walled, consisting of five to ten layers of parenchyma containing yellowish-red oily droplets, with occasional cells containing microsphenoidal crystals of calcium oxalate and an innermost layer of giant cells filled with oil globules; endocarp, a single layer composed of sclereids with unevenly thickened and pitted walls arranged in groups under the cavities of the giant cells of the mesocarp, and separated by thin-walled, unlignified parenchyma; dissepiment with the epidermis on both sides a secreting epithelium, composed of thin-walled, polygonal cells with the cuticle raised, forming large bladders containing oily droplets and occaasional crystals of capsaicin.
Testa epidermis a layer of large, yellowish-green, lignified cells with stongly thickened and striated radial and inner walls, the anticlinal walls markedly wavy and unevenly thickened in surface view, with large, conspicuous, rounded pits; endosperm composed of thin-walled parenchymatous cells containing fixed oil and aleurone grains.
Calyx outer epidermis with anisocytic stomata; numerous glandular trichomes on the inner epidermis with unicellular stalks and ovoid, multicellular heads containing yellowish-brown secretion; epidermis of pedicel with stomata and trichomes similar to those of the calyx; inner tissues of both calyx and pedicel containing idioblasts filled with microsphenoidal crystals of calcium oxalate.

Odour and Taste
Odour slight, characteristic; taste extremely fiery and pungent, strongly sternutatory and irritant to skin and mucous membranes.

IDENTIFICATION

Carry out the method for Thin-layer Chromatography as described in Appendix 1, using ether as the solvent system.

Apply 20 µl of the following solution to the plate: extract 1 g powdered Cayenne Pepper with 10 ml chloroform by heating under reflux for 10-15 minutes, cool and filter.

Spray the plate with Spray Reagent D, heat for 10 minutes at 105° C and examine in daylight.

Major bands relative to the solvent front are approximately as follows: brown 0.95, brown 0.8, brown 0.75, brown 0.35.

QUANTITATIVE STANDARDS

Foreign Matter
Not more than 2% Appendix 3

Total Ash
Not more than 7% Appendix 4

Ash Insoluble in Hydrochloric Acid
Not more than 2% Appendix 5

MATERIAL OF COMMERCE Cayenne Pepper is supplied as whole dried fruits. It is cultivated in many tropical and subtropical countries and obtained mainly from tropical Africa, China and India.

Powdered Cayenne Pepper

Complies with the requirements for Identification and Quantitative Standards stated for Cayenne Pepper.

Characteristic Features
An orange-red powder, strongly sternutatory and irritant, with a very fiery and pungent taste; fragments of the epicarp in surface view, cells polygonal with moderately thickened and beaded walls and a faintly striated cuticle; abundant parenchyma containing reddish oil globules, some with microsphenoidal crystals of calcium oxalate; endocarp fragments composed of large areas of sclereids with thickened and distinctly pitted walls separated by groups of thin-walled parenchyma; conspicuous large, yellow cells of the testa epidermis with wavy, strongly thickened and pitted radial and inner walls; thin-walled parenchyma of the endosperm; very occasional glandular trichomes from the calyx and pedicel.

ACTION Rubefacient, vasostimulant.

CELERY SEED   Umbelliferae

Apii fructus

Synonyms: Apium, Celery Fruit.

Celery Seed consists of the dried ripe fruits of cultivated *Apium graveolens* L.

CHARACTERISTICS

Macroscopical Description
Cremocarps and mericarps; cremocarps roundish-ovoid, laterally compressed, up to 1.5 mm long and 1.5 mm wide sometimes with a slender pedicel; mericarps about 0.5 mm thick, brown with five yellowish, straight primary ridges and a nearly flat commissural surface.

Microscopical Description
Epicarp composed of somewhat elongated cells with slightly sinuous walls in surface view with anomocytic stomata and striated cuticle; papillae seen on fragments of epicarp in side view; six to nine vittae, two in the commissural surface and one to three in each groove of the dorsal surface; occasional lignified sclereids, ovoid to rectangular, in the mesocarp; endocarp consisting of thin-walled parenchymatous cells, elongated in surface view, arranged in groups of six or more and showing parquetry arrangement; endosperm with fixed oil and aleurone grains and small, microspheroidal crystals of calcium oxalate.

Odour and Taste
Odour and taste characteristic of celery.

IDENTIFICATION

Carry out the method for Thin-layer Chromatography as described in Appendix I, using Solvent System A.

Apply 20 µl of each of the following solutions separately to the plate: (1) extract 1 g powdered Celery Seed with 10 ml methanol on a water-bath for 10-15 minutes, cool and filter; (2) 0.025% rutin in methanol.

Spray the plate with Spray Reagent A and examine in ultraviolet light 366 nm.

Major bands relative to rutin are approximately as follows: orange 1.7, broad orange 1.05.

QUANTITATIVE STANDARDS

Foreign Matter
Not more than 2%   Appendix 3

Total Ash
Not more than 10%   Appendix 4

Ash Insoluble in Hydrochloric Acid
Not more than 2%   Appendix 5

Water-soluble Extractive
Not less than 15%   Appendix 7

Volatile Oil

Not less than 1.6%   Appendix 9

MATERIAL OF COMMERCE Celery Seed is supplied as entire cremocarps and mericarps. It is obtained mainly from India, Eastern and Northern Europe.

Powdered Celery Seed

Complies with the requirements for Identification and Quantitative Standards stated for Celery Seed except that the Volatile Oil requirement is 'Not less than 1.0%'.

Characteristic Features

Brown powder, odour and taste characteristic of celery; cells of epicarp somewhat elongated with sinuous walls, striated cuticle and anomocytic stomata; large polygonal cells of vittae; thin-walled elongated cells of endocarp showing parquetry arrangement; endosperm cells with thick walls containing aleurone grains and scattered microspheroidal crystals of calcium oxalate.

ACTION Diuretic.

CENTAURY   Gentianaceae

Centaurii herba

Synonyms: Common Centaury, Centaurium.

Centaury consists of the dried aerial parts of *Centaurium erythraea* Rafn [*Erythraea centaurium* (L.) Pers., *Centaurium minus* Moench, *Centaurium umbellatum* Gilib.], harvested during the flowering period.

CHARACTERISTICS

Macroscopical Description

Stems Yellowish-green, erect, cylindrical, with four indistinct ribs, upper portion branching to form corymb-like cyme.

Leaves Sessile, three to seven-veined, basal rosette; opposite cauline pairs. Lamina, light green, 1-5 cm long and 8-20 mm wide, glabrous, obovate or spathulate, obtuse apex, even base, margin entire.

Flowers Sessile, up to 1 cm long; five green, linear sepals forming keeled, toothed tube; five pink, joined petals, funnel-shaped, longer than calyx; five short stamens attached to corolla tube; unilocular, cylindrical ovary, about 7 mm, with parietal placentation, containing several minute, brown, obovate seeds.

Microscopical Description

Stem Rectangular epidermal cells with sinuous anticlinal walls, intermittently papillose; cuticle smooth; frequent parallel orientated stomata; narrow parenchymatous cortex with chloroplasts, ribs strengthened with collenchyma; stele, narrow outer phloem, areas of normal and intraxylary sieve tissue; ring of lignified xylem containing thin-walled fibres with oblique pits, narrow, pitted tracheids and tracheidal vessels and spirally thickened vessels, up to 20 μm in diameter; parenchymatous pith.

Leaf Lamina, epidermal cells of both surfaces polygonal, with wavy anticlinal walls; stomata, mainly anisocytic, some anomocytic, more frequent on lower surface; marginal cells, elongated and papillose; cuticle, striated, faint and intermittent but stronger around stomata and over margins. Dorsiventral, two indistinct layers of palisade cells, a prism or cluster crystal, 5-10 μm diameter occurs in each cell and adjacent layer of spongy mesophyll. Midrib, collateral bundle containing narrow, 5-10 μm diameter, xylem vessels and tracheids with lignified annular, reticulate or pitted thickening.

Flower Sepal, elongated epidermal cells with straight, anticlinal walls; cuticle striated; infrequent parallel orientated stomata. Petal, inner epidermal cells polygonal, with straight anticlinal walls, papillose with prominent cuticular striations; elongated, outer epidermal cells with crenated anticlinal walls, cuticle transversely striated; mesophyll of petal base contains calcium oxalate clusters. Stamen, lignified fibrous layer of anther wall; yellow pollen grains, about 25 μm diameter, spherical, with three pores, exine distinctly pitted. Bifid stigma with elongated papillae.

Fruit Narrow, elongated, thin-walled epidermal cells containing oil globules; narrow, overlapping cells in parquetry arrangement; whole seeds with large, brown, pitted surface reticulations.

Odour and Taste
Faint and distinctive odour; taste, very bitter.

IDENTIFICATION

Carry out the method for Thin-layer Chromatography as described in Appendix 1, using Solvent System A.

Apply 20 μl of each of the following solutions separately to the plate: (1) extract 1 g powdered Centaury with 10 ml methanol by warming on a water-bath for 10-15 minutes, cool and filter; (2) 0.025% rutin in methanol.

Spray the plate with Spray Reagent A and examine in ultraviolet light 366 nm.

Major bands relative to rutin are approximately as follows: turquoise 1.5*, 1.1-0.3† seven distinct, closely-spaced, yellow/orange bands

* Band may not be visible in low concentration samples.

† Bands remain distinct at lower concentrations but may coalesce as concentration rises.

QUANTITATIVE STANDARDS

Foreign Matter
Not more than 2%   Appendix 3

Total Ash
Not more than 8%   Appendix 4

Ash Insoluble in Hydrochloric Acid
Not more than 2%   Appendix 5

Water-soluble Extractive
Not less than 15%   Appendix 7

MATERIAL OF COMMERCE Centaury is supplied in the cut or broken condition. It is widespread in Europe, North Africa and the Near East and is obtained mainly from southeast Europe and Morocco.

Powdered Centaury

Complies with the requirements for Identification and Quantitative Standards stated for Centaury.

Characteristic Features
Brownish-green powder with a faint odour and bitter taste; fragments of leaf lamina with polygonal, wavy-walled cells, stomata frequent, mainly anisocytic, elongated, papillose cells of margin with strongly striated cuticle; calcium oxalate prisms and clusters in palisade mesophyll; rectangular epidermal cells with parallel orientated stomata; narrow, lignified, xylem conducting elements with annular, reticulate and pitted thickening, some accompanied by thin-walled fibres; fragments of corolla with polygonal, pigmented cells and strongly striated papillae, elongated cells with crenated walls and transverse striations; numerous, yellow pollen grains with pitted exine; fragments of fibrous anther wall; narrow elongated cells containing oil globules; groups of cells with parquetry arrangement; whole seeds with brown surface reticulations.

ACTION Bitter.

CINCHONA BARK Rubiaceae

Cinchonae cortex

Synonyms: Cinchona, Red Cinchona Bark, Peruvian Bark.

Cinchona Bark consists of the dried bark of *Cinchona pubescens* Vahl {*Cinchona succirubra* Pavon} or of its varieties or its hybrids.

This material complies with the requirements of the European Pharmacopoeia for Cinchona Bark and the British Pharmacopoeia

for Cinchona Bark or, when the material is in powder, Powdered Cinchona Bark.

MATERIAL OF COMMERCE Cinchona Bark is supplied as whole or broken quills, or as whole or broken coppiced stems. The former are obtained from Java and other places in the East Indies, and the latter from young coppiced trees grown on plantations in Kenya, Tanzania, Guatemala and Bolivia.

ACTION Bitter.

CINNAMON Lauraceae

Cinnamomi cortex

Synonyms: Cinnamon Bark, Ceylon Cinnamon.

Cinnamon consists of the dried bark, freed from the outer cork and the underlying parenchyma, of the shoots grown on cut stock of *Cinnamomum zeylanicum* Nees.

This material complies with the requirements of the European Pharmacopoeia for Cinnamon.

MATERIAL OF COMMERCE Cinnamon is supplied as whole or broken quills. It is cultivated in many tropical regions and obtained mainly from Sri Lanka (whole quills) but also from the Seychelles, Madagascar and other countries.

ACTION Carminative.

CLIVERS Rubiaceae

Galii aparinis herba

Synonyms: Galium, Goosegrass, Cleavers.

Clivers consists of the dried aerial parts of *Galium aparine* L. collected during the flowering and fruiting period.

CHARACTERISTICS

Macroscopical Description

Stems Usually form the bulk of the herb; quadrangular in cross section and up to about 3 mm wide with a large central hollow; outer

surface dark green to brown with four distinct, more or less equidistant ridges bearing, on the younger stems, conspicuous downward projecting stiff prickles; branches at the nodes with the frequent remains of whorls of leaves and flowering or fruiting stems; fracture short.

Leaves Linear with sharply acute apex and revolute margins, arranged in whorls of eight to twelve; dark green, shining upper surface; pale, felted lower surface showing prominent midrib.

Flowers Small, whitish, arranged in dense terminal panicles, having four elliptical petals.

Fruit Purplish, double achenes with white, hooked bristles.

Microscopical Description

Stem Epidermal cells thin-walled and longitudinally elongated; ridges on young stems bearing at intervals unicellular covering trichomes with moderately thickened walls having faint longitudinal striations arising from several epidermal cells at the base and tapering rapidly downwards to a stiff hooked tip, 70-100 µm long; several layers of collenchyma in the ridges, the remainder of the cortex narrow and parenchymatous; phloem narrow and thin-walled; secondary xylem with lignified vessels and tracheids and a small amount of xylem parenchyma, vessels mostly spirally or annularly thickened, a few with bordered-pitted walls in the older stem; central parenchymous pith usually disintegrated to form a hollow occupying about half the diameter of the stem.

Leaf Dorsiventral; upper epidermal cells sinuous to wavy walled, lower epidermal cells more sinuous; paracytic stomata on both surfaces, more numerous on the lower; downwards projecting, hooked, unicellular, covering trichomes similar to those on the stem ridges occurring along the margins and on the lower surface of the midrib; additional covering trichomes, randomly orientated and frequently not hooked at the tip, found scattered over the upper surface; large idioblasts, up to 250 µm long and 30 µm wide, in the spongy mesophyll containing numerous fine needle crystals of calcium oxalate arranged in a bundle.

Flower Outer epidermis of petals thin-walled with faint longitudinal striations, inner epidermis papillose; calcium oxalate idioblasts similar to those in the leaf present in the mesophyll. Pollen grains spherical, about 30-35 µm in diameter, some showing up to eight pores and a faintly pitted exine.

Fruit Pericarp covered with a dense mass of hooked trichomes similar to those on the stem ridges and leaf margins.

Odour and Taste
Slight odour; bitter taste.

IDENTIFICATION

Carry out the method for Thin-layer Chromatography as described in Appendix 1, using Solvent System A.

Apply 20 µl of each of the following solutions separately to the plate: (1) extract 1 g powdered Clivers with 10 ml methanol on a water-bath for 10-15 minutes, cool and filter; (2) 0.025% rutin in methanol.

Spray the plate with Spray Reagent A and examine in ultraviolet light 366 nm.

Major bands relative to rutin are approximately as follows: intense blue 1.95, blue 1.28, pale green 0.75.

QUANTITATIVE STANDARDS

Foreign Matter
Not more than 2%   Appendix 3

Total Ash
Not more than 13%   Appendix 4

Ash Insoluble in Hydrochloric Acid
Not more than 2%   Appendix 5

Water-soluble Extractive
Not less than 18%   Appendix 7

MATERIAL OF COMMERCE Clivers is usually supplied as the broken or crushed herb. It is obtained from many countries in Europe.

Powdered Clivers

Complies with the requirements for Identification and Quantitative Standards stated for Clivers.

Characteristic Features
Green powder with a slight odour and a bitter taste; unicellular, thick-walled, hooked covering trichomes, free and along margins of leaf or fruit pericarp; epidermal cells of stems with hooked trichomes; epidermal cells of leaves with sinuous anticlinal walls and paracytic stomata; idioblasts of mesophyll containing bundles of needle crystals of calcium oxalate.

ACTION Diuretic.

CLOVE

Caryophylli flos

Synonyms: Caryophyllum, Cloves.

Clove consists of the whole flower buds of *Syzygium aromaticum* (L.) Merill et L. M. Perry *[Eugenia caryophyllus* (C. Spreng.) Bull. et Harr.] dried until they become reddish-brown.

This material complies with the requirements of the European Pharmacopoeia for Clove.

MATERIAL OF COMMERCE Clove is supplied as whole flowerbuds. It is obtained from Indonesia, East Africa and other tropical countries.

ACTION Carminative, topical analgesic.

COCILLANA
Meliaceae

Guareae cortex

Synonyms: Guarea, Guapi Bark, Huapi Bark.

Cocillana is the dried bark of *Guarea rusbyi* (Britton) Rusby and closely related species.

This material complies with the requirements of the British Pharmacopoeia for Cocillana or, when the material is in powder, Powdered Cocillana.

MATERIAL OF COMMERCE Cocillana is supplied as flattened or slightly curved pieces or in the broken condition. It is obtained principally from Bolivia.

ACTION Expectorant.

COLA
Sterculiaceae

Colae semen

Synonyms: Kola Nut, Kola.

Cola consists of the dried cotyledons of *Cola nitida* (Vent.) Schott et Endl. or *Cola acuminata* (Beauv.) Schott et Endl.

CHARACTERISTICS

Macroscopical Description
Reddish-brown, plano-convex pieces about 2.5 cm long and 2 cm wide but frequently somewhat distorted; hard and solid; fracture difficult but short; fractured surface smooth and pale brown.

Microscopical Description
Outer layer of thick-walled cells containing brown tannin; inner portion of thin-walled polyhedral, parenchymatous cells 40-50 µm wide containing simple, ovoid or spherical starch granules 5-10 µm and 20-30 µm in diameter with a protuberance and a two to three radiate hilum.

Odour and Taste
No odour; slightly bitter and astringent taste.

IDENTIFICATION

Carry out the method for Thin-layer Chromatography as described in Appendix 1, using a mixture of ethyl acetate:methanol: water (100:13.5:10) as the Solvent System.

Apply 20 µl of each of the following solutions separately to the plate: (1) extract 1 g powdered Cola with 10 ml methanol on a water-bath for 10-15 minutes, cool and filter; (2) 0.5%, caffeine in methanol.

Spray the plate with Spray Reagent B and examine in daylight.

The chromatogram of Cola shows a band with the same Rf value as caffeine.

QUANTITATIVE STANDARDS

Foreign Matter
Not more than 2%   Appendix 3

Total Ash
Not more than 5%   Appendix 4

Ash Insoluble in Hydrochloric Acid
Not more than 0.5%   Appendix 5

Water-soluble Extractive
Not less than 6%   Appendix 7

MATERIAL OF COMMERCE Cola is supplied in the whole condition. It is obtained from West Africa, Brazil and the West Indies.

Powdered Cola

Complies with the requirements for Identification and Quantitative Standards stated for Cola.

Characteristic Features
Reddish-brown powder with practically no odour and a slightly bitter, astringent taste; yellow, polyhedral, parenchymatous cells; thick-walled cells containing brown tannin; abundant starch granules.

ACTION Central nervous stimulant.

COMFREY ROOT   Boraginaceae

Symphyti radix

Synonym: Symphytum Root.

Comfrey Root consists of the dried rhizome and roots of *Symphytum officinale* L.

CHARACTERISTICS

Macroscopical Description
Rhizomes and Roots Fusiform of variable length, 5-15 mm thick, brownish to greyish-black, deeply longitudinally wrinkled; fracture short, fractured surface hard and waxy, pale grey or brown, exhibiting a greyish cambium line and an indistinctly radiate xylem; rhizome fractured surface shows a pith.

Microscopical Description
Rhizome and Root Several layers of dark brown polyhedral or sub-rectangular cork cells; cortex and phloem of oval, rounded or polygonal thin-walled parenchymatous cells, often containing simple or two to three compound rounded starch granules, 8-13 µm in diameter, with a stellate hilum; lignified vessels chiefly with reticulate thickening but occasionally with bordered pitting; rhizome with pith of thin-walled parenchymatous cells containing starch granules.

Odour and Taste
Slight odour; mucilaginous taste.

IDENTIFICATION

Carry out the method for Thin-layer Chromatography as described in Appendix 1, using Solvent System A.

Apply 20 µl of each of the following solutions separately to the plate: (1) extract 1 g powdered Comfrey Root with 10 ml methanol by warming on a water-bath for 10-15 minutes, cool and filter; (2) 0.025% rutin in methanol.

Spray the plate with Spray Reagent A and examine in ultraviolet light 366 nm.

Major bands relative to rutin are approximately as follows: blue 2.2, whitish 1.85, whitish 1.55.

QUANTITATIVE STANDARDS

Loss on Drying
Not more than 12% when dried in an oven at 100-105°C. Use 2-3 g   Appendix 2

Foreign Matter
Not more than 2%   Appendix 3

Total Ash
Not more than 10% calculated with reference to the oven-dried material   Appendix 4

Ash Insoluble in Hydrochloric Acid
Not more than 4% calculated with reference to the oven-dried material   Appendix 5

Water-soluble Extractive
Not less than 45% calculated with reference to the oven-dried material   Appendix 7

MATERIAL OF COMMERCE   Comfrey Root is usually supplied in the chopped condition. It is obtained from the UK, northern Europe and the USA.

Powdered Comfrey Root

Complies with the requirements for Identification and Quantitative Standards stated for Comfrey Root.

Characteristic Features
Greyish-white powder showing dark brown and black flecks, with a slight odour and a mucilaginous taste; abundant oval and rounded thin-walled parenchymatous cells, dark-brown cork cells, fragments of lignified vessels, occasional starch granules.

STORAGE   Store in a cool, dry, place in well-closed containers.

ACTION   Vulnerary.

CORIANDER   Umbelliferae

Coriandri fructus

Coriander consists of the dried ripe fruits of *Coriandrum sativum* L.

This material complies with the requirements of the British Pharmacopoeia for Coriander or, when the material is in powder, Powdered Coriander.

MATERIAL OF COMMERCE   Coriander is supplied as whole fruits. It is cultivated in many temperate countries and obtained principally from Morocco and eastern Europe.

ACTION   Carminative, stimulant.

CORN SILK

Gramineae

Maidis stigma

Synonym: Zea.

Corn Silk consists of the dried styles and stigmas of *Zea mays* L.

CHARACTERISTICS

Macroscopical Description
Slender, yellow, filamentous styles, 5-20 mm long, exhibiting slender bifid stigmas 0.5-3.0 mm long.

Microscopical Description
Epidermal cells rectangular, often extended into multicellular trichomes 200-800 μm long, the basal portion consisting of two to five cells and the upper portion usually unicellular; purplish red parenchymatous cells containing red colouring matter; two vascular bundles containing narrow tracheids with spiral or annular thickening.

Odour and Taste
Slight odour; insipid taste.

IDENTIFICATION

Carry out the method for Thin-layer Chromatography as described in Appendix 1, using Solvent System B.

Apply 20 μl of each of the following solutions separately to the plate: (1) extract 0.25 g powdered Corn Silk with 10 ml 60% methanol by refluxing on a water-bath for 10-15 minutes, cool, filter and concentrate to about 1 ml; (2) 0.05% aescin in methanol.

Spray the plate with Spray Reagent C, heat at 105°C for 5-10 minutes then observe in daylight.

Major bands relative to aescin are approximately as follows: deep purple 2.7, pale purple 2.6, yellow 1.3, brown-green 0.6.

QUANTITATIVE STANDARDS

Foreign Matter
Not more than 2%   Appendix 3

Total Ash
Not more than 8%   Appendix 4

Ash Insoluble in Hydrochloric Acid
Not more than 2%   Appendix 5

Water-soluble Extractive
Not less than 10%   Appendix 7

MATERIAL OF COMMERCE Corn Silk is supplied as a loose tangled mass. It is obtained from southern Europe and the USA.

Powdered Corn Silk

Complies with the requirements for Identification and Quantitative Standards stated for Corn Silk.

Characteristic Features
Yellow powder with a slight odour and an insipid taste; rectangular epidermal cells often extended into multicellular trichomes; fragments of trichomes; parenchymatous cells containing red contents.

ACTION Diuretic; urinary demulcent.

COUCH GRASS RHIZOME
Gramineae
Agropyri repentis rhizoma

Synonyms: Quackgrass, Triticum, Triticum repens, Graminis rhizoma.

Couch Grass Rhizome consists of the dried rhizomes, largely free from roots, of *Agropyron repens* (L.) P. Beauv. [*Elymus repens* (L.) Gould].

CHARACTERISTICS

Macroscopical Description
Cylindrical or flattened pieces of varying length, 2-4 mm in diameter and slightly swollen at the nodes which occur at intervals of 2-3 cm, internodes hollow; yellowish to straw-coloured, surface hard, lustrous and longitudinally furrowed; fracture tough and fibrous, short at the nodes; occasional remains of slender roots and leaf scars at the nodes, where branching may also occur.

Microscopical Description
Transverse section showing a narrow band of sclerenchyma beneath the epidermis, a wide cortex containing scattered vascular bundles; a distinct endodermis enclosing a continuous band of pericyclic sclerenchyma in which an outer circle of vascular bundles is embedded and an inner circle of larger vascular bundles is partially embedded; pith hollow in the centre. Epidermis composed of parallel rows of cells in which narrow, much elongated cells with thickened, lignified and pitted walls alternate with small, thin-walled twin cells; hypodermis of two or three layers of narrow, fusiform cells with moderately-thickened, lignified walls; cortical cells large, thin-walled, parenchymatous; endodermis strongly lignified with horse-shoe thickening; pericyclic fibres with moderately thickened and pitted walls; vascular bundles each with a small group of phloem, a few large vessels with small, slit-shaped pits and more numerous narrower vessels with spiral and annular thickening; pith parenchymatous, composed of large cells with slightly thickened and pitted walls.

Odour and Taste
Odourless; taste slightly sweetish.

IDENTIFICATION
Thin-layer Chromatographic analysis is unsuitable for this material; macroscopical and microscopical examination should be relied upon for identification.

QUANTITATIVE STANDARDS

Foreign Matter
Not more than 2%   Appendix 3

Total Ash
Not more than 5%   Appendix 4

Ash Insoluble in Hydrochloric Acid
Not more than 3%   Appendix 5

Water-soluble Extractive
Not less than 9%   Appendix 7

MATERIAL OF COMMERCE Couch Grass Rhizome is supplied as cut pieces. It is harvested from the wild and obtained mainly from south eastern Europe, especially Hungary.

Powdered Couch Grass Rhizome
Complies with the requirements for Quantitative Standards stated for Couch Grass Rhizome.

Characteristic Features
Buff to yellowish, odourless with a sweetish taste; fragments of the epidermis, isolated or attached to the underlying hypodermal layers, composed of narrow, elongated cells with undulating, thickened, lignified and distinctly pitted walls alternating with small, sub-circular, thin-walled, unlignified twin cells; occasional fragments of the endodermis showing lignified thickening on three walls; groups of moderately thick-walled fibres and associated vessels with numerous minute, slit-shaped pits or with spiral or annular thickening; rounded or polygonal parenchymatous cells, some with slightly thickened and distinctly pitted walls. Starch and calcium oxalate absent.

ACTION Diuretic.

CRANESBILL ROOT
Geraniaceae

Geranii maculati rhizoma

Synonyms: American Cranesbill Root, Storksbill Root, Wild Geranium Root.

Cranesbill Root consists of the rhizomes of *Geranium maculatum* L. collected in autumn and dried.

CHARACTERISTICS

Macroscopical Description
Rhizomes more or less cylindrical, slightly flattened, simple or occasionally branched, up to 5 cm or more long and about 1.5 cm thick; somewhat knotty and convoluted with numerous small protuberances, and circular, depressed, stem scars; dull brown with a purplish tinge, the surface between the nodules annulated and transversely ridged; fracture tough, short; the transverse surface pinkish-grey, showing a narrow bark; distinct, dark, cambium line with scattered, small groups of vascular tissue and a large central pith.

Microscopical Description
Cork composed of a number of rows of thin-walled cells, polygonal in surface view, with brown contents; phelloderm cells thicker-walled and tangentially elongated; cortex thin-walled, parenchymatous; cambial zone distinct and continuous, separating the secondary phloem and secondary xylem, both of which are very parenchymatous; vascular bundles few and arranged radially at irregular intervals, each with a group of sieve tissue and a small number of lignified vessels, tracheids and tracheidal vessels; the vessels moderately large with reticulately thickened walls; the tracheids and tracheidal vessels smaller, with bordered pits; large area of pith, composed of rounded, thin-walled cells with intercellular spaces; scattered throughout the parenchyma of the cortex, stele and pith, cells containing large cluster crystals of calcium oxalate, the remainder containing starch granules, simple, ovate or ellipsoidal, up to about 35 µm long with a slit hilum near the broader end. Some cells in the outer region with reddish contents.

Odour and Taste
No odour; taste bitter and very astringent.

IDENTIFICATION

Carry out the method for Thin-layer Chromatography as described in Appendix 1, using Solvent System A.

Apply 20 µl of each of the following separately to the plate: (1) extract 1 g powdered Cranesbill Root with 10 ml methanol by warming on a water-bath for 10-15 minutes, cool and filter; (2) 0.025% rutin in methanol.

Spray the plate with Spray Reagent A and examine in ultraviolet light 366 nm.

Major bands relative to rutin are approximately as follows: turquoise 1.8, yellow 1.6, pink 1.4-1.3, royal blue 1.2-0.2.

QUANTITATIVE STANDARDS

Foreign Matter
Not more than 3%   Appendix 3

Total Ash
Not more than 12%   Appendix 4

Ash Insoluble in Hydrochloric Acid
Not more than 4%   Appendix 5

Water-soluble Extractive
Not less than 30%   Appendix 7

MATERIAL OF COMMERCE Cranesbill Root is supplied in the whole or broken condition. It is obtained from the USA.

Powdered Cranesbill Root

Complies with the requirements for Identification and Quantitative Standards stated for Cranesbill Root.

Characteristic Features
Pale pinkish to brown powder with no odour and a very bitter and astringent taste; fragments of reddish-brown cork; abundant parenchyma containing simple starch granules; large cluster crystals of calcium oxalate up to about 120 µm in diameter; groups of lignified tracheids with bordered pits and vessels with reticulate thickening.

ACTION Astringent.

DAMIANA

Damianae folium

Synonym: Turnera.

Damiana consists of the dried leaves and stems of *Turnera diffusa* Willd. var. *aphrodisiaca* Urb. and possibly other species of Turnera.

CHARACTERISTICS

Macroscopical Description

Stems 1-2 mm diameter, varying from markedly hairy and greyish-green to slightly hairy and reddish-brown, finely longitudinally ridged and showing scars spirally arranged at intervals of 8-12 mm.

Leaves Light greyish-green to yellowish-green, under-surface paler; 5-25 mm long and 3-10 mm wide, broadly lanceolate, apex sub-acute, base tapering, margin serrate to dentate, three to six teeth on each margin; venation pinnate, main veins leaving midrib at an acute angle, veins more prominent on lower surface; both surfaces pubescent; petiole, 2-3 mm long.

Microscopical Description

Stems Indistinct dark brown outer layers with many covering trichomes or with four to six layers of yellowish-brown cork cells; cortical parenchyma with numerous cluster crystals of calcium oxalate; pericycle of closely spaced, discrete groups of thick-walled, lignified fibres occasionally associated with prismatic crystals of calcium oxalate; xylem small with pitted vessels up to 20 μm in diameter; pith of lignified parenchyma containing cluster crystals of calcium oxalate.

Leaf Isobilateral with upper palisade cells slightly smaller and more densely packed than the lower; upper epidermal cells with straight or slightly sinuous anticlinal walls, stomata absent; lower epidermal cells with sinuous anticlinal walls and frequent stomata, usually paracytic but some anomocytic; both epidermises have numerous covering trichomes or their scars; trichomes, unicellular up to 900 μm long, often twisted or bent near leaf surface, bluntly pointed, lumen very narrow or absent except near base where walls are lignified; vascular strand with crescent-shaped, dense xylem; little spongy mesophyll but parenchymatous cells surrounding vascular strand filled with cluster crystals of calcium oxalate 10-25 μm in diameter.

Odour and Taste

Pleasant, aromatic odour; bitter and pungent taste.

IDENTIFICATION

Carry out the method for Thin-layer Chromatography as described in Appendix 1, using Solvent System A.

Apply 20 μl of each of the following solutions separately to the plate: (1) extract 1 g powdered Damiana with 10 ml methanol by warming on a water-bath for 10-15 minutes, cool and filter; (2) 0.025% rutin in methanol.

Spray with Spray Reagent A and observe in ultraviolet light 366 nm.

Major bands relative to rutin are approximately as follows: orange 2.15, orange 1.7, broad orange-yellow 1.5, broad orange-yellow 1.33, orange 0.9.

QUANTITATIVE STANDARDS

Stems
Not more than 15%

Foreign Matter
Not more than 3%   Appendix 3

Total Ash
Not more than 10%   Appendix 4

Ash Insoluble in Hydrochloric Acid
Not more than 3%   Appendix 5

Water-soluble Extractive
Not less than 15%   Appendix 7

MATERIAL OF COMMERCE Damiana is usually supplied as the crushed herb. Small, spherical, yellowish-brown fruits may sometimes be present. It is obtained from the south eastern USA and Mexico.

Powdered Damiana

Complies with the requirements for Identification and Quantitative Standards stated for Damiana.

Characteristic Features
Yellowish-green powder with a pleasant, aromatic odour and a bitter, pungent taste; numerous unicellular, very thick-walled trichomes with warty surface; leaf epidermal cells with paracytic stomata and trichome scars; numerous cluster crystals of calcium oxalate; thick-walled fibres; lignified, pitted parenchyma cells.

ACTION Thymoleptic.

DANDELION LEAF   Compositae
Taraxaci folium

Synonym: Taraxacum Leaf.

Dandelion Leaf consists of the dried leaves of *Taraxacum officinale* Weber, collected before flowering.

CHARACTERISTICS

Macroscopical Description
Simple, lanceolate to obovate, almost entire to runcinate, up to 40 cm or more long and about 6 cm wide tapering towards the base to a short petiole, apex obtuse; upper surface dark green and with occasional scattered hairs, particularly over the veins; lower surface paler and nearly glabrous; midrib and main veins light green or frequently purplish-green, raised on the lower surface.

Microscopical Description
Leaf dorsiventral; upper and lower epidermal cells with thin, sinuous anticlinal walls; anomocytic stomata on both surfaces, more frequent on the lower; occasional uniseriate, multicellular trichomes consisting of a basal portion composed of four to six small, square to barrel-shaped cells with brown walls, surmounted by a much collapsed and shrivelled portion composed of thin-walled, elongated cells terminating in a spathulate or slightly swollen apex; in some of these trichomes, especially on the upper epidermis, the basal portion is multiseriate, about four cells wide at the epidermis, tapering to unicellular where the collapsed portion commences; vascular tissue of the petiole and midrib with annularly thickened vessels and associated brown, anastomosing laticiferous tissue.

Odour and Taste
Mild characteristic odour; bitter taste.

IDENTIFICATION

Carry out the method for Thin-layer Chromatography as described in Appendix 1, using Solvent System A.

Apply 20 µl of each of the following solutions separately to the plate: (1) extract 1 g powdered Dandelion Leaf with 10 ml 60% methanol on a water-bath for 15-10 minutes, cool and filter; (2) 0.025% rutin in methanol.

Spray the plate with Spray Reagent A and examine in ultraviolet light 366 nm.

Major bands relative to rutin are approximately as follows: white 2.0, white 1.5, blue 1.1, yellowish 1.0, orange 0.7.

QUANTITATIVE STANDARDS

Foreign Matter
Not more than 2%   Appendix 3

Total Ash
Not more than 15%   Appendix 4

Ash Insoluble in Hydrochloric Acid
Not more than 4%   Appendix 5

Water-soluble Extractive
Not less than 20%   Appendix 7

MATERIAL OF COMMERCE Dandelion Leaf is usually supplied in the broken or crushed condition. It is obtained from European countries including the UK.

Powdered Dandelion Leaf

Complies with the requirements for Identification and Quantitative Standards stated for Dandelion Leaf.

Characteristic Features
Dark green powder with no odour and a bitter taste. Fragments of leaf epidermis with sinuous, anticlinal walls and occasional anomocytic stomata; on some fragments part of the basal portions of the trichomes may very occasionally be attached; narrow, annularly thickened vessels and fragments of brown laticiferous tissue.

ACTION Diuretic; choleretic.

DANDELION ROOT   Compositae
Taraxaci radix

Synonym: Taraxacum Root.

Dandelion Root consists of the dried root and rhizome of *Taraxacum officinale* Weber, collected in the autumn.

CHARACTERISTICS

Macroscopical Description
Roots cylindrical, up to 2.5 cm in diameter, tapering and frequently branched; outer surface brown and longitudinally wrinkled bearing root scars and a branched crown at the apex, often with brownish hairs; fracture short and horny, the fractured surface exhibiting alternate layers of brown laticiferous vessels and white parenchymatous tissue with a lemon-yellow xylem in the centre.

Microscopical Description
Narrow, brown, thin-walled cork layer; phloem characterised by an anastomosing network of laticiferous vessels alternating with groups of sieve tissue, the xylem composed of tracheids and vessels up to 55 μm in diameter with spiral and reticulate thickening, accompanied by non-lignified xylem parenchyma; crystals of inulin occur in the phloem and xylem parenchyma.

Odour and Taste
Slight odour; sweetish taste.

IDENTIFICATION

Carry out the method for Thin-layer Chromatography as described in Appendix 1, using a mixture of chloroform:ethanol (95:5) as the solvent system.

Apply 20 μl of the following solution to the plate: extract 1 g powdered Dandelion Root with 10 ml methanol by warming on a water-bath for 10-15 minutes, cool, filter and concentrate to approximately 2 ml.

Spray the plate with Spray Reagent D, heat at 105°C for 15 minutes and examine in daylight.

Major bands relative to the solvent front are approximately as follows: red 0.85, purple 0.75, purple 0.6, red 0.5, red 0.45.

QUANTITATIVE STANDARDS

Loss on Drying
Not more than 15% when dried in an oven at 100 - 105°C. Use 2-3 g   Appendix 2

Foreign Matter
Not more than 1%   Appendix 3

Total Ash
Not more than 12% calculated with reference to the oven-dried material Appendix 4

Ash Insoluble in Hydrochloric Acid
Not more than 3.5% calculated with reference to the oven-dried material Appendix 5

Water-soluble Extractive
Not less than 40% calculated with reference to the oven-dried material   Appendix 7

MATERIAL OF COMMERCE Dandelion Root may be supplied as broken or chopped pieces. It is obtained from European countries, including the UK.

69

Powdered Dandelion Root

Complies with the requirements for Identification and Quantitative Standards stated for Dandelion Root.

Characteristic Features
Yellowish-brown powder with a slight odour and a sweetish taste; parenchymatous cells containing inulin, brown reticulately thickened vessels and tracheids, fragments of laticiferous tissue and brown cork; occasional fragments of large covering trichomes from the crowns.

STORAGE Store in a cool, dry place in well closed containers.

ACTION Hepatic.

DEVIL'S CLAW   Pedaliaceae
Harpagophyti radix

Synonym: Harpagophytum.

Devil's Claw consists of the dried, transverse slices of the tubers of *Harpagophytum procumbens* DC.

CHARACTERISTICS

Macroscopical Description
Irregularly circular slices of tuber 2-4 cm and sometimes up to 6 cm in diameter and 2-5 mm thick; cork reddish-brown to dark brown, longitudinally wrinkled; transverse surface yellowish-brown to brown, radiate and concentric, central region raised, fracture short.

Microscopical Description
Several rows of large, thin-walled cork cells frequently with yellowish-brown contents; parenchymatous cortex with very occasional sclereids with reddish-brown contents, xylem arranged in concentric rings; reticulately thickened vessels, some with rounded perforations in the end walls (tracheidal vessels); abundant lignified parenchymatous cells associated with the vessels and in the small central pith.

Odour and Taste
No odour; extremely bitter taste.

IDENTIFICATION

A. To 0.1 g powdered Devil's Claw add 0.1 ml Phloroglucinol Solution followed by 0.1 ml hydrochloric acid; on mixing, a dark green colour is produced.

B. Carry out the method for Thin-layer Chromatography as described in Appendix 1, using a mixture of ethyl acetate:methanol: water (77:15:8) as the Solvent System and allowing the solvent front to ascend a distance of 10 cm above the line of application.
Apply 20 µl of each of the following solutions separately to the plate: (1) extract 1 g powdered Devil's Claw with 10 ml 60% methanol on a water-bath for 10-15 minutes, cool and filter; (2) 0.025% rutin in methanol.
Spray the plate with Spray Reagent D, heat at 100°C for 5-10 minutes and observe in daylight.
Major bands relative to rutin are approximately as follows: brown 1.35, brown 1.3, deep purplish-brown 1.1, greenish-brown 0.9.

QUANTITATIVE STANDARDS

Foreign Matter
Not more than 2%   Appendix 3

Total Ash
Not more than 22%   Appendix 4

Ash Insoluble in Hydrochloric Acid
Not more than 5%   Appendix 5

Water-soluble Extractive
Not less than 50%   Appendix 7

MATERIAL OF COMMERCE Devil's Claw is supplied as slices of tuber, sometimes in the broken condition. It is obtained from regions bordering the Kalahari Desert.

Powdered Devil's Claw

Complies with the requirements for Identification and Quantitative Standards stated for Devil's Claw.

Characteristic Features
Brown powder with no odour and an intensely bitter taste; abundant lignified, pitted parenchyma associated with reticulately thickened vessels and vessel tracheids; large, thin-walled cork cells, some with yellowish-brown contents.

ACTION Antirheumatic.

ECHINACEA ROOT Compositae

Echinaceae angustifoliae radix

Synonyms: Coneflower, Narrow-Leaved Coneflower Root, Black Sampson.

Echinacea Root consists of the dried rhizome and roots of *Echinacea angustifolia* DC.

CHARACTERISTICS

Macroscopical Description
Root cylindrical or slightly tapering and sometimes spirally twisted, passing imperceptibly into a rhizome in the upper part; rhizome up to about 15 mm in diameter, roots 4-10 mm in diameter; outer surface pale brown to yellowish-brown; rhizomes crowned with remains of the aerial stem and sometimes showing surface annulations; roots longitudinally wrinkled and deeply furrowed; fracture short when dry but becoming tough and pliable on exposure to the atmosphere.

Microscopical Description
Rhizomes and roots in transverse section showing a thin outer bark separated by a distinct cambium line from a wide xylem; a small circular pith in the rhizome. Cork composed of several rows of thin-walled cells ccntaining yellowish-brown pigment; cortex parenchymatous; rhizome with occasional small groups of thick-walled, lignified fibres in the pericycle; phloem and xylem composed of very narrow strands of vascular tissue separated by wide, nonlignified medullary rays; xylem vessels lignified, 25-75 µm in diameter, usually with reticulate thickening but occasionally with spiral or annular thickening; stone cells, occurring singly or in small groups, varying considerably in size and shape from rounded to rectangular to elongated and fibre-like, up to 300 µm long and 20-40 µm wide, with intercellular spaces containing a dense black deposit; schizogenous oleo-resin canals, 80-150 µm in diameter and containing yellowish-orange oleo-resin, are scattered throughout the parenchyma of the cortex and medullary rays; sphaerocrystalline masses of inulin occur throughout the parenchymatous tissue.

Odour and Taste
Mild, aromatic odour; sweet taste initially, but quickly becoming bitter followed by a tingling sensation on the tongue.

IDENTIFICATION

Carry out the method for Thin-layer Chromatography as described in Appendix 1, using Solvent System A.

Apply 20 µl of each of the following solutions separately to the plate: (1) extract 1 g powdered Echinacea Root with 10 ml methanol on a water-bath for 10-15 minutes, cool and filter; (2) 0.025% rutin in methanol.

Spray the plate with Spray Reagent A and examine in ultraviolet light 366 nm.

Major bands relative to rutin are approximately as follows: pale blue 1.7, pale blue 1.3, pale blue 0.8.

QUANTITATIVE STANDARDS

Foreign Matter
Not more than 3%   Appendix 3

Total Ash
Not more than 9%   Appendix 4

Ash Insoluble in Hydrochloric Acid
Not more than 3%   Appendix 5

Water-soluble Extractive
Not less than 15%   Appendix 7

MATERIAL OF COMMERCE Echinacea Root is supplied as small, broken fragments. It is obtained principally from North America.

Powdered Echinacea Root

Complies with the requirements for Identifi-

cation and Quantitative Standards stated for Echinacea Root.

Characteristic Features
Brown powder with a slight aromatic odour and initially a sweet taste, quickly becoming bitter and leaving a tingling sensation on the tongue. Thin-walled polygonal cork cells with with red-brown contents; lignified reticulately thickened vessels; abundant stonecells of various shapes; fragments of oleo-resin canals with reddish-brown contents; abundant thin-walled parenchyma with sphaerocrystalline masses of inulin.

ACTION Immunostimulant.

ELDER FLOWER   Caprifoliaceae

Sambuci flos

Synonyms: Common Elder Flower, Sambucus.

Elder Flower consists of the dried flowers of *Sambucus nigra* L.

CHARACTERISTICS

Macroscopical Description
Inflorescence, flat-topped terminal cyme; flowers small, 1-3 mm in diameter, creamy-yellow, each composed of a five-toothed calyx, a gamopetalous corolla with five lobes, five epipetalous stamens and a trilocular inferior ovary; calyx lobes very small, brownish-green, ovoid, attached to top of ovary; corolla with a short tube and spreading lobes; stamens, with short filaments and lemon-yellow anthers, attached to corolla tube; ovary sub-ovoid with three capitate stigmas.

Microscopical Description
Epidermal cells of upper surface of sepals polygonal with faintly striated cuticle, those of lower epidermis wavy-walled with strongly striated cuticle and scattered, rounded, anomocytic stomata; unicellular marginal teeth rounded at the apex occur in the basal region; epidermal cells of the upper surface of petals polygonal with slightly

thickened and beaded walls and striated cuticle, those of the lower epidermis distinctly wavy with large, rounded, anomocytic stomata; numerous small globules of volatile oil in both epidermises; mesophyll of sepals and petals contains idioblasts of numerous small, sandy crystals of calcium oxalate; fibrous layer of anthers with characteristic thickening and beading on walls; pollen grains sub-spherical, 17-24 μm in diameter, with smooth exine, three distinct pores and three furrows.

Odour and Taste
Slight, characteristic aromatic odour; slightly bitter and mucilaginous taste.

IDENTIFICATION

Carry out the method for Thin-layer Chromatography as described in Appendix 1, using Solvent System A.
    Apply 20 μl of each of the following solutions separately to the plate: (1) extract 1 g powdered Elder Flower with 10 ml methanol by warming on a water-bath for 10-15 minutes, cool and filter; (2) 0.025% rutin in methanol.
    Spray the plate with Spray Reagent A and examine in ultraviolet light 366 nm.

Major bands relative to rutin are approximately as follows: green 1.6, orange 1.5, blue 1.35, green 1.05, orange 0.95.

QUANTITATIVE STANDARDS

Foreign Matter
Not more than 2%   Appendix 3

Total Ash
Not more than 10%   Appendix 4

Ash Insoluble in Hydrochloric Acid
Not more than 2%   Appendix 5

Water-soluble Extractive
Not less than 25%   Appendix 7

MATERIAL OF COMMERCE Elder Flower is supplied in the whole or broken condition. Pieces of pedicel and fragments of leaf may also be present. It is obtained from European countries, including the UK.

Powdered Elder Flower

Complies with the requirements for Identification and Quantitative Standards stated for Elder Flower.

Characteristic Features
Yellowish-buff powder with a slight aromatic but characteristic odour and a bitter, mucilaginous taste; sub-spherical pollen grains very abundant, occurring scattered or in association with fragments of anther; characteristic fibrous layer of anther; numerous petal fragments containing oil droplets, epidermal cells showing beaded walls, striated cuticle and anomocytic stomata; occasional fragments of sepals showing polygonal to wavy-walled epidermal cells with striated cuticle; sandy crystals of calcium oxalate scattered or in idioblasts in parenchymatous cells.

ACTION Diaphoretic.

ELECAMPANE   Compositae

Helenii rhizoma

Synonym: Inula.

Elecampane consists of the dried roots and rhizomes of *Inula helenium* L., collected in the autumn when the plant is two to three years old.

CHARACTERISTICS

Macroscopical Description
Rhizomes Irregular, dark brown, tapering, 2-8 cm long and 0.5-2.0 cm wide, longitudinally wrinkled and sometimes curved or twisted; crown somewhat annulate and surmounted by a stem scar, remains of stem or occasional buds; fragments of roots sometimes attached or root scars present.
Roots Nearly cylindrical and tapering, frequently twisted, up to 15 cm long and 1.5-3 cm in diameter.

Microscopical Description
Rhizome Narrow dark-brown cork, a parenchymatous cortex and a radiate xylem; parenchymatous cells containing masses of inulin; large, round to oval schizolysigenous oleo-resin glands occur in the cortex, phloem and xylem parenchyma, arranged in interrupted circles of radial rows; lignified vessels and tracheids reticulately thickened or with bordered pits; xylem fibres in the older rhizomes; parenchymatous pith.
Root Similar but without pith.

Odour and Taste
Aromatic and pleasant odour; sweet taste, becoming pungent later.

IDENTIFICATION

Carry out the method for Thin-layer Chromatography as described in Appendix 1, using Solvent System B.

Apply 20 µl of each of the following solutions separately to the plate: (1) extract 1 g powdered Elecampane with 10 ml methanol on a water-bath for 10-15 minutes, cool and filter; (2) 0.05% aescin in methanol.

Spray the plate with Spray Reagent C, heat at 105°C for 5-10 minutes then examine in daylight.

Major bands relative to aescin are approximately as follows: purple 2.0, brownish green 0.65, 0.4 and 0.2.

QUANTITATIVE STANDARDS

Loss on Drying
Not more than 14% when dried in an oven at 100-105°C. Use 2-3 g   Appendix 2

Foreign Matter
Not more than 2%   Appendix 3

Total Ash
Not more than 8% calculated with reference to the oven-dried material   Appendix 4

Ash Insoluble in Hydrochloric Acid
Not more than 1% calculated with reference to the oven dried material   Appendix 5

Water-soluble Extractive
Not less than 27% calculated with reference to the oven-dried material   Appendix 7

MATERIAL OF COMMERCE Elecampane is supplied as broken pieces, frequently with more root than rhizome. It is obtained from Europe, China and the USA.

Powdered Elecampane

Complies with the requirements for Identification and Quantitative Standards stated for Elecampane.

Characteristic Features
Light brown powder with an aromatic odour and a sweet taste which becomes somewhat pungent later; parenchymatous cells containing masses of inulin; yellow to reddish-brown fragments of large, round to oval oleo-resin glands; yellowish-brown oleoresin; lignified vessels and tracheids and some lignified fibres.

STORAGE Store in a cool, dry place in well closed containers.

ACTION Expectorant.

ELEUTHEROCOCCUS   Araliaceae

Eleutherococci radix

Synonym: Siberian Ginseng.

Eleutherococcus consists of the dried roots and rhizomes of *Eleutherococcus senticosus* Maxim. *[Acanthopanax senticosus* (Rupr. et Maxim.) Harms].

CHARACTERISTICS

Macroscopical Description
Roots Cylindrical, up to 0. 5 cm in diameter, straight, occasionally branched, dark brown, smooth surface with bark closely adhering to the xylem.
Rhizomes Up to 4 cm wide, surface pale brown, longitudinally wrinkled, showing root scars and traces of aerial stems; fracture somewhat fibrous; fractured surface pale yellow.

Microscopical Description
Root Five to seven rows of brown cork cells; secondary phloem containing secretory canals in groups of four or five, up to 20 µm in diameter, with brown contents; phloem fibres with thick, lignified walls occurring singly or in small groups; cluster crystals of calcium oxalate in phloem parenchyma; parenchymatous cells surrounding secretory cells and the medullary ray cells containing small starch granules, xylem of reticulately thickened and pitted vessels.

Rhizome Similar to the roots except for larger secretory canals, up to 25 µm in diameter, and the presence of a parenchymatous pith containing starch granules.

Odour and Taste
Faint, aromatic odour; bitter, acrid and persistent taste.

IDENTIFICATION

A. Apply a few drops of Sodium Hydroxide Solution to the cut surface; a bright yellow colour is produced.
B. Extract 0.5 g powdered Eleutherococcus with 5 ml boiling water, cool, filter and add a few drops of Dilute Ferric Chloride Solution; a green colour is produced.
C. Carry out the method for Thin-layer Chromatography as described in Appendix 1, using Solvent System B.

Apply 20 µl of each of the following solutions separately to the plate: (1) extract 1 g powdered Eleutherococcus with 10 ml methanol on a water-bath for 10-15 minutes, cool and filter; (2) 0.05% aescin in methanol.

Spray the plate with Spray Reagent E and observe in daylight.

Major bands relative to aescin are approximately as follows: purplish-brown 0.9, reddish-brown 0.8, reddish-brown 0.7.

QUANTITATIVE STANDARDS

Aerial Parts
Not more than 3%

Foreign Matter
Not more than 1%   Appendix 3

Total Ash
Not more than 6%   Appendix 4

Ash Insoluble in Hydrochloric Acid
Not more than 1.5%   Appendix 5

Water-soluble Extractive
Not less than 4%   Appendix 7

MATERIAL OF COMMERCE Eleutherococcus is supplied as broken pieces of root and rhizome, frequently split longitudinally. It is obtained from the USSR.

Powdered Eleutherococcus

Complies with the requirements for Identification and Quantitative Standards stated for Eleutherococcus.

Characteristic Features
Brown powder with a faint, aromatic odour and a slightly acrid, persistent taste; groups of secretory canals with brown contents, surrounded by parenchymatous cells containing cluster crystals of calcium oxalate; parenchymatous cells with small starch granules, thick-walled lignified fibres, fragments of reticulate and pitted vessels; turns bright yellow when mounted in sodium hydroxide solution.

ACTION Adaptogen; tonic.

EQUISETUM

Equiseti herba

Synonym: Horsetail.

Equisetum consists of the dried, sterile stems of *Equisetum arvense* L.

CHARACTERISTICS

Macroscopical Description
Stems green, erect, 20-80 cm long and 3-5 mm in diameter with six to twenty deep longitudinal grooves, rough to the touch, hollow; grooved, toothed sheaths 3-8 mm long at the internodes, many subulate, acute teeth, green with blackish tips; numerous lateral solid branches arranged in whorls, 5-20 cm long, 1-2 mm in diameter, four grooves and with four pale green, triangular-lanceolate teeth with acuminate apices; fracture short, exposing a large central cavity in the main stems.

Microscopical Description
Epidermis with elongated, wavy-walled cells often thickened and beaded, numerous typical paracytic stomata alternating with epidermal cells and having horizontal striated guard cells; ridged area exhibits numerous two-celled, non-lignified protuberances which glisten when viewed in polarised light; cortex of thin-walled cells with many large lacunae; non-lignified, sclerenchymatous fibrous cells up to 1 mm long with oblique or bifurcate apices in the ridges; xylem of lignified, annularly or spirally thickened vessels occurring singly or in small groups; large central cavity.
No single cell protuberances should be present (absence of *Equisetum palustre* L.).

Odour and Taste
No odour; no taste.

IDENTIFICATION

Carry out the method for Thin-layer Chromatography as described in Appendix 1, using Solvent System A and allowing the solvent front to ascend a distance of 12 cm above the line of application.

Apply 20 µl of each of the following solutions separately to the plate: (1) extract 1 g powdered Equisetum with 10 ml methanol on a water-bath for 15 minutes cool and filter; (2) 0.025% rutin in methanol.

Spray the plate with Spray Reagent A and examine in ultraviolet light 366 nm.

Major bands relative to rutin are approximately as follows: narrow deep red 1.8 deep blue 1.65, blue 1.1, yellow-orange 0.8.

QUANTITATIVE STANDARDS

Foreign Matter
Not more than 2%   Appendix 3

Total Ash
Not more than 20%   Appendix 4

Ash Insoluble in Hydrochloric Acid
Not more than 10%   Appendix 5

Water-soluble Extractive
Not less than 15%   Appendix 7

MATERIAL OF COMMERCE Equisetum is supplied in the broken condition. It is obtained from European countries including the UK.

Powdered Equisetum

Complies with the requirements for Identification and Quantitative Standards stated for Equisetum.

Characteristic Features
Dull green powder with no odour or taste; fragments of epidermis with elongated, wavy-walled cells with anticlinal walls sometimes thickened and beaded, numerous typical paracytic stomata with characteristic guard cells distinguished by transverse curved ridges; fragments of epidermal cells exhibiting numerous two-celled protuberances which glisten when viewed in polarised light, bundles of narrow, brown non-lignified fibres with oblique acuminate or bifurcate apices.

No single cell protuberances should be present (absence of *Equisetum palustre* L.).

ACTION Diuretic; astringent.

EUCALYPTUS LEAF
Myrtaceae

Eucalypti folium

Synonym: Blue Gum Tree Leaf.

Eucalyptus Leaf consists of the dried leaves of *Eucalyptus globulus* Labill., obtained from mature trees.

CHARACTERISTICS

Macroscopical Description
Leaves ensiform, up to 25 cm or more long and 4 cm wide; relatively thick, coriaceous and brittle; margin entire, apex acute, base obtuse to acute, sometimes slightly asymmetric; both surfaces pale greyish-green, glabrous, abundantly punctate and with scattered, small, slightly raised, brown to almost black corky spots; midrib pale fawn, raised only slightly on lower surface; very numerous, straight, pinnately-arranged lateral veins anastomosing about 1-2 mm from margin and forming an almost straight line parallel to it; fracture short, minutely fibrous in midrib; petiole about 1-3 cm, light brown, woody, slightly flattened, grooved, almost always twisted.

Microscopical Description
Isobilateral; upper and lower palisades multilayered with three or four rows of short cells; spongy mesophyll, about four layers of small, loosely-packed rounded cells; large ovoid schizogenous glands in mesophyll and penetrating to epidermises; surface-ruptured glands lined with several layers of cork cells; epidermal cells small, covered by very thick, smooth cuticle; midrib not greatly thicker than lamina; the large oval meristele, slightly depressed above, surrounded by a sheath of fibres in small variable-sized groups of from six to ten, only narrowly separated by thin-walled parenchyma, enclosing two small vascular bundles above the main xylem tissue; vessels narrow, spirally or annularly thickened or bordered-pitted, strongly lignified; fibres very thick-walled, rarely pitted, incompletely lignified and with associated files of slightly elongated prism crystals; spongy and palisade mesophylls with frequent, dark-centred, cluster crystals up to about 30-35 μm; very few prisms; wide areas of small-celled collenchyma above and below meristele. Upper and lower epidermises of small polygonal cells, anticlinal walls almost straight, moderately thickened or inconspicuously beaded; relatively large, sunken, anomocytic stomata, about twice as numerous in lower epidermis.

Odour and Taste
Weakly aromatic, stronger when freshly crushed, characteristic and somewhat camphoraceous to terebinthinate. Taste rather unpleasant, pungent then slightly cooling, bitter and astringent.

IDENTIFICATION

Carry out the method for Thin-layer Chromatography as described in Appendix 1, using Solvent System C.

Apply 60 μl of each of the following solutions to the plate: (1) extract 2 g of powdered Eucalyptus Leaf by shaking with 20 ml of dichloromethane for 20 minutes. Filter, evaporate the filtrate just to dryness and dissolve the residue in 1 ml of toluene; (2) 0.1% cineole in toluene.

Spray the plate with Spray Reagent D, heat at 105°C for 10-15 minutes and examine in daylight.

Major bands relative to cineole are approximately as follows: purple 1.95, blue 1.0, purple 0.5.
Note: This chromatogram is characterised by the dominance of the blue band of cineole (Rf 0.45).

QUANTITATIVE STANDARDS

Foreign Matter
Not more than 2%   Appendix 3

Total Ash
Not more than 6%   Appendix 4

MATERIAL OF COMMERCE Eucalyptus Leaf is supplied as whole or cut leaves. It is obtained from Spain, Morocco, Australia and other countries.

Powdered Eucalyptus Leaf

Complies with the requirements for Identification and Quantitative Standards stated for Eucalyptus Leaf.

Characteristic Features
Light, greyish-green powder with a characteristic aromatic odour and a pungent, bitter and astringent taste; epidermal cells in surface view polygonal, small, straight-walled, thickened; relatively large, sunken, stomata; in sectional view lamina fragments markedly curved, outer wall and cuticle very thick; palisade up to four-layered, often enclosing calcium oxalate crystals; spongy mesophyll narrow, containing numerous, fairly large cluster and cuboid prism crystals; groups of slightly irregular fibres, most thick-walled, lumen narrow, weakly lignified, pits infrequent; some groups with sheath of small, more or less rectangular prisms; isolated, larger cuboid prisms and dark-centred clusters; patches of light brown, thin-walled, corky tissue; fragments of oil glands, curved; lining cells small, thin-walled, colourless; xylem, lignified, narrow tracheidal elements and wider, spirally-thickened vessels.

ACTION Antiseptic.

EUONYMUS BARK   Celastraceae

Euonymi cortex

Synonyms: Euonymus, Wahoo Bark, Spindle Tree Bark.

Euonymus Bark consists of the dried root-bark of *Euonymus atropurpureus* Jacq.

CHARACTERISTICS

Macroscopical Description
Quilled or curved pieces up to about 4 mm thick; outer surface with irregular patches or large areas of soft, spongy, greyish-brown cork, finely fissured longitudinally with transverse ridges or, where the cork has been rubbed off, pale buff and nearly smooth; inner surface yellowish-buff, uneven and slightly porous, with occasional adherent shavings of yellowish wood; fracture short and powdery with fine, silky projecting threads of secretion.

Microscopical Description
Narrow cork of thin-walled, lignified cells; narrow parenchymatous cortex penetrated by wide wedges of phloem; secondary phloem with uniseriate medullary rays and numerous scattered, narrow, elongated and thin-walled laticiferous cells, numerous cells with brown contents occur scattered throughout the cortex and medullary rays; many cells of the cortex and phloem contain simple, rounded starch granules 3-12 µm in diameter; cluster crystals of calcium oxalate 30-40 µm in diameter occur in the cortex but less frequently in the phloem.

Odour and Taste
Faint odour; bitter and acrid taste.

IDENTIFICATION

Carry out the method for Thin-layer Chromatography as described in Appendix 1, using Solvent System B.

Apply 20 µl of each of the following solutions separately to the plate: (1) extract 1 g powdered Euonymus Bark with 10 ml methanol on a water-bath for 10-15 minutes cool, filter and concentrate to 5 ml; (2) 0.05% aescin in methanol.

Spray the plate with Spray Reagent C, heat at 105°C for 5-10 minutes then examine in daylight.

Major bands relative to aescin are approximately as follows: purplish green 1.9, purplish brown 0.7, brownish green 0.4.

QUANTITATIVE STANDARDS

Adhering Wood
Not more than 5%

Foreign Matter
Not more than 2%   Appendix 3

Total Ash
Not more than 14%   Appendix 4

Ash Insoluble in Hydrochloric Acid
Not more than 4%   Appendix 5

Ethanol (45%)-soluble Extractive
Not less than 24%   Appendix 6A

MATERIAL OF COMMERCE Euonymus Bark is supplied as transverse, curved pieces or occasionally as quills, sometimes broken. It is obtained from central and eastern North America.

Powdered Euonymus Bark

Complies with the requirements for Identification and Quantitative Standards stated for Euonymus Bark.

Characteristic Features
Pale greyish-buff powder with a faint odour and a bitter, acrid taste; abundant parenchyma, some cells with brown contents, others containing small, spherical starch granules and cluster crystals of calcium oxalate which may also occur scattered; thin-walled, fibre shaped, laticiferous cells with granular contents; fragments of lignified cork.

ACTION Laxative.

FENNEL, BITTER   Umbelliferae
Foeniculi amari fructus

Bitter Fennel consists of the dry, whole cremocarps and mericarps of *Foeniculum vulgare* Miller, subsp. *vulgare*, var. *vulgare*.

This material complies with the requirements of the European Pharmacopoeia for Bitter Fennel.

MATERIAL OF COMMERCE Bitter Fennel is supplied as whole cremocarps together with separated mericarps. It is cultivated in many countries and obtained particularly from eastern and central Europe.

ACTION Carminative.

FENNEL, SWEET   Umbelliferae
Foeniculi dulcis fructus

Sweet Fennel consists of the dry, whole cremocarps and mericarps of *Foeniculum vulgare* Miller, subsp. *vulgare* var. *dulce* (Miller) Thellung.

This material complies with the requirements of the European Pharmacopoeia for Sweet Fennel.

MATERIAL OF COMMERCE Sweet Fennel is supplied as whole cremocarps together with separated mericarps. It is cultivated in many countries and obtained particularly from Egypt, China, India, Bulgaria, France and Turkey.

ACTION Carminative.

FENUGREEK SEED Leguminosae-Papilionoideae

Foenugraeci semen

Synonyms: Trigonella, Trigonellae semen.

Fenugreek Seed consists of the dried, ripe seeds of *Trigonella foenum-graecum* L.

CHARACTERISTICS

Macroscopical Description
Dense, hard seeds, oblong to rhomboidal in outline and flattened, 4-6 mm long, 2-3 mm wide and about 2 mm thick; surface dull, light brownish-yellow, smooth; towards the end on one of the long narrow sides a depression marks the hilum, in the centre of which the micropyle appears as a whitish point; from the depression a deep furrow runs diagonally across both flat surfaces, separating the radicle from the remainder of the seed. Cut transversely, shows a narrow testa and a rather scanty dark and translucent endosperm surrounding the yellowish-white embyro with two large cotyledons.

Microscopical Description
Epidermis of the testa with a thick cuticle and composed of a layer of palisade cells about five times as long as wide, conical towards the outside and flattened at the base, lumen containing yellowish-brown pigment and walls thickened and striated; in surface view, cells polygonal and, seen from above, with a small lumen and walls with fine, radiating pits, seen from below, lumen larger and walls not pitted; hypodermis a characteristic layer of cells, narrower at the upper end and constricted in the middle, with bar-like thickenings on the radial walls; inner part of the testa composed of several layers of thin-walled parenchyma. Endosperm with an outer layer of tabular cells containing aleurone grains and, in surface view, showing distinct collenchymatous thickening; inner layers parenchymatous and containing mucilage. Embryo composed of parenchyma packed with aleurone grains and globules of fixed oil, the outer layers of the cotyledons differentiated into epidermis and palisade.

Odour and Taste
Odour strong, characteristic and spicy, reminiscent of Slippery Elm; taste mealy and unpleasant.

IDENTIFICATION

Carry out the method for Thin-layer Chromatography as described in Appendix 1, using Solvent System C.

Apply 60 µl of each of the following solutions to the plate: (1) extract 2g of powdered Fenugreek Seed by shaking with 10 ml of dichloromethane for 20 minutes. Filter, evaporate the filtrate just to dryness and dissolve the residue in 1 ml of toluene; (2) 0.1% cineole in toluene.

Spray the plate with Spray Reagent D, heat at 105°C for 10-15 minutes and examine in daylight.

Major bands relative to cineole are approximately as follows: purple 2.1, red 1.65, brown 1.25, purple 0.7, brown 0.45.

QUANTITATIVE STANDARDS

Foreign Matter
Not more than 4%   Appendix 3

Total Ash
Not more than 6%   Appendix 4

Ash Insoluble in Hydrochloric Acid
Not more than 1.5%   Appendix 5

Water-soluble Extractive
Not less than 30%   Appendix 7

MATERIAL OF COMMERCE Fenugreek Seed is supplied as whole seeds. It is harvested from cultivated plants and obtained from Morocco, Turkey, India and China.

Powdered Fenugreek Seed

Complies with the requirements for Identification and Quantitative Standards stated for Fenugreek Seed.

Characteristic Features
Pale yellowish-brown with a strong, characteristic and spicy odour and a mucilaginous, slightly bitter and disagreeable taste; fragments of the testa in sectional view showing the palisade cells of the epidermis and un-

derlying hypodermal cells with characteristic bar-like thickenings on the radial walls; yellowish-brown fragments of the epidermis in surface view composed of small polygonal cells with thickened and pitted walls, frequently attached to part of the hypodermis; viewed from above, the hypodermis walls are circular in outline showing rounded tops of the bars of thickening, viewed from below, the cells are polygonal with the bars of thickening joining the upper and lower walls; parenchyma of the testa, some layers composed of elongated rectangular cells with slightly thickened and beaded walls, others thin-walled and enclosing irregular intercellular spaces; collenchymatous cells of the outer layer of the endosperm, other cells of the endosperm thin-walled and containing mucilage which swells in aqueous mounts; parenchyma of the embryo with aleurone grains and globules of fixed oil.

ACTION Demulcent, hypoglycaemic.

FEVERFEW

Compositae

Tanaceti parthenii herba

Feverfew consists of the dried aerial parts of *Tanacetum parthenium* (L.) Schultz Bip. collected when the plant is in flower.

CHARACTERISTICS

Macroscopical Description

Stems Green, somewhat quadrangular, longitudinally ribbed, much branched, older stems up to 5 mm wide, younger stems sometimes less than 1 mm wide, bearing many alternate, pinnate to bipinnate leaves.

Leaves Yellowish-green, petiolate, usually 2-5 cm long but sometimes up to 10 cm, ovate, deeply divided into five or occasionally seven segments, each with a coarsely crenate margin and obtuse apex; both surfaces downy and the mid-rib prominent on the lower surface.

Flowers Flowering heads up to 2.5 cm wide, arranged in a loose corymb on long pedicels arising from the axils of the leaves; each capitulum with an involucre composed of lanceolate to oblong, downy bracts with pale, scarious margins, a single row of white, short, broad ray florets and numerous yellow disc florets arranged on a hemispherical receptacle.

Microscopical Description

Stem Epidermal cells thin-walled and axially elongated with cuticular striations, occasional anomocytic stomata and scattered uniseriate covering trichomes; cortex narrow, parenchymatous with collenchyma in the ridges; small groups of vascular tissue surrounding a parenchymatous pith; xylem with spirally and annularly thickened vessels.

Leaf Upper and lower epidermal cells with wavy anticlinal walls, striated cuticle and anomocytic stomata, more frequent on the lower epidermis; trichomes, more abundant on lower epidermis, of two types; covering trichomes, uniseriate with up to six small isodiametric basal cells and an elongated, tapering apical cell, often at right angles to the axis of the basal cells; glandular trichomes, slightly sunken, composed of a short, biseriate, two or four-celled stalk and a biseriate head of four cells, around which the cuticle forms a bladder-like covering.

Flower Epidermis of the bracts composed of elongated cells, stomata absent; upper epidermis of ray florets papillose; lower epidermis, cells with sinuous anticlinal walls, striated cuticle and numerous glandular trichomes similar to those on the leaf; upper epidermis of tubular florets with wavy anticlinal walls, striated cuticle, papillose near the margin, sometimes containing pale yellow amorphous masses and with small rosette crystals of calcium oxalate in the mesophyll; spherical pollen grains with spiny exine and three pores.

Odour and Taste

Camphoraceous odour; bitter and acrid taste.

(Caution: may cause blistering on the lips and soft palate.)

IDENTIFICATION

Carry out the method for Thin-layer Chromatography as described in Appendix 1, using Solvent System A.

Apply 20 µl of each of the following solutions separately to the plate: (1) extract 1 g powdered Feverfew with 10 ml methanol on a water-bath for 10-15 minutes, cool and filter; (2) 0.025% rutin in methanol.

Spray the plate with Spray Reagent A and examine in ultraviolet light 366 nm.

Major bands relative to rutin are approximately as follows: whitish-blue 2.25, greenish-blue 2.0, yellowish-green 1.65, yellowish-orange 1.5.

There should be no green band at 2.3 (distinction from Matricaria) nor blue band at 1.1 (distinction from Roman Chamomile).

QUANTITATIVE STANDARDS

Foreign Matter
Not more than 2%   Appendix 3

Total Ash
Not more than 15%   Appendix 4

Ash Insoluble in Hydrochloric Acid
Not more than 3%   Appendix 5

Water-soluble Extractive
Not less than 15%   Appendix 7

MATERIAL OF COMMERCE Feverfew is supplied in the crushed or broken condition. It is collected from the wild in continental Europe but is cultivated in the UK.

Powdered Feverfew

Complies with the requirements for Identification and Quantitative Standards stated for Feverfew.

Characteristic Features
Yellowish-green powder with faint camphoraceous odour and a bitter, acrid taste; fragments of leaf with epidermal cells with wavy anticlinal walls and anomocytic stomata, uniseriate covering trichomes with up to six small basal cells and an elongated apical cell; biseriate glandular trichomes composed of up to eight cells; papillose cells of upper epidermis of ray florets, lower epidermis with sinuous walls and striated cuticle; fragments of disc florets containing pale yellow amorphous masses and small rosette crystals of calcium oxalate; spherical pollen grains with a spiny exine.

ACTION Migraine prophylactic.

FRANGULA BARK   Rhamnaceae

Frangulae cortex

Synonyms: Frangula, Alder Buckthorn Bark.

Frangula Bark consists of the dried bark of the stems and branches of *Rhamnus frangula* L. [*Frangula alnus* Miller].

This material complies with the requirements of the European Pharmacopoeia for Frangula Bark and the British Pharmacopoeia for Frangula Bark or, when the material is in powder, Powdered Frangula Bark.

MATERIAL OF COMMERCE Frangula Bark is supplied as single or double quills, curved or nearly flat pieces or in the broken condition. It is obtained mainly from eastern Europe, especially Poland, former Yugoslavia and the former USSR.

ACTION Stimulant laxative.

FUMITORY

Fumariae herba

Synonyms: Fumaria, Common Fumitory.

Fumitory consists of the dried aerial parts of *Fumaria officinalis* L. collected during the flowering period.

CHARACTERISTICS

Macroscopical Description
Stems Diffusely branched, up to about 70 cm long and 3 mm in diameter, green to brownish, bearing alternate, stalked, greyish-green, glabrous leaves.

Leaves Several times pinnately divided, the ultimate, flattened, lanceolate segments often coarsely three-toothed or lobed.

Flowers Small, tubular, 7-9 mm long, arranged in long racemes opposite the leaves, having four pink petals in two pairs with dark blackish-red tips and six stamens united by their filaments in two groups of three.

Fruits Slightly flattened, obscurely keeled achenes, green and with a finely rugose surface, 2-2.5 mm in diameter with one seed.

Microscopical Description
Stem Roughly polygonal in outline with a number of vascular bundles surrounding a central hollow parenchymatous pith; pericycle consisting of a ring of thin-walled pitted cells of two types, some with thin sinuous anticlinal walls and others with thick sinuous anticlinal walls, with arcs of lignified fibres external to each vascular bundle; xylem with reticulate and bordered-pitted vessels.

Leaf Epidermal cells with wavy, anticlinal walls and anomocytic stomata on both surfaces; small annularly, spirally and reticulately thickened lignified vessels in the veins.

Flower Spherical pollen grains, 35-40 µm in diameter, with pitted exine and six large pores.

Fruit Cells of epicarp have a thick cuticle, coarsely warty or nodular with occasional stomata.

Odour and Taste
Slightly aromatic odour; slightly bitter taste.

IDENTIFICATION

Carry out the method for Thin-layer Chromatography as described in Appendix 1, using Solvent System A.

Apply 20 µl of each of the following solutions separately to the plate: (1) extract 1 g powdered Fumitory with 10 ml methanol on a water-bath for 10-15 minutes, cool and filter; (2) 0.025% rutin in methanol.

Spray with Spray Reagent A and examine in ultraviolet light 366 nm.

Major bands relative to rutin are approximately as follows: narrow pale blue 1.75, blue 1.7, broad yellow 1.25, green 1.1, blue 0.7.

QUANTITATIVE STANDARDS

Foreign Matter
Not more than 2%   Appendix 3

Total Ash
Not more than 16%   Appendix 4

Ash Insoluble in Hydrochloric Acid
Not more than 5%   Appendix 5

Water-soluble Extractive
Not less than 20%   Appendix 7

MATERIAL OF COMMERCE Fumitory is usually supplied as the crushed or broken material. It is obtained from European countries including the UK.

Powdered Fumitory

Complies with the requirements for Identification and Quantitative Standards stated for Fumitory.

Characteristic Features
Olive green powder with a slightly aromatic odour and a slightly bitter taste; epidermal cells of leaf with wavy anticlinal walls and anomocytic stomata; lignified vessels with annular, spiral and reticulate thickening; lignified fibres and elongated lignified parenchyma; spherical pollen grains with pit-

ted exine and six pores; two types of lignified cells from the pericycle of the stem; coarsely warty cells from epicarp and globules of oil

(if fruits present).

ACTION Choleretic.

GALANGAL

Zingiberaceae

Galangae rhizoma

Synonyms: Lesser Galangal, Galanga, East Indian Root.

Galangal consists of the dried rhizomes of *Alpinia officinarum* Hance.

CHARACTERISTICS

Macroscopical Description
Rhizome subcylindrical, slightly curved or angularly bowed; 5-10 cm long, 1-2 cm thick; larger pieces sympodially branched; distal ends with bud or remains of aerial shoot; dull reddish-brown, longitudinally wrinkled; pale creamish-white, slightly raised, encircling scale leaves with crinkled edges, at irregular intervals of 3-10 mm; scars or short remains of adventitious roots on under-surface; fracture tough, fibrous, lighter reddish-brown with numerous scattered darker spots; endodermis well-marked; stele about one third of total diameter.

Microscopical Description
Epidermal cells in section shallow, outer wall with thick, smooth cuticle; in surface view polygonal, anticlinal walls straight, moderately thick, often conspicuously beaded; stomata very infrequent; two or three layers of outer cortex, pigmented, more or less collapsed, small cells; inner cortex ground tissue of larger, rounded to oval parenchymatous cells, varying in size in transverse section, walls slightly thickened, not pitted, small intercellular spaces; axially the cells two to three times longer than wide, have oblique or pointed ends; majority of cells densely starch-filled, grains almost entirely simple, longest up to 50 µm, more or less elongated club-shaped, some with one or more small protuberances, hilum small, towards broader end, striations very faint; smaller grains variable, ovoid, rounded,

muller-shaped; interspersed throughout cortex numerous cells partially or completely filled with dark reddish-brown amorphous masses; fewer with pale yellowish volatile oil; a large number of collateral vascular bundles throughout cortex, most numerous in outer region, few near stele; variable in size but of similar structure; a group of up to eight to ten angular-shaped vessels, with reticulate and spiral thickening, thin-walled, very weakly lignified, most associated with a small, darkly pigmented cell near their outer edge; small area of thin-walled phloem tissue at inner radius or to one side of the xylem; complete, or almost complete, encircling sheath, two to four cells thick, thin-walled fibres, some relatively large diameter, unlignified; in longitudinal view show few, fine, widely-spaced, oblique, slit-shaped pits. Endodermis of small uniform parenchymatous, starch-free cells, walls suberised; pericycle cells smaller, collapsed. Stele ground tissue and cell contents as in cortex; vascular bundles relatively more numerous, structure similar, excepting the large number of bundles adjacent to endodermis lack fibres on the contiguous side.

Odour and Taste
Odour faintly aromatic, spicy, reminiscent of ginger. Taste strong, fiery, aromatic, somewhat bitter and astringent.

IDENTIFICATION

Carry out the method for Thin-layer Chromatography as described in Appendix 1, using Solvent System C.

Apply 60 µl of each of the following solutions to the plate: (1) extract 1 g of powdered Galangal by shaking with 10 ml of dichloromethane for 20 minutes. Filter, evaporate the filtrate just to dryness and dissolve the residue in 1 ml toluene; (2) 0.1% cineole in toluene.

Spray the plate with Spray Reagent D, heat at 105°C for 10-15 minutes and examine in daylight.

Major bands relative to cineole are approximately as follows: purple 1.9, purple 1.0, yellow 0.5, yellow 0.35, grey 0.15.

QUANTITATIVE STANDARDS

Total Ash
Not more than 5%   Appendix 4

Ash Insoluble in Hydrochloric Acid
Not more than 1%   Appendix 5

MATERIAL OF COMMERCE Galangal is supplied as rhizomes sliced transversely. It is harvested from cultivated plants and obtained from southern China, India, Thailand and neighbouring countries.

Powdered Galangal

Complies with the requirements for Identification and Quantiative Standards stated for Galangal.

Characteristic Features
A reddish-brown powder with a faintly aromatic odour and a strong, pungent taste; abundant starch granules, simple, ovoid to irregular with a small circular hilum towards the broader end; thin-walled secretion cells, some containing reddish-brown resin, others with yellowish oil droplets; epidermal cells in surface view, straight-walled and moderately thickened and beaded; groups of vessels with reticulate or spiral thickening, some with associated small pigment cells; thin-walled fibres.

ACTION Carminative.

GARLIC   Alliaceae

Allii sativi bulbus

Synonym: Allium.

Garlic consists of the fresh or dried compound bulbs of *Allium sativum* L.

CHARACTERISTICS

Macroscopical Description
Sub-globular compound bulbs, 3-5 cm broad, consisting of eight to twenty cloves, the whole surrounded by two to five layers of white scale leaves attached to a flattened, circular base; cloves ovoid and three to four-sided, summit acute, narrowed into a thread-like portion of fibre, base truncate; each clove covered with a white scale leaf and a pinkish-white epidermis, easily separated from the solid portion, consisting of two flaky scale leaves and two yellowish-green conduplicate foliage leaves.

Microscopical Description
Covering scale leaves have outer epidermis of elongated, sub-rectangular cells with thickened, beaded walls frequently lignified; elongated hypodermal cells with pitted, thick walls arranged with their long axes at right angles to the epidermal cells; hypodermal cells contain a prismatic crystal of calcium oxalate, 20-30 µm long; inner epidermis similar to the outer epidermis and a hypodermal layer of thick-walled, elongated cells with triangular intercellular spaces. The fleshy leaves have thin-walled upper and lower epidermises and a mesophyll of parenchymatous cells with small groups of slightly lignified annular and spiral vessels.

Odour and Taste
Strongly aromatic and characteristic odour; pungent and persistent taste.

MATERIAL OF COMMERCE Garlic is supplied as fresh or dried, whole bulbs. It is cultivated in many temperate zones, particularly in Mediterranean countries and in China, the USA and Argentina.

STORAGE Whole Garlic should be stored in a cool, dry place with free access to air.

Powdered Garlic

Characteristic Features
Whitish-cream powder with a strongly aromatic, characteristic odour and a pungent, persistent taste; fragments of covering scale leaves with elongated, subrectangular cells with thickened, beaded walls, frequently lignified, associated with elongated, thick-walled cells of hypodermis, having their long axes at right-angles to the epidermal cells; prismatic crystals of calcium oxalate; thin-walled epidermal cells of fleshy leaves; occasional slightly lignified annular and spiral vessels.

IDENTIFICATION

Carry out the method for Thin-layer Chromatography as described in Appendix 1, using a mixture of butan-1-ol: propan-1-ol: glacial acetic acid: water (3:1:1:1) as the Solvent System.

Apply 20 µl of each of the following solutions separately to the plate: (1) extract 1 g powdered Garlic with 10 ml 80% methanol by refluxing on a water-bath for 15 minutes, cool and filter; (2) 0.025% L-methionine in methanol.

Spray the plate with Ninhydrin Reagent and heat to 105°C for 20-30 minutes, then examine in daylight.

Major bands relative to L-methionine are approximately as follows: pinkish-yellow 0.9, broad orange 0.8, pinkish-orange 0.6, orange 0.38.

QUANTITATIVE STANDARDS

Note: Commercial methods for the production of Powdered Garlic are variable and in some cases the scale leaves may be removed, utilising only the cloves. Consequently, analytical criteria may vary according to source. Standards for two typical materials are as follows:

Powdered Garlic from Egypt

Generally prepared from entire bulbs.

Loss on Drying
Not more than 8% when dried in an oven at 100-105°C. Use 2-3 g   Appendix 2

Foreign Matter
Not more than 1%   Appendix 3

Total Ash
Not more than 12% calculated with reference to the oven-dried material   Appendix 4

Ash Insoluble in Hydrochloric Acid
Not more than 3% calculated with reference to the oven-dried material   Appendix 5

Water-soluble Extractive
Not less than 70% calculated with reference to the oven-dried material   Appendix 7

Powdered Garlic from China

Generally prepared from the cloves only.

Loss on Drying
Not more than 7% when dried in an oven at 100-105°C. Use 2-3 g   Appendix 2

Foreign Matter
Not more than 1%   Appendix 3

Total Ash
Not more than 5% calculated with reference to the oven-dried material   Appendix 4

Ash Insoluble in Hydrochloric Acid
Not more than 1% calculated with reference to the oven-dried material   Appendix 5

Water-soluble Extractive
Not less than 80% calculated with reference to the oven-dried material   Appendix 7

STORAGE Store in well-sealed containers in a cool, dry place.

ACTION   Hypolipidaemic; antimicrobial.

GENTIAN

Gentianaceae

Gentianae radix

Synonym: Gentiana.

Gentian consists of the dried underground organs of *Gentiana lutea* L.

This material complies with the requirements of the European Pharmacopoeia for Gentian Root and the British Pharmacopoeia for Gentian or, when the material is supplied in powder, Powdered Gentian.

MATERIALS OF COMMERCE Gentian is supplied as fairly large portions of root and rhizome or in the broken condition. It is generally obtained from mountain regions of Southern Europe.

ACTION Bitter.

GINGER

Zingiberaceae

Zingiberis rhizoma

Synonyms: Zingiber, Unbleached Ginger.

Ginger is the rhizome of *Zingiber officinale* Roscoe, scraped or unscraped.

This material complies with the requirements of the British Pharmacopoeia for Ginger or, when the material is in powder Powdered Ginger.

MATERIAL OF COMMERCE Ginger is supplied as completely scraped or partially scraped rhizomes or as chopped pieces. Completely scraped rhizomes are obtained from Jamaica and partially scraped rhizomes are obtained from West Africa, India, China South-East Asia and Australia.

ACTION Carminative; anti-emetic.

GINKGO LEAF

Ginkgoaceae

Ginkgo folium

Synonym: Maidenhair Tree Leaf.

Ginkgo Leaf consists of the dried leaves of *Ginkgo biloba* L.

CHARACTERISTICS

Macroscopical Description
Yellowish-green to olive green, under surface slightly paler, both surfaces glabrous; papery, flexible, easily split; up to 10 cm wide and 8 cm long; typically fan-shaped but occasionally sub-reniform, sides straight or somewhat concave, entire, termination of lamina curved, slightly undulate, sinuous-crenate or more markedly irregular crenate; base tapering; venation open dichotomous, veins very closely spaced, appearing to radiate from the base, almost equally prominent on both surfaces; petiole up to 8 cm long, 1-1.5 mm thick, flexible, finely grooved. Only leaves from young stems are deeply lobed.

Microscopical Description
Leaf Dorsiventral, palisade not well-differentiated, loosely-packed, relatively large cells; upper epidermal cells more or less rectangular, two to three times long as wide, anticlinal walls not thickened, longer sides irregularly sinuous, short sides straight, stomata absent; lower epidermal cells smaller, polygonal to sub-rectangular, thin-walled, only slightly wavy, very numerous stomata with guard cells large and deeply sunken and the stomatal chamber overhung by the

projecting papillae of the subsidiary cells; outer walls of both epidermises considerably thickened and convex forming, in the lower epidermis, short papillae; mesophyll containing numerous, regularly-spaced vascular bundles with narrow xylem elements and partially lignified fibres; abundant, large cluster crystals of calcium oxalate adjacent to the vascular bundles; brownish schizogenous cavities in the mesophyll between the vascular strands.

Petiole Epidermal cells with thickened outer wall, forming short papillae, infrequent stomata; completely lignified fibres in small, variable groups, beneath the epidermis, in part forming a more continuous band; cortex containing secretion cavities and large cluster crystals; vascular tissue with narrow, lignified tracheary elements, enclosed in a sheath, two to three cells thick, of lignified, pitted parenchymatous cells; smaller cluster crystals within the vascular tissue.

Odour and Taste
Slight odour, faintly reminiscent of tobacco; taste very slightly bitter and astringent.

IDENTIFICATION

Carry out the method for Thin-layer Chromatography as described in Appendix 1, using Solvent System A.

Apply 20 µl of each of the following solutions separately to the plate: (1) extract 1 g powdered Ginkgo Leaf with 10 ml methanol on a water-bath for 10-15 minutes, cool and filter; (2) 0.025% rutin in methanol.

Spray the plate with Spray Reagent A and examine in ultraviolet light 366 nm.

Major bands relative to rutin are approximately as follows: turquoise 2.2, yellow 1.4, yellow 1.2, turquoise 1.1, yellow 1.1, orange 1.0, turquoise 0.90, orange 0.8, yellow 0.75, orange 0.65.

QUANTITATIVE STANDARDS

Foreign Matter
Not more than 3%   Appendix 3

Total Ash
Not more than 15%   Appendix 4

Ash Insoluble in Hydrochloric Acid
Not more than 3.5%   Appendix 5

Water-soluble Extractive
Not less than 18%   Appendix 7

MATERIAL OF COMMERCE Ginkgo Leaf is supplied in whole or broken condition. It is obtained from China, Japan and Korea, and from plantations in France and the southeastern USA.

Powdered Ginkgo Leaf

Complies with the requirements for Identification and Quantitative Standards stated for Ginkgo Leaf.

Characteristic Features
Greyish-green powder with a faint odour and slight, bitter, astringent taste; rectangular epidermal cells with sinuous walls and no stomata; smaller epidermal cells with numerous stomata; very abundant, large cluster crystals, up to 120 µm; parenchyma with short files of smaller cluster crystals; lignified, narrow, spirally-thickened vessels and tracheids with numerous closely-spaced, large bordered pits; rectangular, lignified parenchyma cells; thick-walled fibres, some incompletely lignified.

ACTION Vasoactive; platelet aggregation inhibitor.

GINSENG

Araliaceae

Ginseng radix

Synonym: Korean Ginseng.

Ginseng consists of the dried roots of *Panax ginseng* C.A. Meyer.

CHARACTERISTICS

Macroscopical Description
Fusiform or cylindrical roots, sometimes branched, 5-12 cm or sometimes up to 20 cm long and up to 2.5 cm in diameter at the crown, with one or more stem scars; pale yellow or cream surface, smooth in the upper part but with fine longitudinal ridges and root scars in the lower parts; some fine rootlets may be attached; fracture short; fractured surface light yellowish-brown, exhibiting a ring of secretory canals in the cortex and a distinct brownish-yellow cambium .

Microscopical Description
Traces of cork composed of thin-walled polygonal cells but mainly with phelloderm on the outside; wide cortex of parenchymatous cells with numerous secretory canals arranged in concentric zones; parenchymatous xylem with non-lignified tracheids and slightly lignified vessels with spiral and reticulate thickening, isolated or in small groups; small granules of starch 0.5-1.0 μm in diameter in all the parenchymatous cells and occasional cluster crystals of calcium oxalate in the cells of the central region.

Odour and Taste
Slightly aromatic odour; initially sweet taste, becoming bitter.

IDENTIFICATION

A. To 0.1 g powdered Ginseng add 0.1 ml concentrated sulphuric acid; a red colour is produced after 1-2 minutes.
B. Carry out the method for Thin-layer Chromatography as described in Appendix 1, using Solvent System B.

Apply 20 μl of each of the following solutions separately to the plate: (1) extract 0.5 g powdered Ginseng with 10 ml 60% methanol on a water-bath for 10-15 minutes cool and filter; (2) 0.05% aescin in methanol.

Spray the plate with Spray Reagent C, heat at 105°C for 5-10 minutes then examine in daylight.

Major bands relative to aescin are approximately as follows: brown 1.2, purple 0.9, greenish-purple 0.65, greenish-purple 0.5.

QUANTITATIVE STANDARDS

Loss on Drying
Not more than 10% when dried in an oven at 100-105°C. Use 2-3 g.   Appendix 2

Foreign Matter
Not more than 2%   Appendix 3

Total Ash
Not more than 8% calculated with reference to the oven-dried material   Appendix 4

Ash Insoluble in Hydrochloric Acid
Not more than 2% calculated with reference to the oven-dried material   Appendix 5

Ethanol (70%)-soluble Extractive
Not less than 20% calculated with reference to the oven-dried material   Appendix 6A

MATERIAL OF COMMERCE Ginseng is supplied in the whole or broken condition. It is obtained from Korea, China and North America. Red Ginseng is also available commercially from Korea. It is obtained by first steaming, then drying the root without scraping off the outer layer of cork.

Powdered Ginseng

Complies with the requirements for Identification and Quantitative Standards stated for Ginseng.

Characteristic Features
Pale yellowish-brown powder with a slightly aromatic odour and a sweetish taste which

later becomes bitter; oval parenchymatous cells packed with starch granules, occasional cluster crystals of calcium oxalate, yellowish-brown secretory vessels with yellowish-brown contents.

STORAGE Store in a cool, dry place in well closed containers.

ACTION Adaptogen; tonic.

GOLDEN ROD Compositae

Solidaginis virgaureae herba

Golden Rod consists of the dried flowering tops of *Solidago virgaurea* L.

CHARACTERISTICS

Macroscopical Description

Stems Very variable, up to 1 m long and 4 mm thick, almost cylindrical, little branched, finely longitudinally ridged; lower part often reddish-violet; sometimes entirely glabrous or with short, bent, apically directed hairs, more numerous on upper part.

Leaves Spirally arranged; lower leaves largest, up to 10 cm long, 2 cm wide, petiolate; upper leaves progressively smaller, sessile to amplexicaul, with small stipules; shape varying from narrowly lanceolate, obovate to oblanceolate; apex tapering, acute; base of petiolate leaves tapering; margin more or less entire in upper leaves, widely and finely serrate in lower; tapering base smooth; very short hairs along margins; venation pinnate with very fine network between; surfaces entirely glabrous or sparsely hairy, usually on paler lower surface.

Flowers A lax panicle of small clusters of up to six heads on short, sometimes hairy pedicels in leaf axils; each head 6-10 mm diameter; involucre of up to five rows of imbricate bracts, greenish-yellow, narrow, pointed, inner surface smooth and shiny, outer with hairs near apex or glabrous, margins scarious; outermost bracts shorter and wider; florets all golden yellow; six to twelve spreading, widely separated ray florets, twice as long as bracts, strap elongated ovoid, finely three or five- notched at apex; numerous hermaphrodite tubular florets opening into five more or less recurved lobes.

Fruits Brown achenes, up to 3 or 4 mm, surface minutely hairy; pappus short, filaments in a single row.

Microscopical Description

Stem Section almost circular, often with irregularly spaced, multicellular outgrowths of varying size; some bearing long, uniseriate trichomes; epidermal cells rectangular, outer wall thickened, slightly convex, cuticle coarsely ridged; cortex cells collenchymatous, larger and thinner-walled towards pericycle; groups of thick-walled, sparsely pitted fibres; phloem narrow; xylem a continuous ring of lignified tissue with protuberances into pith opposite rows of strongly lignified bordered-pitted vessels; parenchyma of pith weakly lignified, few small pits.

Leaf Dorsiventral; palisade single or double layered, the cells short; upper epidermal cells more or less polygonal, isodiametric or slightly elongated, anticlinal walls thin, almost straight or gently wavy, stomata absent or very infrequent; lower epidermal cells similar to upper, some smaller, short walls straight, longer more sinuous, numerous stomata, three or four subsidiary cells, mainly anisocytic, few anomocytic; trichomes of two forms may occur on both epidermises; long usually curved, uniseriate with up to twelve short cells, walls more thickened in the lower, larger cells; few quite small, thin-walled with a swollen, more or less ovoid head, terminating in a short, narrow, whip-like extension, the stalk of one or two slightly swollen cells.

Flower Epidermal cells of bracts, thin-walled with small pits, elongated, ends oblique; marginal cells long, colourless, at intervals one, two or three cells break away forming apically directed projections, longer towards apex, some with swollen terminal cells; central epidermis with covering trichomes, curved, with up to five cells, conspicuously thickened and enlarged at joints. Epidermal cells of both tubular and ligulate florets similar; most are elongated, straight-walled or slightly sinuous; smaller, polygonal near apices; inner slightly papillose at tips of tubular florets; epidermis of both corollas striated, the outer longitudinally, inner transversely. Stigma of tubular florets deeply bifid, papillose along entire length; papillae longest in mid region. Pollen grains spherical, about 30 μm, three indistinct pores, the exine spiny. Ovary with appressed, apically directed, biseriate hairs, each of two cells, slightly unequal in length, thin-walled, pitted along contiguous wall, bifurcating near apices. Pappus, slender, multiseriate, apices of cells free from surface, forming acutely pointed projections; some cells weakly lignified.

Odour and Taste
Slight odour; taste somewhat aromatic and bitter.

IDENTIFICATION

Carry out the method for Thin-layer Chromatography as described in Appendix 1, using Solvent System A.

Apply 20 μl of each of the following solutions separately to the plate: (1) extract 1 g powdered Golden Rod with 10 ml methanol by warming on a water-bath for 10-15 minutes, cool and filter; (2) 0.025% rutin in methanol.

Spray the plate with Spray Reagent A and examine in ultraviolet light 366 nm.

Major bands relative to rutin are approximately as follows: turquoise 2.3, yellow 2.0, yellow 1.8, yellow 1.5, yellow 1.0.

QUANTITATIVE STANDARDS

Foreign Matter
Not more than 3%   Appendix 3

Total Ash
Not more than 8%   Appendix 4

Ash Insoluble in Hydrochloric Acid
Not more than 2%   Appendix 5

Water-soluble Extractive
Not less than 11%   Appendix 7

MATERIAL OF COMMERCE Golden Rod is supplied in the whole or cut condition. It is obtained mainly from eastern European countries.

ACTION Diuretic; anticatarrhal, diaphoretic.

GOLDEN SEAL ROOT   Ranunculaceae

Hydrastis rhizoma

Synonym: Hydrastis.

Golden Seal Root consists of the dried rhizomes and roots of *Hydrastis canadensis* L.

CHARACTERISTICS

Macroscopical Description
   Rhizomes Horizontal or oblique, subcylindrical, 1-6 cm long and 2-10 mm in diameter, occasionally with stem bases; numerous short upright branches terminating in cup-shaped scars and bearing encircling cataphyllary leaves; externally, brown to greyish or yellowish-brown, deeply longitudinally wrinkled, marked by numerous stem scars and more or less annulate scars of scale leaves, from the lower and lateral surfaces many long, slender, brittle, curved, wiry roots which are frequently broken off to leave short protuberances or circular, yellow scars; fracture short and resinous; fractured surface yellowish-orange at centre and greenish-yellow at margin with thick, dark yellow to yellowish-brown bark; twelve to twenty radially elongated, bright yellow, narrow xylem bundles separated by wide medullary rays; large pith.
   Roots Numerous, filiform up to 35 mm long, 1 mm in diameter, curved or twisted; fracture short and brittle, fractured surface yellowish-orange to greenish-yellow.

Microscopical Description
   Rhizome Cork, yellowish-brown, po-

lygonal with thin lignified walls; abundant thin-walled, polygonal to round or elongated, parenchymatous cells and some collenchyma in the secondary cortex containing abundant starch granules, simple or rarely two to four compound, spherical or ovoid with small, round or slit-like hilum; numerous masses of granular, orange-brown matter in the parenchyma; lignified tracheidal-vessels, usually small with slit-like pits, occasionally large vessels with reticulate thickening.

Root Cork, single layer of cells, irregularly elongated; very occasional fragments of piliferous layer from young roots with root hairs; few thin-walled, lignified fibres associated with vessels; occasional fragments of epidermis of stem bases composed of cells with thick, lignified, beaded walls, slightly elongated in surface view.

Odour and Taste
Faint, unpleasant odour; bitter and persistent taste.

IDENTIFICATION

Carry out the method for Thin-layer Chromatography as described in Appendix 1, using a mixture of propan-l-ol: anhydrous formic acid: water (90:1:9) as the Solvent System and allowing the solvent front to ascend a distance of 12 cm above the line of application.

Apply 20 µl of each of the following solutions separately to the plate: (1) extract 1 g powdered Golden Seal Root with 10 ml methanol and 1 ml 18M ammonia by refluxing on a water-bath for 10-15 minutes, cool and filter; (2) 0.01% berberine chloride in methanol; (3) 0.01% hydrastine hydrochloride in methanol.

Spray the plate with Dragendorff's Reagent followed by Sodium Nitrite Solution and examine in daylight.

The chromatogram of Golden Seal Root shows bands with the same Rf values as the berberine and hydrastine.

QUANTITATIVE STANDARDS

Foreign Matter
Not more than 3%   Appendix 3

Total Ash
Not more than 10%   Appendix 4

Ash Insoluble in Hydrochloric Acid
Not more than 4%   Appendix 5

Water-soluble Extractive
Not less than 14%   Appendix 7

MATERIAL OF COMMERCE Golden Seal Root is supplied as entire rhizomes with roots free and attached or in the chopped condition. It is obtained mainly from eastern North America.

Powdered Golden Seal Root

Complies with the requirements for Identification and Quantitative Standards stated for Golden Seal Root.

Characteristic Features
Dull yellow powder with a faint, unpleasant odour and a bitter, persistent taste; abundant, thin-walled parenchymatous cells, polygonal to round, containing numerous starch granules and masses of orange-brown granular matter; yellowish-brown cork with thin, lignified walls; small, lignified tracheidal-vessels with small slit-like pits; abundant starch granules; ovoid to spherical masses of granular, orange-brown matter.

ACTION Anti-inflammatory.

GRINDELIA Compositae

Grindeliae herba

Synonyms: Gumweed, Gum Plant, Tar Weed.

Grindelia consists of the dried flowering tops of *Grindelia robusta* Nutt., *G. squarrosa* (Pursh) Dunal, *G. camporum* Greene or *G. humilis* Hook. et Arn.

CHARACTERISTICS

Macroscopical Description

Stems Form the major part of the commercial material. Sub-cylindrical or flattened, sometimes split longitudinally, up to about 4 mm wide; surface smooth or with fine longitudinal striations, pale yellowish-brown to green, occasionally with a pinkish tinge; fracture fibrous, the fractured surface showing a large, white, central pith.

Leaves Brittle and frequently broken in commercial material; up to about 5 cm long but usually smaller; oblong or spathulate, apex acute, margin serrate, base sessile or amplexicaul; both surfaces pale green or brownish, glabrous but covered with a reticulum of very numerous, minute pits.

Capitula Terminal and solitary; subconical, up to about 15 mm in diameter, very hard and resinous, each composed of a flat receptacle with four or five rows of small, lanceolate to acuminate, imbricated bracts, recurved at the tips, a single row of ligulate florets and a large central group of numerous disc florets; ligulate florets about 12 mm long, corolla orange-yellow with a three-lobed apex; disc florets about 5 mm long, corolla tubular, pale yellow, five lobed with five protruding stamens; ovary on both types of floret surmounted by two small calyx lobes from which emerge several narrow, bristle-like awns, 2-3 mm long.

Microscopical Description

Stem Epidermis composed of longitudinally elongated cells with thickened outer and inner walls, occasional scattered stomata and large glandular trichomes similar to those on the leaf; cortex with outer collenchyma of several layers of cells and a narrow parenchymatous region in which, adjacent to the endodermis, schizogenous resin ducts occur at intervals; pericycle with small, lignified, very thick-walled fibres, densely packed and forming a wide band partially enclosing a ring of closely-packed vascular bundles; vascular bundles with a small group of phloem and lignified xylem composed of vessels embedded in small-celled parenchyma; pith parenchymatous, some of the cells in the outer region lignified with slightly thickened and pitted walls.

Leaf Isobilateral with a single-layered palisade under both epidermises; epidermal cells polygonal with straight or slightly wavy walls; stomata numerous, occurring in groups on both epidermises, anomocytic, broadly elliptical and projecting above the epidermis; large, sessile, multicellular, ovoid glandular trichomes up to 100 μm in diameter, occurring in depressions in the epidermis, the cells each containing a microrosette crystal of calcium oxalate; very occasional covering trichomes, uniseriate, conical, composed of two or three cells.

Capitulum Bracts one cell thick at the margins with teeth formed by the projection of two or more adjacent cells; central region multilayered containing narrow vascular strands and, near the base, cells containing microrosette crystals of calcium oxalate; outer epidermis in the central region with very numerous multicellular glandular trichomes similar to those on the leaf, and occasional groups of stomata; inner epidermis composed of longitudinally-elongated cells. Corolla of the ligulate florets papillose at the tip; outer epidermal cells longitudinally elongated with finely pitted walls and narrow bands of cellulosic thickening; corolla of the disc florets with narrow, thin-walled, elongated epidermal cells; in both types of corolla microrosette crystals and prisms of calcium oxalate occur in the basal region. Epidermis of the anther filaments composed of small, square to rectangular cells with slightly thickened walls; pollen grains spherical, about 35 μm in diameter, with three pores and a markedly spiny exine. Apices of the stigmas with long, finger-like papillae. Awns composed of thick-walled cells extended at the margins to form projecting teeth.

Odour and Taste

Odour balsamic, taste aromatic, bitter and resinous.

IDENTIFICATION

Carry out the method for Thin-layer Chromatography as described in Appendix 1, using Solvent System A.

Apply 40 µl of each of the following solutions separately to the plate: (1) extract 1 g powdered Grindelia with 10 ml methanol by warming on a water-bath for 10-15 minutes, cool, filter and concentrate the filtrate to 2 ml; (2) 0.025% rutin in methanol.

Spray the plate with Spray Reagent A and examine in ultraviolet light 366 nm.

Major bands relative to rutin are approximately as follows: yellow 2.4, turquoise 2.3, yellow 1.6, yellow 1.35.

There are a series of faint bands from 1.0-0.7.

Due to the relatively low concentration of Grindelia's constituents, the chromatogram may not be well resolved. For this reason, samples should be analysed against an authenticated specimen.

QUANTITATIVE STANDARDS

Foreign Matter
Not more than 3%   Appendix 3

Total Ash
Not more than 10%   Appendix 4

Ash Insoluble in Hydrochloric Acid
Not more than 2%   Appendix 5

MATERIAL OF COMMERCE Grindelia is supplied whole or cut. It is obtained from California and arid regions of the western USA.

Powdered Grindelia

Complies with the requirements for Identification and Quantitative Standards stated for Grindelia.

Characteristic Features
Light yellowish to greenish-brown with a slightly aromatic, balsamic odour and a somewhat bitter and resinous taste; abundant groups of narrow fibres from the stems, some associated with vessels with spiral or annular thickening or with small, closely-packed bordered pits; fragments of the epidermises of the leaves and bracts with groups of anomocytic stomata and large multicellular, glandular trichomes containing microrosette crystals of calcium oxalate; occasional fragments of the corollas containing microrosette and elongated prism crystals; characteristic fibrous layer of the anthers; pollen grains typical of the Compositae with three pores and a spiny exine; infrequent groups of parenchyma containing brown, schizogenous resin ducts.

ACTION Expectorant.

GROUND IVY   Labiatae

Glechomae hederaceae herba

Synonym: *Nepeta hederacea.*

Ground Ivy consists of the dried aerial parts of *Glechoma hederacea* L., collected during the flowering period.

CHARACTERISTICS

Macroscopical Description
Stems Quadrangular, hairy, up to 3 mm wide, pale green to purplish-green, bearing numerous pairs of opposite leaves.

Leaves Petiolate, 1-3 cm wide or occasionally larger, reniform ovate-cordate with a crenate margin; upper surface dark green, lower surface paler green and punctate, both surfaces distinctly hairy.

Flowers In groups of two to four in the axils of the upper leaves, with a green, hairy, tubular calyx and a purplish-blue, two-lipped corolla.

Fruit Capsules up to about 2 mm long, each containing three or four smooth, oval nutlets.

Microscopical Description

Stem Epidermal cells rectangular in surface view with scattered covering and glandular trichomes similar to those on the leaf; vascular tissue with small groups of small, lignified vessels having spiral and annular thickening or occasionally with bordered pits; central pith composed of slightly lignified, longitudinally elongated parenchymatous cells with moderately thickened and pitted walls.

Leaf Dorsiventral; upper epidermal cells sinuous to wavy in surface view with a striated cuticle, those of the lower epidermis more wavy-walled, cuticle not striated; diacytic stomata abundant on lower surface only; covering trichomes of two types on both epidermises, those occurring most abundantly uniseriate, multicellular from two to six cells long, often with a collapsed cell and with a warty and sometimes striated cuticle; others, occurring less frequently, unicellular, conical with a warty wall; glandular trichomes also very abundant particularly on the lower epidermis, some small with a unicellular stalk and a unicellular or occasionally bicellular head, the majority being larger and of the Labiatae type with a unicellular stalk and a six to eight-celled head.

Flower Epidermal cells of the calyx wavywalled in surface view and on the outer epidermis abundant covering and scattered glandular trichomes similar to those on the leaf, occasional diacytic stomata; epidermal cells of the corolla distinctly papillose and on the inner epidermis in the central region very long covering trichomes with brown granular contents; pollen grains spherical to ovoid, 55-60 µm in diameter with a smooth exine.

Odour and Taste

Aromatic, pungent odour; slightly bitter and astringent taste.

IDENTIFICATION

Carry out the method for Thin-layer Chromatography as described in Appendix 1, using Solvent System A.

Apply 20 µl of each of the following solutions separately to the plate: (1) extract 1 g powdered Ground Ivy with 10 ml ethanol (70%) by refluxing on a water-bath for 10-15 minutes, cool, filter and evaporate to 2 ml; (2) 0.025% rutin in methanol.

Spray the plate with Spray Reagent A and examine in ultraviolet light 366 nm.

Major bands relative to rutin are approximately as follows: bluish-green 2.75, narrow green 2.4.

QUANTITATIVE STANDARDS

Foreign Matter
Not more than 5%   Appendix 3

Total Ash
Not more than 10%   Appendix 4

Ash Insoluble in Hydrochloric Acid
Not more than 2%   Appendix 5

Water-soluble Extractive
Not less than 10%   Appendix 7

MATERIAL OF COMMERCE Ground Ivy is supplied in the broken or chopped condition. It is obtained from many of the countries of Europe.

Powdered Ground Ivy

Complies with the requirements for Identification and Quantitative Standards stated for Ground Ivy.

Characteristic Features

Greyish-green powder with a characteristic pungent odour and a slightly bitter, astringent taste; fragments of leaf showing wavy-walled epidermal cells, some with striated cuticle, others with diacytic stomata and numerous covering and glandular trichomes, the covering trichomes often detached and occurring scattered; vascular tissue from the stems with groups of lignified vessels slightly lignified, elongated parenchymatous cells from the pith; very occasional fragments of papillose cells of the corolla; scattered spherical to ovoid pollen grains.

ACTION Expectorant.

GUAIACUM RESIN Zygophyllaceae

Guaiaci resina

Guaiacum Resin is obtained from the heart-wood of *Guaiacum officinale* L. or *Guaiacum sanctum* L., either by heating the cut wood and collecting the liquid resin or by evaporating to dryness an alcoholic extract of the wood.

CHARACTERISTICS

Description
Large, rounded blocks or ovoid tears, frequently covered with a dull, green powder; breaks easily leaving a clear, brown, glassy surface; thin pieces somewhat transparent and appearing yellowish-green to reddish-brown.

Odour and Taste
Aromatic odour when warmed; acrid taste.

IDENTIFICATION

A. To 10 ml of 1% ethanolic (96%) solution of Guaiacum Resin add 0.2 ml Ferric Chloride Solution; a blue colour is produced.
B. Carry out the method for Thin-layer Chromatography as described in Appendix 1, using a mixture of chloroform: ethyl acetate (95:5) as the Solvent System.
Apply 20 µl of each of the following solutions separately to the plate: (1) extract 0.1 g powdered Guaiacum Resin with 10 ml methanol by warming gently for 3-4 minutes, cool and filter; (2) 0.025% methyl red in methanol.
 Expose the plate to ultraviolet light 366 nm for one or two minutes and examine in daylight.
 Major bands relative to methyl red are approximately as follows: blue 1.6, blue 0.3.

Absence of Colophony Shake 1 g powdered Guaiacum Resin with 5 ml petroleum spirit (boiling range 50° to 70°) for 5 minutes then filter; the filtrate is colourless. Shake the filtrate with an equal volume of Copper Acetate Solution; no green colour develops.

QUANTITATIVE STANDARDS

Total Ash
Not more than 5% Appendix 4

Ash Insoluble in Hydrochloric Acid
Not more than 2% Appendix 5

Ethanol (96%)-insoluble Residue*
Not more than 15% Appendix 6B

* Guaiacum Resin obtained by alcoholic extraction with a filtration stage will yield much less Ethanol-insoluble Residue: not more than 3%.

MATERIAL OF COMMERCE Guaiacum Resin is usually supplied as large blocks but sometimes the blocks may be broken into smaller pieces. It is obtained from Colombia, Venezuela and the West Indies.

Powdered Guaiacum Resin

Complies with the requirements for Identification and Quantitative Standards stated for Guaiacum Resin.

Characteristic Features
Greyish-brown powder becoming green on exposure to light with an aromatic odour when warmed and an acrid taste.

ACTION Anti-inflammatory.

HAMAMELIS BARK

Hamamelidaceae

Hamamelidis cortex

Synonym: Witch Hazel Bark.

Hamamelis Bark consists of the dried bark from stems and branches of *Hamamelis virginiana* L. collected in the spring.

CHARACTERISTICS

Macroscopical Description
Channelled, slightly curved or almost flat pieces, up to 2 mm thick and 1.5-2 cm wide, length variable up to 20 cm; outer surface, depending on age, dull, almost smooth to minutely scaly or fissured, cork dark grey, frequent, paler, lichen cover; inconspicuous tangentially elongated lenticels; few areas of smooth to slightly granular, pale reddish-brown, exposed cortex; inner surface distinctly longitudinally striated, light pink-tinged tan, occasional strips of off-white adhering wood; fracture short and granular in cork and cortex, shortly fibrous in phloem.

Microscopical Decription
Several layers of thin-walled cork cells, alternating in places with rows of cells, filled with amorphous brown contents, more thickened, especially the inner tangential wall; outer phelloderm of fairly thick-walled, finely-pitted cells, inner layers more tangentially elongated and collenchymatously thickened; outer cortex cells smaller, ovoid, with intercellular spaces; almost uniformly wide, continuous pericycle, mainly small sclereids, variable in shape and wall thickness, numerous pits, at irregular intervals single, or small groups of, thick-walled fibres, lignified and infrequently pitted, cells of outer and inner margins of pericycle band contain prism crystals; parenchymatous outer phloem with few, irregular groups of larger sclereids, pits few and narrow, walls conspicuously striated; medullary rays numerous, straight or slightly sinuous, uniseriate or, very infrequently, biseriate, small groups of fibres, more or less irregularly arranged, occasionally a few adjacent groups appear as short tangential bands, narrow innermost phloem devoid of fibres; sieve tubes with oblique sieve plates and slightly thickened walls, phloem parenchymatous cells smaller, less thickened, many with amorphous brown contents.

Odour and Taste
Virtually odourless; taste very astringent, only slightly bitter.

IDENTIFICATION

Carry out the method for Thin-layer Chromatography as described in Appendix 1 using Solvent System E.

Apply 20 µl of the following solution to the plate. Extract 5 g of Hamamelis Bark with 20 ml methanol by warming on a water-bath for 20 minutes, cool and filter.

Spray the plate with Spray Reagent F solution, followed by a separate application of 5 ml potassium hydroxide solution; inspect in daylight.

Major bands relative to the solvent front are approximately as follows: brown 0.7, brown 0.6, brown 0.55, brown 0.4, brown 0.3, brown 0.25.

QUANTITATIVE STANDARDS

Foreign Matter
Not more than 2%   Appendix 3

Total Ash
Not more than 6%   Appendix 4

Ash Insoluble in Hydrochloric Acid
Not more than 1.5%   Appendix 5

Ethanol (45%)-soluble Extractive
Not less than 20%   Appendix 6A

MATERIAL OF COMMERCE Hamamelis Bark is supplied as broken quills. It is obtained from the eastern USA and Canada.

Powdered Hamamelis Bark

Complies with the requirements for Identification and Quantitative Standards stated for Hamamelis Bark.

Characteristic Features
Light pinkish-buff, odourless, taste slightly

bitter, markedly astringent; numerous sclereids usually in groups, some quite large, thick-walled, markedly pitted and striated, others smaller and fairly thin-walled; abundant lignified fibres, lumen narrow, seldom pitted, usually in groups with associated prism crystal sheath; thin-walled cork cells, sometimes in association with small

sclereids; uniseriate medullary rays, seen in longitudinal section; parenchyma containing brown amorphous matter, infrequent, isolated, larger prism crystals; lignified medullary rays and narrow bordered-pitted elements from adhering wood.

ACTION Astringent.

HAMAMELIS LEAF
Hamamelidaceae

Hamamelidis folium

Synonym: Witch Hazel Leaf.

Hamamelis Leaf consists of the dried leaves of *Hamamelis virginiana* L.

This material complies with the requirements of the European Pharmacopoeia for

Hamamelis Leaf.

MATERIAL OF COMMERCE Hamamelis Leaf is supplied as whole or broken leaf. It is obtained from eastern USA and Canada.

ACTION Astringent.

HAWTHORN BERRY
Rosaceae

Crataegi fructus

Synonyms: May, Whitethorn, Haw.

Hawthorn Berry consists of the dried, ripe false fruits of *Crataegus monogyna* Jacq. emend Lindm., *Crataegus laevigata* (Poir.) DC. [*C. oxyacantha* L.] or their hybrids.

CHARACTERISTICS

Macroscopical Description
Ovoid false fruits, 6-13 mm long, 4-10 mm wide, each consisting of a much swollen receptacle surmounted by the remains of five reflexed calyx lobes surrounding a shallow, circular opening, with a dense covering of hairs on the exposed inner surface and the remains of the style and stigma in the centre; outer surface of the receptacle red to dark red or brown, glabrous, much shrunken and wrinkled; at the base a short

length of pedicel or, more usually, a small, pale circular scar where the pedicel was attached; receptacle mealy, enclosing one or two hard, yellowish-brown, ovoid fruits up to about 7 mm long, each containing a small, slightly flattened, elongated-ovoid seed with a pale brown, smooth and shiny testa.

Microscopical Description
Outer epidermal cells of the receptacle polygonal with slightly thickened walls, filled with red colouring matter; remainder of receptacle composed of loosely-arranged, thin-walled parenchymatous cells, some containing isolated small cluster crystals of calcium oxalate and, in the inner region, interspersed with small groups of sclereids with moderately thickened, pitted walls; narrow vascular strands occur scattered, composed of a few vessels with annular or spiral thicken-

ing, usually associated with elongated sclereids and a file of small cells each containing a prism crystal of calcium oxalate; covering trichomes from the inner surface long, unicellular, frequently repeatedly bent, tapering to a point at the apex, walls smooth, much thickened and lignified. Pericarp with thin-walled parenchyma containing cluster crystals of calcium oxalate and several dense layers of large, thick-walled sclereids with numerous, sometimes conspicuously branched, pits; as in the receptacle, prism crystals of calcium oxalate sometimes occur associated with the vascular strands. Testa with an epidermal layer of thin-walled cells filled with mucilage and a collapsed, yellowish-brown pigment layer containing abundant elongated crystals of calcium oxalate. Parenchyma of the endosperm and cotyledons thin-walled and densely packed with aleurone grains and globules of fixed oil.

Odour and Taste
Odour slight, somewhat fruity; taste mealy, faintly acidulous and bitter.

IDENTIFICATION

Carry out the method for Thin-layer Chromatography as described in Appendix 1, using Solvent System A.

Apply 20 µl of each of the following solutions separately to the plate: (1) extract 1 g powdered Hawthorn Berry with 10 ml methanol by warming on a water-bath for 10-15 minutes; cool and filter; (2) 0.025% rutin in methanol.

Spray the plate with Spray Reagent A and examine in ultraviolet light 366 nm.

Major bands relative to rutin are approximately as follows: turquoise 2.25, orange 1.65, turquoise 1.5, orange 1.0.

The chromatogram exhibits similar characteristics to that of Hawthorn Flowering Top. Major bands have the same Rf value, but may differ in hue and intensity.

QUANTITATIVE STANDARDS

Foreign Matter
Not more than 2%   Appendix 3

Total Ash
Not more than 5%   Appendix 4

MATERIAL OF COMMERCE Hawthorn Berry is supplied as wrinked dried 'fruits'. It is obtained from the UK and other European countries.

Powdered Hawthorn Berry

Complies with the requirements for Identification and Quantitative Standards stated for Hawthorn Berry.

Characteristic Features
Light reddish brown to tan with a slight odour and a bitter, mucilaginous taste; fragments of parenchyma from the receptacle, those from the outer layers red in colour, some cells containing small cluster crystals of calcium oxalate and occasional fragments including groups of sclereids with moderately-thickened walls; vascular strands with associated files of cells containing calcium oxalate prisms; very abundant sclereids from the pericarp, occurring singly and in dense groups, individual cells with strongly thickened walls and conspicuous, frequently branched, pits; scattered thick-walled, unicellular covering trichomes; occasional fragments of brown pigment layer containing elongated prism crystals of calcium oxalate; parenchyma containing aleurone grains and globules of fixed oil.

ACTION Cardiotonic.

HAWTHORN FLOWERING TOP   Rosaceae

Crataegi folium cum flore

Synonyms: May, Whitethorn, Haw.

Hawthorn Flowering Top consists of the dried flower-bearing tips, up to about 7 cm long, of branches of *Crataegus monogyna* Jacq. emend Lindm., *Crataegus laevigata* (Poir.) DC. [*C. oxyacantha* L.] or their hybrids.

CHARACTERISTICS

Macroscopical Description
Leaves Broadly ovate or obovate, 1.5-3.5 cm long, 2.5-3 cm wide, tapering at the base, petiolate; lamina deeply divided into three or five tapering lobes which are irregularly toothed near their apices and sometimes divided into smaller lobes; apices of the lobes acute or subobtuse; upper surface dark green and with occasional scattered hairs, especially along the margins, lower surface paler with patches of hairs in the axils of the veins.

Flowers Up to about 1.5 cm in diameter, in corymbs of up to twelve or more, pedicels and receptacles very hairy, sometimes distinctly woolly; sepals five, free, pale green, triangular and reflexed; petals five, free, white or brownish, broadly ovate; stamens about twenty with purple anthers; style, usually one.

Stems Up to about 2 mm in diameter, pale green or more frequently greyish-brown and woody, sometimes bearing thorns up to about 1 cm long.

Microscopical Description
Leaf Dorsiventral; cells of the upper epidermis polygonal, straight-walled with a striated cuticle, those of the lower epidermis more sinuous; anomocytic stomata on the lower epidermis only; covering trichomes on both epidermises but more numerous on the lower, long, tapering, unicellular or very occasionally uniseriate with two cells, walls moderately thickened; cluster crystals of calcium oxalate in the spongy mesophyll and sometimes in the palisade, also groups of small prism crystals along the veins.

Flower Epidermis of the pedicel and of the receptacle with abundant covering trichomes similar to those on the leaf but longer and more undulating; calyx with numerous anomocytic stomata on the outer epidermis, inner epidermis with a striated cuticle; epidermal cells of the corolla distinctly papillose; fibrous layer of the anther with characteristic thickenings; pollen grains spherical or ellipsoid, about 35 μm in diameter with three pores and a faintly granular exine.

Stem Epidermal cells with thickened outer and anticlinal walls replaced in older stems by several layers of brown cork cells; cortex parenchymatous with prisms and cluster crystals of calcium oxalate; dense groups of small, tightly-packed pericyclic fibres with much thickened and lignified walls; xylem completely lignified, composed of scattered vessels, thick-walled fibres and parenchyma separated by distinct medullary rays containing brown colouring matter; larger vessels with bordered pits, smaller elements with annular or spiral thickening; central pith parenchymatous and lignified, the cells with moderately thickened walls and numerous pits.

Odour and Taste
Odour leaf-like and not characteristic; taste somewhat bitter.

IDENTIFICATION

Carry out the method for Thin-layer Chromatography as described in Appendix 1, using Solvent System A.

Apply 20 μl of each of the following solutions separately to the plate: (1) extract 1 g powdered Hawthorn Flowering Top with 10 ml methanol by warming on a water-bath for 10-15 minutes, cool and filter; (2) 0.025% rutin in methanol.

Spray the plate with Spray Reagent A and examine in ultraviolet light 366 nm.

Major bands relative to rutin are as follows: turquoise 2.25, yellow 1.65*, turquoise 1.5*, yellow 1.0.

* These bands may coalesce in high concentration to give the appearance of a green band at their overlap.

QUANTITATIVE STANDARDS

Foreign Matter
Not more than 2%   Appendix 3

Total Ash
Not more than 10%   Appendix 4

MATERIAL OF COMMERCE Hawthorn Flowering Top is supplied in the whole or cut form. It is obtained from the UK and other European countries.

Powdered Hawthorn Flowering Top

Complies with the requirements for Identification and Quantitative Standards stated for Hawthorn Flowering Top.

Characteristic Features
Dull, greenish-brown with a leafy odour and a bitter and lingering taste; abundant long, unicellular and tapering covering trichomes, scattered and attached to epidermal fragments of the leaves, receptacles and pedicels; upper epidermis of the leaf with straight-walled cells and a striated cuticle, lower epidermis with sinuous walled cells and numerous anomocytic stomata; calcium oxalate cluster crystals in the mesophyll and small prism crystals along the veins; numerous spherical to ellipsoidal pollen grains with three pores; purple fragments of the fibrous layer of the anthers; corolla with papillose epidermis; occasional fragments of cork with associated cortical parenchyma containing prism and cluster crystals, also groups of fibres, vascular tissue and pitted and lignified parenchyma from the stems.

ACTION Cardiotonic.

HEARTSEASE   Violaceae

Violae tricoloris herba

Synonym: Wild Pansy.

Heartsease consists of the dried aerial parts of *Viola tricolor* L., harvested during the flowering period.

CHARACTERISTICS

Macroscopical Description
   Stems Pale green, glabrous, cylindrical, up to 5 mm wide, branching from the base.
   Leaves Alternate, stipulate, dark green; lamina 1.5-2.5 cm long and 1-2 cm wide, glabrous; lower leaves ovate, apex obtuse, upper leaves ovate-lanceolate, apex subacute; rounded base, crenate or crenate-dentate margin. Petiole up to 3 cm; stipules often palmately lobed.
   Flowers Solitary, 2-2.5 cm diameter; pedicel 2-8 cm long. five green, lanceolate sepals, acute apex, base extended to flat appendage; five ovate, blue-violet and/or yellow petals, overlapping at base, lower one spurred; stamens five, filaments short; ovary, globular with parietal placentation containing numerous light brown obovate seeds,

about 2 mm long.

Microscopical Description
   Stem Elongated epidermal cells with straight, slightly thickened anticlinal walls; cuticle strongly striated; infrequent parallel orientated stomata; covering trichomes, if present, unicellular with distinct cuticular striations; narrow cortex, collenchymatous near epidermis; stele, ring of collateral vascular bundles linked by areas of lignified, pitted parenchyma; parenchymatous pith. Cortical parenchyma may contain an occasional cluster crystal of calcium oxalate.
   Leaf Lamina, epidermal cells of both surfaces polygonal with sinuous anticlinal walls, more wavy on lower surface; stomata anisocytic, slightly more frequent on lower surface; cuticle striated, more prominently adjacent to stomata; over larger veins and margins, elongated, slightly thickened epidermal cells; frequent papillae or short, thickened, unicellular covering trichomes, up to 200 µm long, with distinct, cuticular striations; an occasional glandular trichome with multicellular, multiseriate stalk and head. Dorsiventral, two layers of palisade

cells; spongy mesophyll cells contain clusters of calcium oxalate, 30-35 μm in diameter, in groups of two to six. Midrib with collateral bundle containing narrow, 5 μm diameter, lignified, xylem conducting elements with spiral or annular thickening.

Flower Characteristics of sepal resemble those of leaf. Petal short, rectangular or elongated, outer epidermal cells with sinuous, occasionally beaded, anticlinal walls, cuticle striated; inner epidermal cells, polygonal, mainly papillose with faintly striated cuticle; unicellular covering trichomes, 350-500 μm in length with longitudinal, cuticular striations and acute apices or distinctive wavy walled upper areas, occur at base of petals and particularly within the spur. Stamen, lignified fibrous layer of anther wall; spherical or squarish pollen grains, with three to five pores, up to 65 μm in diameter, exine smooth or finely warty. Pedicel, rectangular, slightly beaded epidermal cells; cuticle smooth; frequent parallel orientated stomata.

Fruit Polygonal, yellow, collenchymatous epidermal cells with occasional anisocytic stomata; testa epidermis yellow, thin-walled, polygonal cells interspersed with two or three reticulate, slightly lignified cells; sclerenchyma layer composed of narrow, thick walled, lignified fibres accompanied by parenchyma layer, each cell containing a prism of calcium oxalate, 7-12 μm long.

Odour and Taste
Leafy odour; taste slightly bitter and astringent.

IDENTIFICATION

Carry out the method for Thin-layer Chromatography as described in Appendix 1 using Solvent System A.

Apply 20 μl of each of the following solutions separately to the plate: (1) extract 1 g powdered Heartsease with 10 ml methanol on a water-bath for 10-15 minutes, cool and filter; (2) 0.025% rutin in methanol.

Spray the plate with Spray Reagent A and examine in ultraviolet light 366 nm.

Major bands relative to rutin are approximately as follows: yellow 1.2, orange 1.0, yellow 0.9, yellow 0.85, yellow 0.7.

QUANTITATIVE STANDARDS

Foreign Matter
Not more than 2%   Appendix 3

Total Ash
Not more than 15%   Appendix 4

Ash Insoluble in Hydrochloric Acid
Not more than 2.5%   Appendix 5

Water-soluble Extractive
Not less than 20%   Appendix 7

MATERIAL OF COMMERCE Heartsease is supplied in cut or broken condition. It is obtained from European countries and is cultivated in the Netherlands and France.

Powdered Heartsease

Complies with the requirements for Identification and Quantitative Standards stated for Heartsease.

Characteristic Features
Light green powder with leafy odour and slightly bitter taste; fragments of leaf lamina with polygonal, wavy-walled cells accompanied by anisocytic stomata; cluster crystals of calcium oxalate, free and embedded in spongy mesophyll; unicellular trichomes with distinctive cuticular striations, free and attached to elongated and polygonal epidermal cells, some with striated cuticle; narrow, lignified xylem conducting elements with spiral, annular, reticulate and pitted thickening; pollen grains with smooth or finely warty exine; papillose, polygonal epidermal cells of corolla; polygonal and reticulate cells of testa epidermis; lignified sclerenchyma accompanied by prisms of calcium oxalate; lignified fibrous anther wall; an occasional distinctive floral covering trichome; small groups of square, lignified, pitted parenchyma.

ACTION Expectorant; dermatological agent.

Chamaelirii rhizoma

Synonyms: Chamaelirium, False Unicorn Root.

Helonias consists of the dried rhizomes and roots of *Chamaelirium luteum* (L.) A. Gray.

CHARACTERISTICS

Macroscopical Description
Rhizomes Vertical or oblique, occasionally slightly curved, sub-cylindrical and somewhat constricted at intervals, 3-5 cm long and up to 1 cm in diameter; externally greyish-brown to pale yellowish-brown; two or three circular stem scars, about 5-7 mm in diameter, along the length of the rhizome; numerous close annulations and either abundant, attached roots or small crater-like root scars; roots more numerous on one side of oblique rhizomes; remains of leaf bases enclosing a small bud at apex; fracture short and horny; smoothed transverse surface light yellow-brown, showing a central stele sharply demarcated from a wide cortex and three or four concentric rings of small vascular bundles.
Roots Numerous, 7-8 cm long and 1-2 mm in diameter, wiry and slightly curved; externally yellowish-orange to pale yellowish-brown and wrinkled; some without cortex, up to 0.5 mm in diameter and pale fawn.

Microscopical Description
Rhizome Outer epidermis sometimes present, more frequently replaced by colourless to pale brown, tangentially elongated, slightly thickened, lignified metaderm; cortex of fairly uniform, large, ovoid, thin-walled parenchymatous cells, many starch-free but containing bundles of calcium oxalate needle crystals 40-45 μm long, embedded in a water-soluble matrix; remainder containing simple, ovoid to spherical starch granules 7-8 μm in diameter; fine leaf traces of narrow, lignified, spirally and annularly thickened vessels occurring radially in varying degrees of obliqueness; outer region of stele with three or four rings of isolated collateral vascular hundles; xylem of very small vessels in a crescent-shaped mass almost enclosing the small phloem; parenchyma of stele densely filled with starch; a few cells containing bundles of calcium oxalate crystals.
Root Epidermis of thin-walled, pale brown cells, many with remains of root hairs attached; cortical parenchyma ovoid and thin-walled; stele enclosed by well-marked endodermis with cells thickened and lignified on inner and radial walls; passage cells absent; vascular tissue polyarch with up to six or eight xylem groups alternating with small phloem groups in a matrix of lignified fibrous cells.

Odour and Taste
Faint odour; slightly astringent taste at first, becoming soapy and intensely bitter and persistent.

IDENTIFICATION

Carry out the method for Thin-layer Chromatography as described in Appendix 1 using Solvent System B.

Apply 20 μl of each of the following solutions separately to the plate: (1) extract 1 g powdered Helonias with 10 ml methanol on a water-bath for 10-15 minutes, cool and filter; (2) 0.05% aescin in methanol.

Spray the plate with Spray Reagent C, heat at 105°C for 5-10 minutes then examine in daylight.

Major bands relative to aescin are approximately as follows: purple 1.4, greenish brown 1.15, purple 1.05, brownish green 0.65.

QUANTITATIVE STANDARDS

Foreign Matter
Not more than 2%   Appendix 3

Total Ash
Not more than 8%   Appendix 4

Ash Insoluble in Hydrochloric Acid
Not more than 3.5%   Appendix 5

Water-soluble Extractive
Not less than 10%   Appendix 7

MATERIAL OF COMMERCE Helonias is supplied in the whole or chopped condition.

It is obtained from North America.

Powdered Helonias

Complies with the requirements for Identification and Quantitative Standards stated for Helonias.

Characteristic Features
Fawn powder with a faint odour and a taste slightly astringent at first, becoming bitter and persistent; abundant, simple starch granules usually clumped together; frequent and often complete bundles of calcium oxalate needle crystals; pale yellow-brown, elongated ovoid, lignified metaderm cells; thick-walled, irregular-lumened, blunt ended, lignified root endodermal cells pitted vessels and moderately thickened tapering fibres.

ACTION Uterine tonic.

HOLY THISTLE   Compositae

Cnici benedicti herba

Synonym: Blessed Thistle.

Holy Thistle consists of the dried aerial parts of *Cnicus benedictus* L. collected when the plant is in flower.

CHARACTERISTICS

Macroscopical Description
Stems Larger stems hollow, irregularly angular, dark green with closely spaced, fine, reddish-brown longitudinal ribs; covered with numerous long, white hairs; younger stem similar but not hollow.

Leaves Dark green, thin and brittle alternate, oblong-lanceolate, deeply pinnately lobed, the lobes spreading or somewhat backwardly directed, bases of incisions rounded, apices terminating in a spine, margin spinous ciliate, apex sharply acute with prominent spine; lower leaves with acute base tapering on to a petiole, upper leaves more closely approximated, cordate at base, sessile to amplexicaul; veins fine, whitish and more prominent on the lower surface, both surfaces pubescent.

Flowers Solitary, terminal, yellow flower-head, capitulum about 3 cm high, 2 cm in diameter; involucre, almost spherical, of several ranks of imbricated, coriaceous bracts, pale green and lustrous on the inner surface, dull outer surface; outer bracts short, ovate with tapering spine; inner bracts longer and narrower, acuminate with an outwardly curving, divided spine; spines clothed with a cobweb-like mass of fine hairs; receptacle flat with numerous, shiny, filiform paleae; florets yellow, disc florets numerous, complete, pappus in three circles, brim with ten very short teeth, ten long outer and ten short inner bristles; corolla pentamerous, sympetalous, zygomorphic with one long, two medium and two short lobes, tube white, lobes yellow; five epipetalous, syngenesious stamens, anthers yellow with purple brown margin; ovary of two fused carpels, ribbed, containing a single ovule; single, shortly branched style with bifid stigma; marginal ray florets small, neuter, with three linear yellow lobes inserted on a rudimentary ovary.

Fruit A finely-ribbed, yellow-brown achene with a woody pappus longer than the achene.

Microscopical Description
Stem Epidermal cells cuboid with slightly thickened and convex outer wall; larger basal cells of trichomes at intervals; thin, finely-ridged cuticle; cortex of fairly large, thin-walled parenchyma within several layers of smaller collenchymatous cells; stele with ring of alternating larger and smaller vascular bundles separated by parenchymatous rays; xylem composed of vessels with spiral, annular and pitted thickening; larger bundles capped with moderately thickened, lignified, pericyclic fibres, groups of pericyclic fibres absent or much reduced outside the smaller bundles; in the inner cortex, outside the larger bundles, up to three or four tangentially arranged schizogenous glands having four or more lining cells and containing reddish-brown secretion; pith of parenchymatous cells, some

near the xylem being lignified .

Leaf Isobilateral, upper and lower palisade mesophyll each of two layers of cells; both epidermises similar, with thin, markedly sinuous, anticlinal walls and numerous anomocytic stomata; numerous trichomes of three main types all with thin, smooth, non-lignified walls - uniseriate and conical, up to twenty cells, uppermost cells may be flattened, 120 μm wide at base, up to 3 mm long, many terminating in fine, filamentous projections several millimetres long; capitate, uniseriate, six to ten cells long, apical cell enlarged to 30-60 μm in diameter and up to 300 μm long; glandular trichomes with short uni- or biseriate stalk and multistoried head of single tabular cells, of width greater than length, enclosed in a thin cuticular bladder.

Bract Inner layer of almost straight, moderately thick-walled, non-pitted, fibre-like cells, slightly lignified and with tapering ends; outer layer with wider cells, variable in size and shape, oblique or bluntly pointed, moderately thickened, lignified with few pits; small cuboid or hexagonal crystals present in some cells. Paleae composed of a small number of files of non-lignified, thin-walled, elongated fusiform cells, bluntly pointed at the apex.

Flower Pappus, spines dense and strongly lignified, the longer spines with thick-walled, conspicuously pitted, fibrous sclereids and having short, upwardly projecting teeth; short spines with similar sclereids but teeth absent, both with numerous club-shaped trichomes near the base. Inner and outer epidermises of corolla similar, composed of longitudinal rows of cells, straight-walled near the base becoming sinuous near the apex; along the margins some cells papillose; thin-walled glandular trichomes present. Pollen grains 40-45 μm in diameter, ovate to subspherical with exine closely and minutely spiny.

Odour and Taste
No odour; bitter and astringent taste.

IDENTIFICATION

Carry out the method for Thin-layer Chromatography as described in Appendix 1, using a mixture of chloroform : methanol (9:1) as the Solvent System.

Apply 20 μl of each of the following solutions separately to the plate: (1) extract 1 g powdered Holy Thistle with 10 ml methanol by refluxing on a water-bath for 10-15 minutes, cool, filter and concentrate to about 3 ml; (2) 0.025% methyl red in methanol.

Spray the plate with Spray Reagent C, heat at 105°C for 5-10 minutes then examine in daylight.

Major bands relative to methyl red are approximately as follows: purple 2.2, pink 1.75, purple 0.8, light green 0.75.

QUANTITATIVE STANDARDS

Foreign Matter
Not more than 3%   Appendix 3

Total Ash
Not more than 15%   Appendix 4

Ash Insoluble in Hydrochloric Acid
Not more than 3%   Appendix 5

Water-soluble Extractive
Not less than 20%   Appendix 7

MATERIAL OF COMMERCE Holy Thistle is supplied in the whole or broken condition. It is obtained from northern and eastern European countries.

Powdered Holy Thistle

Complies with the requirements for Identification and Quantitative Standards stated for Holy Thistle.

Characteristic Features
Dark green powder with no odour but a bitter and astringent taste; yellow pollen grains; thin-walled trichomes often with collapsed cells; fine, structureless, tangled filaments; leaf epidermis with numerous anomocytic stomata; narrow files, slightly twisted, of non-lignified cells of the paleae; narrow pitted vessels and relatively wide spirally and annularly thickened vessels; lignified, fibre-like cells from the bracts; parenchyma with separate, narrow, reddish-brown secretion ducts; sclerenchymatous cells from the pappus; fragments of spines, dense, often pigmented, some with terminal filaments.

ACTION Bitter.

HOPS

Cannabaceae

Lupuli strobilus

Synonyms: Humulus, Lupulus.

Hops consist of the dried strobiles of *Humulus lupulus* L.

CHARACTERISTICS

Macroscopical Description
Yellowish-green, ovoid, cone-like, compound fruits, 3-4 cm long, consisting chiefly of stipules and bracteoles enclosing a small achene. Stipules are flat, ovate and symmetrical, 10-20 mm long and 5-10 mm wide; bracteoles ovate and markedly asymmetrical, 15-30 mm long and 7-10 mm wide, folded along one margin with the fruit at the base of the fold; bracteoles and fruit covered with minute, glistening, yellow glands.

Microscopical Description
Epidermal cells of stipules and bracteoles irregularly polygonal with sinuous anticlinal walls, usually thin, occasionally slightly beaded and thickened; rare anomocytic stomata and cicatrices; mesophyll seen in sectional view shows small cluster crystals of calcium oxalate; glandular trichomes having a two-celled stalk and a spherical glandular head of eight cells; numerous large yellow glands, 100-250 µm in diameter, each consisting of thin-walled cells with a dome-shaped cuticle, circular in surface view and cup shaped in side view, attached to the stipule or bracteole by a short two-celled stalk. Epicarp of fruit consists of sclerenchymatous cells, irregularly elongated, pale brown with thick walls showing numerous small pits and striations.

Odour and Taste
Freshly dried material has a slight, characteristic odour which becomes more pronounced with age; slight but characteristically bitter taste.

IDENTIFICATION

Carry out the method for Thin-layer Chromatography as described in Appendix 1, using Solvent System A.
Apply 20 µl of each of the following solutions separately to the plate: (1) extract 1 g powdered Hops with 10 ml methanol on a water-bath for 5 minutes, cool and filter; (2) 0.025% rutin in methanol.
Spray the plate with Spray Reagent A and examine in ultraviolet light 366 nm.
Major bands relative to rutin are approximately as follows: yellowish-green 1.56, orange 1.4, blue 1.3, dull orange 0.96, blue 0.88.

QUANTITATIVE STANDARDS

Foreign Matter
Not more than 2%   Appendix 3

Total Ash
Not more than 10%   Appendix 4

Ash Insoluble in Hydrochloric Acid
Not more than 3%   Appendix 5

Water-soluble Extractive
Not less than 18%   Appendix 7

MATERIAL OF COMMERCE Hops are supplied as whole or crushed strobiles. The cultivars commonly available are North Downs, Challenger and Fuggles. They are cultivated in the British Isles and in western Europe.

Powdered Hops

Complies with the requirements for Identification and Quantitative Standards stated for Hops.

Characteristic Features
Buff-coloured powder with a characteristic odour and a slightly bitter taste; numerous large, yellow glands free and attached to epidermal cells of stipules and bracteoles; irregularly polygonal cells of epidermises of stipules and bracteoles, glandular trichomes with spherical head of eight cells on two-celled stalk; sclerenchymatous cells of epicarp.

ACTION Sedative; bitter.

HORSE-CHESTNUT SEED   Hippocastanaceae

Hippocastani semen

Horse-chestnut Seed consists of the dried seeds of *Aesculus hippocastanum* L.

CHARACTERISTICS

Macroscopical Description
Dense, hard seeds, up to 2.5-3 cm, irregularly ovoid or subspherical, a few somewhat hemispherical, with an almost plane facet; surface smooth, dark, marbled reddish-brown, a little uneven and with dull lustre; large, nearly circular, rough, greyish-brown scar of hilum; larger seeds show a narrowish V-shaped ridge, marking the position of the radicle of the embryo, extending approximately one fifth of the circumference, the point terminating near a minute perforation in the testa close to the hilum. In section, testa 1-1.5 mm, dark brown, hard and brittle, closely surrounding the embryo of two large, horny, off-white cotyledons and radicle; endosperm absent.

Microscopical Description
Testa epidermis in surface view, yellowish-brown cells of fairly uniform size, majority rounded to polygonal, a few squarish to obscurely triangular; walls considerably, but rather unevenly, thickened; pits absent. In sectional view the cells are columnar, approximately three to four times as high as wide, outer periclinal wall markedly thickened, anticlinal walls less thickened, uneven, becoming thinner towards the base; beneath the epidermis a few layers of small, rounded, collenchymatously thickened cells with small intercellular spaces; the greater part of the testa is of larger, loosely-packed parenchymatous cells forming a spongy tissue; the walls are variably and unevenly thickened, intercellular and large circular spaces are well-marked; inner testa, a narrow zone, ill-defined, thinner-walled cells. All the parenchymatous cells of the testa are darkly pigmented. Embryo, an outer layer of small colourless cells, almost square in sectional view, outer and side walls thickened; in surface view only the irregular, more or less polygonal, lumens are discernible, giving a reticulate pitted appearance.

Cotyledons of moderately-thickened, indistinctly-pitted, round to ovoid, parenchymatous cells, densely filled with starch; granules mainly simple, two size ranges; 15-35 μm most numerous, varying from almost circular, ovoid, bluntly polygonal to pyriform, majority with well-marked cleft or stellate hilum, striations absent; 3-10 μm, less variable, spherical to ovoid, hilum more often a point; very infrequent compound granules of two, three or four small components, occasionally of one larger and one or two small components.

Odour and Taste
Odourless; the taste is somewhat mealy and disagreeably bitter and lingering.

IDENTIFICATION

Carry out the method for Thin-layer Chromatography as described in Appendix 1, using Solvent System B and allowing the solvent to ascend 13.5 cm.

Apply 40 μl of the following solutions to the plate: (1) extract 2 g powdered Horse-chestnut Seed by heating under reflux with 10 ml ethanol (70%) for 10 minutes, cool and filter. Evaporate the clear filtrate to approximately 5 ml; (2) 0.1% aescin in methanol.

Spray the plate with Spray Reagent D, heat at 105°C for 10 minutes and examine in daylight.

Major bands relative to aescin are approximately as follows: purple 1.0, brown 0.4, brown 0.2, brown 0.1.

There is an area of light purple fine detail from approximately 1.7 to 1.2.

QUANTITATIVE STANDARDS

Total Ash
Not more than 5%   Appendix 4

Ash Insoluble in Hydrochloric Acid
Not more than 1%   Appendix 5

Water-soluble Extractive
Not less than 20%   Appendix 7

MATERIAL OF COMMERCE Horse-chestnut Seed is supplied in whole, sliced or powdered form. It is obtained from many temperate countries and particularly from eastern Europe.

Powdered Horse-chestnut Seed

Complies with the requirements of Identification and Quantitative Standards for Horse-chestnut Seed.

ACTION Venoactive.

HYDRANGEA
Hydrangeae arborescentis radix

Hydrangeaceae

Synonyms: Wild Hydrangea, Seven Barks.

Hydrangea consists of the dried rhizomes, with or without roots, of *Hydrangea arborescens* L.

CHARACTERISTICS

Macroscopical Description
Pieces of cylindrical rhizome up to about 8 mm in diameter, the thicker pieces frequently split longitudinally; outer surface yellowish to greyish brown, sometimes pinkish, with distinct longitudinal ridges and occasional elliptical lenticels; bark readily removed, exposing the yellowish-white to buff wood; fracture tough and splintery, the transversely-cut surface showing a narrow bark, a wide area of dense yellowish-white, finely radiate wood, and a small, reddish-brown central pith. A few thin, wiry roots may be present.

Microscopical Description
Cork composed of several layers of yellowish-brown, radially compressed cells, thin-walled and polygonal in surface view; phelloderm and secondary phloem mostly parenchymatous, composed of large, thin-walled cells, some developed as idioblasts, densely filled with bundles of needle crystals of calcium oxalate, the remainder containing starch granules; scattered stone cells, singly or in groups of two or three, in the secondary phloem, the individual cells rectangular, varying in size and frequently much elongated longitudinally, with heavily thickened and pitted walls; secondary xylem completely lignified with narrow strands of vascular tissue separated by med-ullary rays one to three cells wide; vessels isolated and with distinct scalariform thickening, accompanied by tracheids with bordered pits and abundant thick-walled and pitted parenchyma; pith lignified and composed of small, rectangular cells with thickened and pitted walls.

Odour and Taste
No odour; taste slightly sweet, then acrid.

IDENTIFICATION

Carry out the method for Thin-layer Chromatography as described in Appendix 1, using Solvent System A.

Apply 20 µl of each of the following solutions separately to the plate: (1) extract 1g powdered Hydrangea Root with 10 ml methanol on a water-bath for 10-15 minutes, cool, filter and concentrate to approximately 2 ml; (2) 0.025% rutin in methanol.

Spray the plate with Spray Reagent A and examine in ultraviolet light 366 nm.

Major bands relative to rutin are approximately as follows: turquoise 2.1, turquoise 2.0, turquoise 1.4, turquoise 0.9.

The chromatogram exhibits turquoise and blue fine detail, but the above constitute the most prominent bands.

QUANTITATIVE STANDARDS

Foreign Matter
Not more than 2%   Appendix 3

Total Ash
Not more than 6%   Appendix 4

Ash Insoluble in Hydrochloric Acid
Not more than 2%   Appendix 5

Water-soluble Extractive
Not less than 10%   Appendix 7

MATERIAL OF COMMERCE Hydrangea is supplied as broken or chopped pieces. It is obtained from the USA.

Powdered Hydrangea

Complies with the requirements for Identification and Quantitative Standards stated for Hydrangea.

Characteristic Features
A sandy to buff-coloured powder with a slight odour and a taste sweetish at first, then acrid; starch granules, variable in size and shape, but the majority rounded to ovoid and up to about 15 μm in diameter, mostly simple, sometimes with two or three components, the larger granules occasionally showing a prominent hilum as a central cleft; fragments of lignified xylem tissue composed of vessels with scalariform thickening; bordered-pitted tracheids and thick-walled parenchyma, crossed by pitted parenchyma of the medullary rays; thin-walled parenchymatous cells, some containing bundles of calcium oxalate needle crystals which also occur broken and scattered; large, elongated rectangular stone cells with thick walls and large, conspicuous pits; groups of small, rectangular and pitted cells of the pith; occasional brown fragments of cork.

ACTION Diuretic.

HYOSCYAMUS LEAF   Solanaceae

Hyoscyami folium

Synonym: Henbane.

Hyoscyamus Leaf consists of the dried leaf or the dried leaf and flowering, and occasionally fruit-bearing, tops of *Hyoscyamus niger* L.

This material complies with the requirements of the European Pharmacopoeia for Hyoscyamus Leaf and the British Pharmacopoeia for Hyoscyamus Leaf, or, when the material is in powder, Powdered Hyoscyamus Leaf.

MATERIAL OF COMMERCE Hyoscyamus Leaf is supplied in the whole or broken condition. It is obtained principally from the countries of eastern Europe.

ACTION Antispasmodic.

HYSSOP

Hyssopi herba

Hyssop consists of the dried leaves and flowering tops of *Hyssopus officinalis* L.

CHARACTERISTICS

Macroscopical Description

Stems Quadrangular, branched, about 1.5 mm wide bearing numerous pairs of opposite leaves, pale green or brownish and covered with downy hairs, particularly between the longitudinal ridges.

Leaves Linear to oblong, lanceolate, up to 2.5 cm long and 5-8 mm wide, sessile with an entire margin, subacute apex and tapering base; upper surface dark green with scattered hairs, lower surface paler and more pubescent, especially along the margins and the conspicuously raised midrib; both surfaces markedly punctuate.

Flowers In one-sided whorls in the axils of the leaves and as a dense terminal inflorescence up to about 10 cm long; calyx pinkish-brown, tubular, 4-5 mm long, finely pubescent with fifteen longitudinal ribs and five lobes, each terminating in a sharply pointed tooth; corolla dark blue-violet, 10-12 mm long, with two lips.

Microscopical Description

Stem Epidermal cells thin-walled and polygonal in surface view, with occasional diacytic stomata and abundant covering and glandular trichomes; covering trichomes short, conical, mostly unicellular but occasionally uniseriate with two or three cells, walls thickened and conspicuously warted; glandular trichomes of two types, multicellular and capitate, the multicellular type large with a unicellular stalk and a head composed of eight radiating cells with the common cuticle raised to form a bladder, the capitate type smaller with a unicellular stalk and a spherical or ovoid head composed of one or two cells; cortex narrow, mostly parenchymatous with collenchyma in the ridges; small groups of pericyclic fibres with moderately thickened walls; phloem and xylem a complete cylinder surrounding the parenchymatous pith, with a central hollow; xylem lignified with fibres and small spirally or annularly thickened vessels.

Leaf Dorsiventral with a palisade composed of two layers of fairly large, loosely packed cells; epidermal cells sinuous to wavy walled in surface view with abundant diacytic stomata on both surfaces; hesperidin, in the form of sphaerocrystalline masses of fine, radiating crystals in the cells of both epidermises but especially in those of the upper; glandular trichomes of both multicellular and capitate types very abundant; scattered unicellular, warty, covering trichomes, more numerous on the lower epidermis.

Flower Calyx outer epidermis with infrequent stomata and numerous warty covering trichomes, many composed of two or three cells, and scattered multicellular and capitate glandular trichomes; cells of the inner epidermis with very sinuous walls showing thickening at the angles; corolla with purple-violet pigment and, on the outer epidermis, uniseriate covering trichomes composed of two or three cells with thin, smooth walls and glandular trichomes with a two or three-celled, uniseriate stalk and a unicellular, ovoid head; cells of the inner epidermis papillose; pollen grains spherical, about 35 μm in diameter with six pores and furrows and a finely pitted exine.

Odour and Taste

Odour very strong and aromatic; taste aromatic, camphoraceous and bitter.

IDENTIFICATION

Carry out the method for Thin-layer Chromatography as described in Appendix 1, using Solvent System C.

Apply 60 μl of each of the following solutions to the plate: (1) extract 1 g powdered Hyssop by shaking with 10 ml of dichloromethane for 20 minutes. Filter, evaporate the filtrate just to dryness and dissolve the residue in 1 ml toluene; (2) 0.1% cineole in toluene.

Spray the plate with Spray Reagent D, heat at 105°C for 10-15 minutes and examine in daylight.

Major bands relative to cineole are approximately as follows: purple 2.05, red/brown 1.7, pink 1.1, green 0.85, brown 0.7, green 0.55.

QUANTITATIVE STANDARDS

Foreign Matter
Not more than 2%   Appendix 3

Total Ash
Not more than 10%   Appendix 4

Ash Insoluble in Hydrochloric Acid
Not more than 2.5%   Appendix 5

Water-soluble Extractive
Not less than 10%   Appendix 7

MATERIAL OF COMMERCE Hyssop is usually supplied as the cut herb. It is obtained from European countries, particularly France, Hungary and the Netherlands.

Powdered Hyssop

Complies with the requirements for Identification and Quantitative Standards stated for Hyssop.

ACTION Expectorant.

ICELAND MOSS   Parmeliaceae
Lichen islandicus

Synonym: Cetraria.

Iceland Moss consists of the dried thalli of *Cetraria islandica* L. Ach. sensu latiore.

CHARACTERISTICS

Macroscopical Description
Pieces of foliaceous lichen about 6-12 cm long, composed of numerous erect branches about 6 mm or more broad, in an unevenly developed dichotomy; branches flat or curled, thin, about 0.5 mm thick, the margins fringed with minute, brownish projections, each with a slightly swollen, rounded apex; upper surface dark greenish-brown, smooth; lower surface pale greyish, with scattered small, white, ovoid, depressed spots; occasional, dark reddish-brown, cup-shaped, fruiting bodies (apothecia), about 6 mm in diameter, on the upper surface near the margins; texture harsh, springy and brittle.

Microscopical Description
Cut transversely, branches show upper and lower colourless cortical regions composed of closely-packed hyphae, appearing as small-celled pseudoparenchyma; below the upper cortex, the algal or gonidial layer containing numerous yellowish-green, subspherical cells of the alga *Chlorococcum*

humicola; a central medulla with more loosely-packed, greyish-brown hyphae filaments. Sections through an apothecium showing an hymenium layer in the upper cortex with flask-shaped asci, each containing eight ascospores, separated by numerous, narrow, thread-like paraphyses.

Odour and Taste
Odourless; taste mucilaginous and distinctly bitter.

IDENTIFICATION

Thin-layer Chromatographic analysis is unsuitable for this material. Macroscopic and microscopic examination should be relied upon for identification together with the following test.
Boil 1 g of powdered Iceland Moss with 10 ml of water for 3 minutes. On cooling a jelly is produced which gives a blue colour with Iodine Solution (distinction from Irish Moss).

QUANTITATIVE STANDARDS

Foreign Matter
Not more than 5%   Appendix 3

Total Ash
Not more than 3%   Appendix 4

111

Ash Insoluble in Hydrochloric Acid
Not more than 1.5%   Appendix 5

MATERIAL OF COMMERCE Iceland Moss is supplied as pieces of lichen "branches". It is collected from the wild in subarctic or mountainous regions of Europe and obtained mainly from Scandinavian and Balkan countries, Russia and also Canada.

Powdered Iceland Moss

Complies with the requirements for Quantitative Standards stated for Iceland Moss.

Characteristic Features
A greyish-brown powder, odourless, with a mucilaginous and bitter taste; abundant fragments of pseudoparenchyma, some containing ovoid, yellowish-green algal cells about 15 μm long; groups of colourless or pale brown, intertwining, branched hyphae. Many of the particles stain blue-black with iodine water.

ACTION Demulcent.

IPECACUANHA   Rubiaceae

Ipecacuanhae radix

Synonyms: Matto Grosso, Ipecacuanha (*Cephaelis ipecacuanha*); Costa Rica Ipecacuanha (*C. acuminata*).

Ipecacuanha consists of the fragmented and dried underground organs of *Cephaelis ipecacuanha* (Brot.) A. Rich. or of *Cephaelis acuminata* Karsten or of a mixture of both species.

This material complies with the requirements

of the European Pharmacopoeia for Ipecacuanha Root and the British Pharmacopoeia for Ipecacuanha or, when the material is in powder, Powdered Ipecacuanha.

MATERIAL OF COMMERCE Ipecacuanha is supplied as slender, tortuous pieces or in the broken condition. It is obtained from Brazil, Colombia and Central America.

ACTION Expectorant; emetic.

IRISH MOSS   Gigartinaceae

Chondri thallus

Synonym: Chondrus, Carrageen.

Irish Moss consists of the dried, partially bleached, red algae *Chondrus crispus* (L.) Stackh. alone or mixed with *Gigartina mamillosa* (Gooden. et Woodw.) J. Agardh [*G. stellata* (Stackh.) Batt.].

CHARACTERISTICS

Macroscopical Description
Thallus is light yellowish-brown, opaque, occurring in crisp and springy masses. Indi-

vidual thallus 5-30 cm long; subcylindrical stalk with flattened, dichotomous branches which terminate in a rounded emarginate or deeply forked apex. Surface exhibits ovoid perforations or intact rounded or papillae-like fruiting bodies (cystocarps).

Microscopical Description
Transverse section of thallus surrounded by thick, outer layer with positive reaction to ruthenium red; cortex consists of several outer rows of small, thick-walled cells with slight radial elongation and yellowish-green cell content and inner more-rounded cells;

medulla cells, thick-walled mucilaginous aerenchyma with occasional cystocarps, about 20 μm, containing rounded bodies with granular surface, giving blue-violet reaction with 0.01M Iodine Solution.

Odour and Taste
Odour slight, of seaweed; taste mucilaginous and saline.

IDENTIFICATION

Thin-layer Chromatographic analysis is unsuitable for this material. Macroscopic and microscopic examination should be relied upon for identification, together with the following test.
Boil 1 g of powdered Irish Moss with 10 ml of water for 3 minutes. On cooling a jelly is produced which gives no blue colour with Iodine Solution (distinction from Iceland Moss).

QUANTITATIVE STANDARDS

Foreign Matter
Not more than 2%   Appendix 3

Total Ash
Not more than 16%   Appendix 4

Ash Insoluble in Hydrochloric Acid
Not more than 5%   Appendix 5

MATERIAL OF COMMERCE Irish Moss is supplied as whole or cut pieces. It is obtained from North Atlantic shores of Europe and North America.

Powdered Irish Moss

Complies with the requirements for Quantitative Standards stated for Irish Moss.

Characteristic Features
Light reddish-brown/yellow powder with mucilaginous saline taste; fragments of thallus, some distinctly pink-mauve in chloral hydrate; groups of small, thick-walled cells with yellowish-green contents; fragments of thick-walled aerenchyma; isolated sporangia or spores turning blue-violet in 0.01M iodine solution.

ACTION Demulcent.

ISPAGHULA HUSK   Plantaginaceae

Plantaginis ovatae testa

Ispaghula Husk consists of the epidermis and the collapsed adjacent layers removed from the dried ripe seeds of *Plantago ovata* Forssk.

This material complies with the requirements of the British Pharmacopoeia for Ispaghula Husk.

MATERIAL OF COMMERCE Ispaghula Husk is supplied as pale buff, brittle flakes. It is obtained from India, Pakistan and Iran.

ACTION Bulk-forming laxative.

ISPAGHULA SEED

Plantaginaceae

Plantaginis ovatae semen

Synonyms: Blond or Pale Psyllium Seed, Indian Plantago Seed.

Ispaghula Seed consists of the dried, ripe seeds of *Plantago ovata* Forssk. [*P. ispaghula* Roxb.].

CHARACTERISTICS

Macroscopical Description
Seeds boat-shaped, 1.5-3.5 mm long and 1-1.5 mm wide, colour variable, but usually pale, greyish-brown with a pinkish tinge, dull and hard; on the convex surface a central, glossy reddish-brown, elongated oval spot; the concave surface deeply grooved with the hilum a brown spot in the centre of the hollow, more or less covered with a whitish membrane. Transversely-cut surface showing a narrow testa and a wide area of endosperm surrounding the embryo situated near the convex surface, the two large cotyledons with their flattened, contiguous upper surfaces lying in the median plane. The mucilaginous epidermis swells in water, forming a thick, translucent and colourless envelope surrounding each seed.

Microscopical Description
Epidermal cells of the testa large, polyhedral, thin-walled and filled with mucilage which swells in contact with water, rupturing the outer and radial walls; the mucilage stains with Ruthenium Red; occasional small starch granules, simple or compound with four or more components, embedded in the mucilage; inner pigment layer of testa usually composed of thick-walled palisade cells, inner cells irregularly polygonal and thick-walled with numerous large, very conspicuous rounded pits; embryo cells small and thin-walled, those of the cotyledons rounded and surrounding three strands of the vascular tissue running longitudinally, those of the tips of the radicle more regularly arranged and uniform; the cells of both the endosperm and embryo containing fixed oil and aleurone grains.

Odour and Taste
Odour slight; taste bland and very mucilaginous.

IDENTIFICATION

Carry out the method for Thin-layer Chromatography as described in Appendix 1 using Solvent System C.

Apply 60 µl of each of the following solutions to the plate: (1) extract 1 g crushed Ispaghula Seed by shaking with 10 ml dichloromethane for 20 minutes. Filter, evaporate the filtrate just to dryness and dissolve the residue in 1 ml toluene; (2) 0.1% cineole in toluene.

Spray the plate with Spray Reagent D, heat at 105°C for 10-15 minutes and examine in daylight.

Major bands relative to cineole are approximately as follows: red/violet 2.0, red 1.6, yellow 1.35, red/brown 0.4.

Note: The macroscopical description should be used to differentiate between Ispaghula Seed (Blond Psyllium Seed) and Psyllium Seed (Dark Psyllium Seed).

QUANTITATIVE STANDARDS

Foreign Matter
Not more than 3%   Appendix 3

Total Ash
Not more than 6%   Appendix 4

Ash Insoluble in Hydrochloric Acid
Not more than 2%   Appendix 5

MATERIAL OF COMMERCE Ispaghula Seed is supplied as whole seeds. It is obtained from the Indian subcontinent.

Powdered Ispaghula Seed

Powdered Ispaghula Seed complies with the requirements for Identification and Quantitative Standards stated for Ispaghula Seed.

ACTION Bulk-forming laxative.

JAMAICA DOGWOOD Leguminosae-Papilionoideae

Piscidiae radicis cortex

Synonym: Piscidia.

Jamaica Dogwood is the dried root-bark of *Piscidia piscipula* (L.) Sarg. [*Piscidia erythrina* L.].

CHARACTERISTICS

Macroscopical Description
Curved or channelled pieces, 5-10 cm long, 2-6 cm wide and up to 0.5 cm thick; outer surface reddish-orange to greyish-brown where cork is exfoliated; longitudinally ridged and furrowed; inner surface paler and longitudinally striated; fracture tough and fibrous.

Microscopical Description
Narrow reddish-brown cork composed of thin-walled tabular cells; wide, reddish-brown phloem containing groups of long, narrow, lignified fibres surrounded by a crystal sheath of prismatic crystals of calcium oxalate; groups of thick-walled, ovoid sclereids also present; phloem parenchymatous cells with thick, pitted walls and containing small, simple or 2-4 compound spherical starch granules; medullary rays 1-3 cells wide.

Odour and Taste
Faint odour; bitter and acrid taste.

IDENTIFICATION

Carry out the method for Thin-layer Chromatography as described in Appendix 1, using Solvent System A.

Apply 20 µl of each of the following solutions separately to the plate: (1) extract 1 g powdered Jamaica Dogwood with 10 ml 60% methanol on a water-bath for 10-15 minutes, cool and filter; (2) 0.025% rutin in methanol.

Spray the plate with Spray Reagent A and examine in ultraviolet light 366 nm.

Major bands relative to rutin are approximately as follows: blue 2.4, blue 1.95, green 1.55, blue 1.4.

QUANTITATIVE STANDARDS

Foreign Matter
Not more than 2%   Appendix 3

Total Ash
Not more than 14%   Appendix 4

Ash Insoluble in Hydrochloric Acid
Not more than 2%   Appendix 5

Water-soluble Extractive
Not less than 15%   Appendix 7

MATERIAL OF COMMERCE Jamaica Dogwood is supplied as curved or channelled pieces or in the broken or chopped condition. It is obtained from Central America and the West Indies.

Powdered Jamaica Dogwood

Complies with the requirements for Identification and Quantitative Standards stated for Jamaica Dogwood.

Characteristic Features
Reddish-brown powder with a faint odour and a bitter, acrid taste; narrow lignified phloem fibres with crystal sheath containing prismatic crystals of calcium oxalate; thick-walled ovoid sclereids; small starch granules.

ACTION Analgesic.

JAVA TEA

Labiatae

Orthosiphonis folium

Synonym: Orthosiphon.

Java Tea consists of the dried leaves and stem tips of *Orthosiphon aristatus* (Blume) Miq. [*O. stamineus* Benth.; *O. spicatus* (Thunb.) Backer, Bakh. f. et Steenis] harvested shortly before the flowering period.

CHARACTERISTICS

Macroscopical Description

Leaves Lanceolate to ovate, about 2-6 cm long, apex acuminate, cuneate at the base with a short petiole; margin coarsely dentate, venation pinnate and often purplish, especially on the lower surface; upper surface usually dark greyish or yellowish-green, lower surface paler; some leaves much darker with a distinctly purplish tint; both surfaces markedly punctate and with occasional whitish hairs, particularly along the veins on the lower surface.

Stems Up to about 2 mm thick, four-angled with a deep longitudinal groove down two opposite sides; dark purplish-brown, surface smooth or finely ridged longitudinally with scattered hairs along the margins of the grooves; fracture fibrous, inner surface pale brown or cream.

Microscopical Description

Leaf Dorsiventral, the palisade cells small and densely packed; epidermal cells wavy-walled in surface view with slight beading at the angles; diacytic stomata, more numerous on the lower surface; both surfaces with abundant large glandular trichomes of the labiate-type with a unicellular stalk and a radiate head composed of four cells containing brown secretion; occasional, conical, covering trichomes, uniseriate, multicellular, with up to four or more cells, but usually two or three, broad at the base and tapering rapidly to the tip, with thin, distinctly warty walls and reddish contents.

Stem Epidermal cells polygonal to elongated in surface view with scattered stomata and glandular and covering trichomes similar to those of the leaf; underlying groups of collenchyma in the ridges, remainder of cortex narrow and parenchymatous with brownish walls; endodermis distinct; dense groups of narrow pericyclic fibres with moderately thickened and lignified walls; phloem narrow and thin-walled; xylem completely lignified and composed of vessels, singly or in small groups, in radial rows and associated with fibres and xylem parenchyma, separated by narrow medullary rays; larger vessels reticulately thickened, smaller with spiral or annular thickening; small central pith of thin-walled cells with brown walls.

Odour and Taste

Odour slightly aromatic; taste aromatic, somewhat bitter and salty, later astringent.

IDENTIFICATION

Carry out the method for Thin-layer Chromatography as described in Appendix 1, using a mixture of chloroform:ethyl acetate (60:40) as the solvent system.

Apply 40 µl of the following solution to the plate: extract 1 g powdered Java Tea with 10 ml dichloromethane by shaking for 15 minutes, filter.

Examine the plate in ultraviolet light 366 nm.

Major bands relative to the solvent front are approximately as follows: red 0.85, red 0.8, light blue 0.4, light blue 0.35, light blue 0.2, red 0.15, red 0.05.

The prominent light blue bands in the Rf range 0.4-0.2 are indicative of the flavone aglycones present in this plant. In this system strong fluctuations in Rf value are observed with differing levels of chamber saturation.

QUANTITATIVE STANDARDS

Foreign Matter
Not more than 2%   Appendix 3

Total Ash
Not more than 12%   Appendix 4

MATERIAL OF COMMERCE Java Tea is supplied in the whole or broken condition. It is obtained mainly from Indonesia.

Powdered Java Tea

Complies with the requirements for Identifi-

cation and Quantitative Standards stated for Java Tea.

ACTION Diuretic.

JUNIPER BERRY

Juniperi fructus

Juniper Berry consists of the dried, ripe fruits (female cones) of *Juniperus communis* L., collected in the second year of growth.

CHARACTERISTICS

Macroscopical Description
Purplish-black or red purple, subspherical fruits, 5-9 mm in diameter, glabrous with greyish-white bloom; apex with three-radiate furrow, base with remains of pale brown bracts. Transversely cut fruits exhibit yellowish-green, fleshy interior with large oil cavities and three embedded hard, brown, triangular-ovate seeds.

Microscopical Description
Fruit wall Cells of outer epidermis are polygonal with straight, thickened, anticlinal walls and brown amorphous contents. Fruit pulp consists of two to three rows of hypodermal collenchyma and a large area of parenchyma, some cells containing a few oval starch grains, interspersed with numerous airspaces; fibrovascular bundles some with associated rectangular, pitted sclereids; large, isolated, yellow ovoid or rectangular, slightly lignified, pitted iodioblasts up to 300 µm in length and large schizogenous oil glands are embedded in the parenchymatous area. Inner epidermis of polygonal collenchyma, some walls may be beaded.
Seed Testa composed of two to ten rows of thick-walled, irregularly elongated and rectangular, pitted sclereids about 75-90 µm long; perisperm layer of yellow, elongated cells with slightly thickened, sometimes with sinuous or beaded, anticlinal walls; thin-walled cells of endosperm and embryo contain numerous spherical aleurone grains and globules of fixed oil.

Odour and Taste
Aromatic and terebinthinate odour; taste sweet and slightly resinous.

IDENTIFICATION

Carry out the method for Thin-layer Chromatography as described in Appendix 1 using Solvent System C.

Apply 60 µl of each of the following solutions separately to the plate: (1) extract 1 g of powdered Juniper Berry by shaking with 10 ml dichloromethane for 20 minutes. Filter, evaporate the filtrate just to dryness and dissolve the residue in 1 ml toluene; (2) 0.1% cineole in toluene.

Spray the plate with Spray Reagent D, heat for 10-15 minutes at 105°C and examine in daylight.

Major bands relative to cineole are approximately as follows: purple 2.0, red 1.75, brown 1.4, pink 1.2, pink 0.5.

Extraction using dichloromethane, as specified above, removes fixed oils from Juniper Berry, which will appear on the chromatogram as a large elongated purple band extending from the start to approximately Rf 0.4. This band may obscure bands corresponding to components of the essential oil. If, instead, the essential oil is extracted by steam distillation and 40 µl of a 10% solution in toluene is applied to the plate, the elongated band is eliminated.

In this case, the following additional bands relative to cineole are approximately as follows: blue 1.0, purple/red 0.8.

QUANTITATIVE STANDARDS

Foreign Matter
Not more than 2%   Appendix 3

Total Ash
Not more than 5%   Appendix 4

Ash Insoluble in Hydrochloric Acid
Not more than 0.5% Appendix 5

Water-soluble Extractive
Not less than 30% Appendix 7

MATERIAL OF COMMERCE Juniper Berry is supplied as whole globular fruits. They are obtained from European countries, especially Italy, Hungary, Rumania, Albania and former Yugoslavia.

Powdered Juniper Berry

Complies with the requirements for Identification and Quantitative Standards stated for Juniper Berry.

Characteristic Features
Dark brown, fragments adhesive when freshly powdered; aromatic terebinthinate odour and sweet resinous taste; numerous globules of fixed and volatile oil in undefatted powder; fragments of thick-walled cells containing brown pigment; abundant parenchyma with numerous intercellular airspaces; narrow, lignified vessels with annular or reticulate thickening accompanied by isolated, thick-walled, lignified fibres with blunt apices; large, yellow, oval or rectangular, slightly lignified and pitted iodioblasts; embedded circular and fragmented schizogenous oil cells; groups of thick-walled, rectangular sclereids containing prisms of calcium oxalate; thin-walled cells containing numerous spherical aleurone grains.

ACTION Diuretic.

KAVA-KAVA
Piperaceae

Piperis methystici rhizoma

Synonyms: Kava, Kawa.

Kava-Kava consists of the rhizome, usually free from roots and sometimes scraped, of *Piper methysticum* G. Forst., cut into pieces and dried.

CHARACTERISTICS

Macroscopical Description
Irregular, cubical or wedge-shaped pieces or transverse slices of rhizome about 1-5 cm thick, but varying considerably in size and shape; outer surface dark greyish-brown, very unevenly wrinkled with occasional, large, whitish, circular root scars; inner surface pale yellowish or greyish-brown, fracture coarsely fibrous and starchy; transverse surface showing a thin cork, narrow bark and a wide, distinctly radiate xylem surrounding a large, sunken pith; pieces cut longitudinally, showing numerous fibrous strands in the xylem. Roots, when present, dark brown, thin and fibrous.

Microscopical Description
Cork composed of thin-walled cells, polygonal in surface view; underlying phelloderm and cortex parenchymatous, endodermis distinct; secondary phloem narrow, with wide medullary rays separating areas of crushed sieve tissue; secondary xylem distinctly radiate with strands of lignified vascular tissue, alternating with wide medullary rays; vascular groups composed of large vessels with reticulate thickening, abundant parenchymatous cells with moderately thickened walls and numerous pits, and groups of thicker-walled fibres with bluntly tapering ends; pith parenchymatous; some of the parenchymatous cells of the cortex, medullary rays and pith containing dense masses of reddish-brown oleo-resin, the remainder filled with starch granules, simple or two or three compound; individual granules spherical or slightly ovoid, up to about 25 µm in diameter, with a central split or deeply-cleft hilum.

Odour and Taste
Odour slight and agreeable; taste pungent and somewhat bitter at first, then producing a sensation of numbness.

IDENTIFICATION

Carry out the method for Thin-layer Chromatography as described in Appendix I using ether as the solvent system.

Apply 20 µl of the following solution to the plate; extract 1 g powdered Kava-Kava with 10 ml chloroform by heating under reflux for 10-15 minutes, cool and filter.

Spray the plate with Spray Reagent D, heat for 10 minutes at 105°C and examine in daylight.

Major bands relative to the solvent front are approximately as follows: purple 0.9, orange 0.7, orange 0.65, pink 0.6, purple 0.3, brown 0.2.

The chromatogram exhibits much fine detail between Rf 0.7-0.4 but is dominated by a purple zone at approximately Rf 0.3.

QUANTITATIVE STANDARDS

Foreign Matter
Not more than 2%   Appendix 3

Total Ash
Not more than 8%   Appendix 4

Ash Insoluble in Hydrochloric Acid
Not more than 1.5%   Appendix 5

Water-soluble Extractive
Not less than 5%   Appendix 7

MATERIAL OF COMMERCE Kava-Kava is supplied in sliced or broken form. It is obtained from the South Pacific islands, particularly from the regions of Western Samoa, Tonga, Fiji and Vanuatu.

Powdered Kava-Kava

Complies with the requirements for Identification and Quantitative Standards stated for Kava-Kava.

Characteristic Features
A pale yellowish-brown powder with a slight, agreeable odour and a bitter, pungent and numbing taste; abundant starch granules, simple or two or three compound; parenchymatous cells containing reddish or yellowish-brown oleo-resin; elongated, lignified and pitted parenchyma of the xylem and medullary rays; fragments of vessels with reticulate thickening; groups of moderately thickened, slightly lignified fibres; large, thin-walled parenchymatous cells of the pith; occasional fragments of thin-walled cork.

ACTION Anxiolytic.

LADY'S MANTLE   Rosaceae

Alchemillae herba

Lady's Mantle consists of the dried aerial parts of *Alchemilla xanthochlora* Rothm. or *Alchemilla vulgaris* L. sensu latiore, harvested during the flowering period.

CHARACTERISTICS

Macroscopical Description
Very variable in size, hairiness and leaf shape, depending on the microspecies. Leaves mostly radical on long petioles, large, up to about 10 cm in diameter, orbicular or reniform, green on both sides, palmately divided to less than half their depth into seven or nine broad, serrate lobes, each edged with long, white hairs; petioles hairy with a groove on the adaxial surface; flowering stems hollow, branched, up to about 15 cm long, bearing few smaller leaves on short petioles with large green or brownish, toothed stipules; flowers small, 3-4 mm in diameter, green to yellowish, in loose compound terminal cymes with short pedicels; calyx free, double, with four small segments of the epicalyx alternating with four larger sepals; petals absent; stamens four; a single carpel with a capitate stigma.

Microscopical Description
Leaf Dorsiventral, the cells of the palisade layer small and closely-packed; upper epidermal cells sinuous to slightly wavy in surface view with unevenly thickened and beaded walls, lower epidermal cells more wavy and more evenly thickened, with bead-

ing only at the angles; stomata anomocytic and distinctly sunken, more numerous on the lower epidermis; covering trichomes abundant on the lower epidermis and along the margins, each arising from the centre of a group of six or eight small, radiating thick-walled cells; individual trichomes unicellular, very long, narrow and tapering to a bluntly pointed apex, with thick lignified walls and an enlarged, rounded and pitted base; spongy mesophyll with fairly large cluster crystals of calcium oxalate containing few components in many of the cells adjacent to the veinlets.

Stem and Petiole Epidermis composed of longitudinally elongated thin-walled cells with occasional stomata and long, unicellular trichomes similar to those on the leaf; several layers of underlying collenchyma gradually merging into the large, thin-walled parenchyma of the cortex and ground tissue, with some of the cells containing cluster crystals of calcium oxalate; in the stem, about six separate concentric vascular bundles embedded in the ground tissue, each with a central pith and surrounded by an endodermis, individual bundles with a pericycle composed of several layers of small, closely-packed, thick-walled fibres, a wide area of thin-walled phloem and a lignified xylem composed of fibres, parenchyma and small vessels with spiral thickening; three such bundles in the petiole, where the parenchymatous ground tissue is continuous, whereas in the stem the central area breaks down forming a hollow.

Flower Epicalyx and sepals of the calyx with small, wavy-walled epidermal cells and calcium oxalate cluster crystals in the underlying mesophyll; fibrous layer of the anther with typical beaded walls; pollen grains spherical, about 20 µm in diameter, with three distinct pores and a finely pitted exine.

Odour and Taste
Odour faint; taste slightly astringent.

IDENTIFICATION

Carry out the method for Thin-layer Chromatography as described in Appendix 1, using Solvent System A.

Apply 20 µl of each of the following solutions separately to the plate: (1) extract 1 g powdered Lady's Mantle with 10 ml methanol by warming on a water-bath for 10-15 minutes, cool and filter; (2) 0.025% rutin in methanol.

Spray the plate with Spray Reagent A and examine in ultraviolet light 366 nm.

Major bands relative to rutin are approximately as follows: turquoise 2.0, turquoise 1.8-1.7, yellow 1.6, yellow 1.3*, yellow 0.9.

* This is the prominent band of the chromatogram.

QUANTITATIVE STANDARDS

Foreign Matter
Not more than 3%   Appendix 3

Total Ash
Not more than 7%   Appendix 4

Ash Insoluble in Hydrochloric Acid
Not more than 1.5%   Appendix 5

Water-soluble Extractive
Not less than 18%   Appendix 7

MATERIAL OF COMMERCE Lady's Mantle is supplied in the cut or broken condition. It is obtained from Great Britain and other European countries, especially Poland, Hungary, Bulgaria and former Czechoslovakia.

Powdered Lady's Mantle

Complies with the requirements for Identification and Quantitative Standards stated for Lady's Mantle.

Characteristic Features
Yellowish-brown powder with a faint odour and a slightly bitter and astringent taste; fragments of the leaves in surface view with sinuous to wavy epidermal cells, the anticlinal walls unevenly thickened and beaded; stomata anomocytic; cluster crystals of calcium oxalate in the spongy mesophyll; abundant thick-walled, lignified, unicellular covering trichomes, some attached to the epidermises, but the majority broken off at the base; groups of lignified fibres and vascular tissue from the petioles and stems, the vessels spirally thickened or with bordered pits; thin-walled parenchyma containing cluster crystals; occasional, small, spherical pollen grains and fragments of the fibrous layer of the anther.

ACTION Astringent.

LILY OF THE VALLEY LEAF Convallariaceae

Convallariae folium

Synonyms: Muguet Leaf, May Lily Leaf.

Lily of the Valley Leaf consists of the dried leaves of *Convallaria majalis* L.

CHARACTERISTICS

Macroscopical Description
Leaves paired, bases surrounded by convoluted sheath, 5-12 cm long. Leaf green, glabrous, ovate-lanceolate or elliptical, 8-20 cm long and 3-5 cm wide, with entire margin, acute apex and parallel venation.

Microscopical Description
Lamina epidermal cells of both surfaces thin-walled, elongated and ovoid with smooth cuticle and frequent parallel-orientated stomata; epidermal cells of veins and sheath rectangular, and papillose on margins. Isobilateral, undifferentiated mesophyll cells, some packed with fine needle crystals of calcium oxalate about 50-60 µm in length, others containing several elongated prisms up to 120 µm long; parallel row of equal-sized collateral bundles containing only phloem and xylem.

Odour and Taste
Distinctive sharp odour and bitter taste.

IDENTIFICATION

Carry out the method for Thin-layer Chromatography as described in Appendix 1, using Solvent System A.

Apply 20 µl of each of the following solutions separately to the plate: (1) extract 1 g powdered Lily of the Valley Leaf with 10 ml methanol by warming on a water-bath for 10-15 minutes, cool and filter; (2) 0.025% rutin in methanol.

Spray the plate with Spray Reagent A and examine in ultraviolet light 366 nm.

Major bands relative to rutin are approximately as follows: turquoise 2.2, turquoise 1.6, turquoise 1.4, orange 1.0, turquoise 0.85, green/yellow 0.65, orange 0.55.

QUANTITATIVE STANDARDS

Foreign Matter
Not more than 3%   Appendix 3

Total Ash
Not more than 10%   Appendix 4

Ash Insoluble in Hydrochloric Acid
Not more than 3%   Appendix 5

Water-soluble Extractive
Not less than 20%   Appendix 7

MATERIAL OF COMMERCE Lily of the Valley Leaf is supplied whole or cut. It is obtained from Great Britain and Europe, particularly the Balkan countries.

Powdered Lily of the Valley Leaf

Complies with the requirements for Identification and Quantitative Standards stated for Lily of the Valley Leaf.

Characteristic Features
Brownish-green powder with a distinctive odour and a bitter taste; fragments of leaf with elongated epidermal cells, smooth cuticle and frequent parallel-orientated stomata; transverse sections with undifferentiated spongy mesophyll; calcium oxalate needles and elongated prisms free and embedded in mesophyll cells; narrow, lignified xylem vessels with annular and reticulate thickening; occasional spherical pollen grains about 35 µm in diameter, with smooth or finely granular exine and a single pore.

ACTION Cardioactive.

LIME FLOWER Tiliaceae

Tiliae flos

Synonyms: *Tilia cordata* is Small-leaved Lime; *T. platyphyllos* Large-leaved Lime; *T. × vulgaris* Common Lime.

Lime Flower consists of the whole, dried inflorescence of *Tilia cordata* Mill., *of Tilia platyphyllos* Scop., of *Tilia × vulgaris* Hayne or a mixture of these.

This material complies with the requirements of the European Pharmacopoeia for Lime Flower.

MATERIAL OF COMMERCE Lime Flower is usually supplied whole but may be broken up. It is obtained mainly from south-eastern Europe, Turkey and China.

ACTION Antispasmodic; diaphoretic.

LINSEED Linaceae

Lini semen

Synonym: Flaxseed.

Linseed consists of the dried, ripe seeds of *Linum usitatissimum* L.

This material complies with the requirements of the European Pharmacopoeia for Linseed.

MATERIAL OF COMMERCE Linseed is supplied as whole seeds or powder. It is obtained from Argentina, Morocco, India and other countries.

ACTION Bulk forming laxative; demulcent.

LIQUORICE ROOT Leguminosae-Papilionoideae

Liquiritiae radix

Synonyms: Glycyrrhiza, Licorice.

Liquorice Root consists of the dried, unpeeled roots and stolons of *Glycyrrhiza glabra* L.

This material complies with the requirements of the European Pharmacopoeia for Liquorice Root and the British Pharmacopoeia for Liquorice, or, when the material is in powder, Powdered Liquorice.

MATERIAL OF COMMERCE Liquorice Root is supplied as cylindrical pieces or in the chopped condition. It is obtained mainly from Southern Europe, the Middle East and China .

ACTION Anti-inflammatory; expectorant.

LOBELIA

Campanulaceae

Lobeliae herba

Synonym: Indian Tobacco.

Lobelia consists of the dried aerial parts of *Lobelia inflata* L.

This material complies with the requirements of the British Pharmacopoeia 1988 for Lobelia, or, when the material is in powder,

Powdered Lobelia.

MATERIAL OF COMMERCE Lobelia is supplied in the broken or crushed condition. It is obtained from eastern North America and the Netherlands.

ACTION Respiratory stimulant.

LOVAGE ROOT

Umbelliferae

Levistici radix

Lovage Root consists of the dried roots and rhizomes of *Levisticum officinale* Koch.

CHARACTERISTICS

Macroscopical Description
Root-stock short, up to 5 cm or more thick, upper part, often with remains of hollow stem bases and leaves, coarsely and irregularly transversely wrinkled; small number of adventitious roots, up to 2-3 cm thick, often long, little branched, small wiry rootlets and scattered wart-like excrescences; few irregular, faint, usually incomplete, transverse wrinkles and ridges; surface almost smooth, light greyish-brown; cut surface almost white in bark with abundant droplets of yellowish secretion, outer zone variably lacunose; xylem, irregular outline comprising about one third of total diameter, pale yellow, densest near cambium; variable-sized central parenchymatous region, containing secretion ducts.

Microscopical Description
Root Outer zone of up to about eight layers of thin-walled cork cells, pale yellowish-brown, in surface view relatively large, variable in shape from squarish to shortly rectangular, to somewhat narrow and elongated; internally a few layers of slightly thick-walled, tangentially elongated, parenchyma followed by thinner, rounded parenchyma containing oval to round secretion ducts; phloem wide, medullary rays multiseriate, varying in length, numerous, somewhat wavy, especially in outer phloem; sieve tissue of small, thin-walled rounded cells; frequent secretion ducts, up to about 220 µm total diameter, lined with relatively few almost colourless cells; narrow cambiform zone. Xylem with unlignified medullary rays; elongated wedge-shaped xylem bundles, comprising larger reticulately thickened vessels, singly or in groups of up to four, up to 125 µm diameter, surrounded by small-celled unlignified parenchyma; groups, usually radial, of smaller reticulately thickened vessels, up to 55-60 µm, embedded in unlignified parenchyma; central xylem, thin-walled parenchyma with secretion canals and scattered groups of very small vessels. Starch abundant in bark, central parenchyma and medullary rays, simple rounded to ovoid granules, of variable size, up to about 12 µm; numerous compound grains, somewhat larger, many with several components.

Odour and Taste
Odour strong, penetrating, characteristic, reminiscent of Celery; taste slightly sweet at first, spicy, becoming burning and numbing, rather unpleasant and lingering.

123

IDENTIFICATION

Carry out the method for Thin-layer Chromatography as described in Appendix 1, using Solvent System D with non-saturated conditions.

Apply 40 µl of the following solution to the plate: extract 1 g powdered Lovage Root with 10 ml methanol by warming on a water bath for 30 minutes, cool, filter and concentrate to approximately 2 ml.

Examine the plate under ultraviolet light 366 nm.

Major bands relative to the solvent front are approximately as follows: large, intense white 0.85*, white 0.65, white 0.4. Fine detail exists in the areas of Rf 0.55-0.45 and 0.35-0.25.

* This strong white band is characteristic of *Levisticum officinale*.

QUANTITATIVE STANDARDS

Foreign Matter
Not more than 5%   Appendix 3

Total Ash
Not more than 8%   Appendix 4

Ash Insoluble in Hydrochloric Acid
Not more than 1%   Appendix 5

Water-soluble Extractive
Not less than 45%   Appendix 7

MATERIAL OF COMMERCE Lovage Root is supplied sliced or broken. It is harvested from cultivated plants and obtained mainly from Poland, eastern Germany, the Netherlands and Balkan countries.

Powdered Lovage Root

Complies with the requirements for Identification and Quantitative Standards stated for Lovage Root.

Characteristic Features
Pale creamish-yellow; odour characteristic, aromatic; taste pleasantly aromatic, slightly sweet; abundant thin-walled parenchyma, unpitted, small intercellular spaces; few, small starch granules; reticulately thickened lignified vessels, up to 60-70 µm diameter, singly or in small groups, vessel segments short, ends oblique; very few, much narrower, spiral vessels; in some parenchyma, scattered small, colourless or pale yellowish droplets of oil; ill-defined, pale yellowish secretion canals.

ACTION Carminative; mild diuretic.

LUCERNE   Leguminosae-Papilionoideae

Medicaginis herba

Synonym: Alfalfa.

Lucerne consists of the dried aerial parts of *Medicago sativa* L., harvested during the flowering period.

CHARACTERISTICS

Macroscopical Description
Stems Up to 90 cm, branched, cylindrical or slightly angled, longitudinally striated, almost glabrous.

Leaves Trifoliate, parts equal; leaflets up to 3 cm, narrowly obovate, apex acute, base tapering; margin very finely serrate to dentate in upper part, entire below point of narrowing; long tangled hairs on lower margin; venation pinnate, veins numerous, closely spaced; upper surface dark green, few hairs; lower surface lighter, hairs more frequent, especially on veins; stipules small, linear-lanceolate, joined to petiole, toothed, glabrous or hairy.

Flowers Racemes up to 4 cm long, seven

to ten papilionate flowers 8 mm long, purple; pedicel about 2 mm, shorter than calyx tube; calyx divided almost to middle with five nearly equal teeth.

Fruits Open-centred, spirally twisted pods with two to four turns, sharply beaked, surface glabrous or hairy; calyx persistent; ten to twenty greenish-brown angular seeds, about 2 mm.

Microscopical Description

Stem Section irregularly four or five-sided to almost circular, slightly undulate; epidermal cells subrectangular, outer wall more thickened, cuticle ridged; small areas of collenchyma in angles; large number of vascular bundles more or less united by completely lignified interfascicular sclerenchyma, each bundle having up to five rows of vessels and a group of incompletely lignified pericycle fibres; pith outer cells thin-walled, with small pits, lignified; epidermal cells in surface view, straight, elongated, thin-walled, cuticle finely striated; stomata few, pore axially orientated, subsidiary cells small; twinned prism crystals, in short files or groups, in sub-epidermal tissue; larger vessels bordered-pitted.

Leaf Dorsiventral, palisade single or double; upper epidermal cells more or less rectangular, thin-walled, slightly sinuous, occasional beads; stomata, anisocytic or anomocytic, with three or four subsidiary cells; lower epidermal cells, similar in shape and size, walls distinctly sinuous, beads numerous, stomata abundant, few covering trichomes with two very short basal cells and one long, often bent or undulate, terminal cell, very thick-walled and coarsely warted; infrequent small glandular trichomes with one to four-celled uniseriate stalk and one, two or four-celled head.

Flower Epidermal cells of sepals similar to leaf, variable in shape and outline; stomata present; trichomes more numerous, the covering longer, distinctly bent near base, markedly undulate; inner epidermal cells of petals with short papillae, tips thickened, cuticle striated; outer epidermal cells thin-walled, shortly rectangular, slightly beaded or infolded; pollen grains spherical, about 35 μm, three pores and furrows, exine smooth.

Odour and Taste

Faint, grass-like, odour and little taste.

IDENTIFICATION

Carry out the method for Thin-layer Chromatography as described in Appendix 1, using Solvent System A.

Apply 20 μl of each of the following solutions separately to the plate: (1) extract 1 g powdered Lucerne with 10 ml methanol by warming on a water-bath for 10-15 minutes, cool, filter and concentrate to approximately 2 ml; (2) 0.025% rutin in methanol.

Spray the plate with Spray Reagent A and examine in ultraviolet light 366 nm.

Major bands relative to rutin are approximately as follows: turquoise 2.2, blue 1.9, yellow 1.5, yellow 1.1 , yellow 0.75.

QUANTITATIVE STANDARDS

Foreign Matter
Not more than 2%   Appendix 3

Total Ash
Not more than 10%   Appendix 4

Ash Insoluble in Hydrochloric Acid
Not more than 2%   Appendix 5

Water-soluble Extractive
Not less than 20%   Appendix 7

MATERIAL OF COMMERCE Lucerne is supplied in crushed or cut condition. It is obtained from European countries.

Powdered Lucerne

Complies with the requirements for Identification and Quantitative Standards stated for Lucerne.

Characteristic Features

Mid greenish-brown with slight odour and bland taste; unicellular trichomes with warty walls and narrow lumen, straight or undulate, usually acutely bent at base; leaf epidermal cells sinuous, finely beaded, numerous anisocytic or anomocytic stomata; slender groups of lignified fibres associated with files of prism crystals; narrow bordered-pitted and spirally thickened vessels; lignified, pitted parenchyma of pith; papillose cells of petals with striated cuticle; infrequent small glandular trichomes; spherical pollen grains with three pores and furrows.

ACTION Tonic.

125

MARIGOLD

Compositae

Calendulae flos

Synonym: Calendula.

Marigold consists of the dried ligulate florets or dried composite flowers of *Calendula officinalis* L.

CHARACTERISTICS

Macroscopical Description

Flower Capitulum somewhat flattened dorsiventrally, concave below, under surface greyish-green with central bos bearing short, ribbed pedicel, or scar, densely pubescent; involucre 1.5-2 cm diameter of numerous tough, strongly curved, acutely pointed, linear-lanceolate bracts, 8-15 mm long and up to 2 mm wide, in two rows; narrow, fawn margins with long, tangled trichomes; outer surface veined, dark greyish-green, bearing abundant trichomes, inner surface paler green, smooth; disc florets very numerous, closely-packed, orange-yellow to dull brown, hermaphrodite, corolla funnel-shaped with five spreading, pointed lobes 3-4 mm long, tube of approximately equal length, bearing few trichomes near the base; five epipetalous stamens, anthers sometimes exerted, style shorter, obscurely bifid; corolla easily separated from the fawn-coloured, hairy, sterile ovary; ray florets female, numerous, in two or three rows, yellow to dull orange-brown, oblanceolate with three or four short teeth, strap of corolla glabrous, 12-35 mm long, 3-6 mm wide, corolla tube 1.5-2 mm long, numerous long hairs without, slightly projecting, bifid stigma.

Fruit An achene, dark brownish-green, 1-2 mm thick, tapering towards base and apex, inwardly curved to greater or lesser degree, dorsal surface with two or three rows of minute, bluntly conical to spiny projections and numerous long hairs, most fruits with pale lateral wings; larger fruits with fawn, arcuate, beak-like extensions at both ends on the concave side; ventral surface smooth and lighter coloured.

Microscopical Description

Bract Inner epidermal cells rectangular, anticlinal walls straight or slightly sinuous; numerous anisocytic stomata; epidermal cells near apex pigmented and impart a brownish-red colour to solution of Chloral Hydrate; trichomes abundant, especially along the margins; covering predominate; the most characteristic are long with from two to eight short basal cells and an extremely long, slender, more or less convoluted, whip-like terminal portion; others with up to six uniform cells, with a bluntly rounded apical cell, or with a large number of components and a more pointed apex; biseriate covering trichomes also occur, varying in length from about three to six cells per row; glandular trichomes less numerous, having a three to four-celled uniseriate stalk and a clavate head of up to six cells; in the non-marginal area there are frequent very short-stalked glandular trichomes. Outer epidermal cells isodiametric, walls straight to sinuous, stomata as on the inner epidermis; large, very long, biseriate covering trichomes and glandular trichomes with biseriate stalks and multicellular, clavate heads, some very large with up to eight heads per row.

Ray floret Inner epidermal cells elongated rectangular and almost straight-walled, cuticle faintly striated; stomata absent; outer epidermal cells similar, but with three or four anomocytic stomata present very close to the apices of the teeth; trichomes very numerous on the tube, majority are covering, biseriate, a few terminating in a blunt-ended single cell; some of the larger ones with more than two cells in the base; fewer glandular trichomes, with multicellular, uni- or biseriate stalks and clavate heads; stigma epidermal cells straight-walled, polygonal, prolonged into short, thin-walled, bulbous papillae.

Disc floret Outer epidermal cells elongated, straight or slightly sinuous-walled, stomata absent; abundant trichomes on area below point of insertion of the stamens, mainly glandular, uni - or biseriate, fewer covering, uni- or biseriate types; inner epidermal cells similar to outer; cells at apices of corolla lobes extended, to form thicker-walled, acuminate projections; at the position of insertion of stamens an area of square to rectangular, lignified cells with well defined beads of thickening at cell junctions; fibrous layer cells with well defined beads of thickening at the junctions; cells of the fibrous layer of anther with slender thickening; within the upper part of the anthers a layer of isodiametric to elongated, moderately thick-walled, lignified and pitted cells; pollen grains up to 45 μm, spherical, with three pores, exine finely granular with numerous short spines; apex of stigma covered by fairly large, thin-walled projections.

Achene Epidermal cells polygonal, anticlinal walls straight; outer periclinal walls markedly convex or forming short papillae; numerous covering trichomes, very long, biseriate, or shorter and uniseriate; glandular trichomes with biseriate stalks and multicellular heads; lignified internal tissue containing rounded to ovoid cells, thin-walled and distinctly pitted, also groups of elongated, narrow, pitted, fibre-like cells.

Odour and Taste
Odour faint and pleasantly aromatic; taste rather bitter.

IDENTIFICATION

Carry out the method for Thin-layer Chromatography as described in Appendix 1, using Solvent System A.

Apply 20 μl of each of the following solutions separately to the plate: (1) extract 1 g powdered Marigold with 10 ml methanol by warming on a water-bath for 10-15 minutes, cool and filter; (2) 0.025% rutin in methanol.

Spray the plate with Spray Reagent A and examine in ultraviolet light 366 nm.

Major bands relative to rutin are approximately as follows: turquoise 2.2, turquoise 2.1, turquoise 1.4, yellow 1.1, yellow 1.0, yellow 0.7.

QUANTITATIVE STANDARDS

Foreign Matter
Not more than 2%   Appendix 3

Total Ash
Not more than 10%   Appendix 4

Ash Insoluble in Hydrochloric Acid
Not more than 2%   Appendix 5

Water-soluble Extractive
Not less than 20%   Appendix 7

MATERIAL OF COMMERCE Marigold is supplied as whole capitula or as separated ligulate florets. It is usually harvested from cultivated crops and is obtained mainly from eastern Europe, especially Poland and Hungary; also from Egypt.

Powdered Marigold

Complies with the requirements for Identification and Quantitative Standards stated for Marigold.

ACTION Anti-inflammatory, vulnerary.

MARSHMALLOW LEAF   Malvaceae

Althaeae folium

Marshmallow Leaf consists of the dried leaves of *Althaea officinalis* L. harvested before the flowering period.

CHARACTERISTICS

Macroscopical Description
Greyish-green, both surfaces velvety with a felt-like pubescence; lamina thin and brittle; 4-8 cm long and 3-10 cm wide; typically triangular to ovate with three or five dentate lobes, sometimes not well accentuated; some leaves more rounded, others rather narrowly ovate; apex acute, base equal and usually more or less cordate; margin dentate to serrate-dentate; main venation palmate with five or, infrequently, three large veins terminating in the lobes, less prominent pinnately arranged veins terminating in the larger marginal dentations; petiole up to 3 or 4 cm, occasionally longer.

Microscopical Description
Dorsiventral, palisade occupying nearly half the thickness of the lamina, single-layered

or, in places, two layers of shorter cells, the inner less well differentiated; occasional cluster crystals in the palisade layer, more frequent crystals in the spongy mesophyll, particularly beneath the lower epidermis, and somewhat larger crystals in short files alongside the veinlets; outer periclinal wall of cells of both epidermises only slightly thickened, flat or slightly convex, cuticle smooth; raised stomata in both epidermises. Upper epidermal cells more or less polygonal, isodiametric, anticlinal walls straight or gently curved, some sinuous; stomata numerous, with up to four subsidiary cells, anomocytic or less obviously anisocytic; lower epidermal cells similar to upper, often with more sinuous walls; stomata as in upper epidermis, more numerous, and some with two subsidiary cells, paracytic. Both epidermises densely covered with stellate trichomes of two to six, infrequently up to eight, almost-straight, thick-walled, weakly lignified, unicellular components, smooth and slenderly tapering to a point; lumen usually with brownish contents in the lower part, almost occluded towards the apex; few, often longer, single, straight trichomes and, less frequently, shorter, bent or undulate trichomes. Glandular trichomes not numerous, on both surfaces over veins and in interneural regions, small with very short unicellular stalk, rounded to ovoid head with four to eight very thin-walled cells; basal cell somewhat thickened, surrounding epidermal cells in rosette arrangement. Randomly scattered in the epidermises isolated cells filled with mucilage which stains with Ruthenium Red. Entrapped in the dense trichome covering occasional spherical pollen grains, about 90 μm diameter, exine relatively thick, finely reticulate and covered with short spines, pink in Chloral Hydrate mount. The dull, brownish, elongated-ellipsoidal two-celled spores of *Puccinia malvacearum* also often present on the leaf surface.

Odour and Taste
Almost odourless; taste insipid and somewhat mucilaginous.

IDENTIFICATION

Carry out the method for Thin-layer Chromatography as described in Appendix 1, using Solvent System A.

Apply 20 μl of each of the following solutions separately to the plate: (1) extract 1 g powdered Marshmallow Leaf with 10 ml methanol by warming on a water-bath for 10-15 minutes, cool and filter; (2) 0.025% rutin in methanol.

Spray the plate with Spray Reagent A and examine in ultraviolet light 366 nm.

Major bands relative to rutin are approximately as follows: turquoise 2.3, yellow 2.2, turquoise 2.1, yellow 1.8, orange/yellow 1.7, turquoise 1.1, yellow 0.75, blue 0.6, yellow 0.5.

QUANTITATIVE STANDARDS

Foreign Matter
Not more than 2%   Appendix 3

Total Ash
Not more than 16%   Appendix 4

Ash Insoluble in Hydrochloric Acid
Not more than 3%   Appendix 5

Water-soluble Extractive
Not less than 15%   Appendix 7

MATERIAL OF COMMERCE Marshmallow Leaf is supplied in large felted masses or as cut leaf. It is usually harvested from cultivated crops and obtained mainly from Eastern Europe.

Powdered Marshmallow Leaf

Complies with the requirements for Identification and Quantitative Standards stated for Marshmallow Leaf.

ACTION Demulcent.

MARSHMALLOW ROOT
Malvaceae
Althaeae radix

Synonym: Althaea Root.

Marshmallow Root consists of the dried, peeled roots of *Althaea officinalis* L.

CHARACTERISTICS

Macroscopical Description
Scraped, yellowish-white roots, straight or slightly tapering with deep longitudinal furrows; up to 20 cm long and 2 cm wide at the upper end; brownish circular root scars often present; fracture short, granular and fibrous; transverse surface exhibiting a moderately wide, finely radiate outer region separated by a brown cambium line from the cream-yellow wood.

Microscopical Description
Phloem with numerous long, thin-walled, non-lignified fibres arranged in tangential groups alternating with groups of sieve tissue, with a ground tissue of thin-walled parenchyma; xylem containing reticulately or scalariformly thickened or bordered pitted vessels accompanied by lignified tracheids, a small amount of lignified parenchyma and occasional small groups of fibres with only the middle lamella lignified; xylem and phloem traversed by numerous non-lignified medullary rays, mostly uniseriate; the majority of the parenchymatous cells of the phloem and medullary rays containing abundant small starch granules, mostly simple, spherical to ovoid, occasionally two to three compound, with a well-marked circular or slit-shaped hilum, some cells containing cluster crystals of calcium oxalate 20-40 µm diameter, others developed as idioblasts containing mucilage which stains pink with Ruthenium Red Solution.

Odour and Taste
Faint, aromatic odour; mucilaginous taste.

IDENTIFICATION

Carry out the method for Thin-layer Chromatography as described in Appendix 1, using Solvent System A.

Apply 20 µl of each of the following solutions separately to the plate: (1) extract 1 g powdered Marshmallow Root with 10 ml methanol on a water-bath for 10-15 minutes, cool and filter; (2) 0.025% rutin in methanol. Spray with Spray Reagent A and examine in ultraviolet light 366 nm.

Major bands relative to rutin are approximately as follows: narrow blue 2.55, pale blue 2.5, blue 2.4, blue 0.9, blue 0.65.

QUANTITATIVE STANDARDS

Loss on Drying
Not more than 12% when dried in an oven at 100-105°C. Use 2-3 g   Appendix 2

Foreign Matter
Not more than 2%   Appendix 3

Total Ash
Not more than 8% calculated with reference to the oven-dried material   Appendix 4

Ash Insoluble in Hydrochloric Acid
Not more than 3% calculated with reference to the oven-dried material   Appendix 5

Water-soluble Extractive
Not less than 22% calculated with reference to the oven dried material   Appendix 7

Swelling Index
Not less than 10, with powdered root sieved through 710 µm   Appendix 8

MATERIAL OF COMMERCE Marshmallow Root is supplied as broken or chopped pieces of root. The root is collected from cultivated plants at least two years old, scraped and dried. It is obtained from European countries.

Powdered Marshmallow Root

Complies with the requirements for Identification and Quantitative Standards stated for Marshmallow Root.

Characteristic Features
Creamish-white powder with a faint, aro-

matic odour and a bland, mucilaginous taste; abundant non-lignified fibres often associated with lignified xylem parenchyma; abundant starch granules; abundant thick-walled phloem parenchymatous cells, some containing cluster crystals of calcium oxalate; scattered cluster crystals of calcium oxalate and amorphous masses of mucilage which stain pink with Ruthenium Red Solution; fragments of lignified vessels; very occasional fragments of cork with thin, lignified walls may be present.

STORAGE Store in a cool, dry place in well closed containers.

ACTION Demulcent.

MATÉ

Aquifoliaceae

Mate folium

Synonyms: Yerba Maté, Paraguay Tea.

Maté consists of the leaves of *Ilex paraguariensis* A. St.-Hil., briefly cured by strong heating then more gently dried.

CHARACTERISTICS

Macroscopical Description
Leaves simple, oblong-lanceolate, ovate or obovate, up to 10 cm or more long and 2-3 cm wide; relatively thick, coriaceous and brittle; margin with widely-spaced fine serrations or obscurely dentate, apex subacute to rounded, sometimes indistinctly emarginate; base acute, tapering; both surfaces glabrous, smooth, yellowish-green to grey-green or light brown, very infrequent small black spots; midrib prominent on lower surface, lateral veins pinnately arranged, curved somewhat towards apex, anastomosing near margin; fracture short; petiole woody, grooved, up to 1 cm long.

Microscopical Description
Dorsiventral, palisade two to four layers, cells quite short; spongy mesophyll wider, air-spaces large, well defined, infrequent cluster crystals up to about 50 μm, less obvious smaller prism crystals randomly in spongy and midrib parenchyma; in section upper and lower epidermal cells similar, almost square, periclinal wall thickened, cuticle finely serrated; upper epidermis, anticlinal walls almost straight, slightly thickened, indistinctly beaded, iso-diametric to sub-rectangular or polygonal, fine sinuous striations, stomata absent; lower epidermis, cells similar in shape, smaller, thin-ner-walled, cuticular striations more well-marked, numerous stomata with up to six small subsidiary cells; epidermal cells over veins, more uniformly subrectangular; very infrequent, short, thick-walled, unicellular trichomes; midrib, meristele with numerous rows of small-diameter xylem elements, endodermis moderately thick-walled, lignified, pitted rectangular cells; pericycle, one or more layers, lignified, smaller diameter, moderately thickened, elongated, pitted fibres; upper and lower areas of subepidermal collenchyma.

Odour and Taste
Odour aromatic, faintly of wood smoke; taste bitter and similarly aromatic and empyreumatic, slightly astringent.

IDENTIFICATION

Carry out the method for Thin-layer Chromatography as described in Appendix I, using Solvent System A.

Apply 20 μl of each of the following solutions separately to the plate: (1) extract 1 g powdered Maté with 10 ml methanol by warming on a water bath for 10-15 minutes, cool and filter; (2) 0.025% rutin in methanol.

Spray the plate with Spray Reagent A and examine in ultraviolet light 366 nm.

Major bands relative to rutin are approximately as follows: turquoise 2.2, yellow 2.0, yellow 1.6, yellow 1.45, yellow 1.0.

The chromatogram for Maté generally displays a turquoise hue throughout, except for the intense yellow band corresponding to rutin. Bands may coalesce in high concentration.

QUANTITATIVE STANDARDS

Foreign Matter
Not more than 2%   Appendix 3

Total Ash
Not more than 8%   Appendix 4

Ash Insoluble in Hydrochloric Acid
Not more than 2%   Appendix 5

Water-soluble Extractive
Not less than 20%   Appendix 7

MATERIAL OF COMMERCE Maté is supplied as broken or cut leaves. It is harvested mainly from the wild, although cultivation is rapidly increasing, and obtained from southern Brazil, Argentina and Paraguay.

Powdered Maté

Complies with the requirements for Identification and Quantitative Standards stated for Maté.

ACTION Stimulant.

MATRICARIA FLOWER Compositae

Matricariae flos

Synonyms: Matricaria, German Chamomile.

Matricaria Flower consists of the dried flower-heads of *Matricaria recutita* L. [*Chamomilla recutita* (L.) Rauschert].

This material complies with the requirements of the European Pharmacopoeia for Matricaria Flower.

MATERIAL OF COMMERCE Matricaria Flower is supplied in the whole or partially broken condition. It is obtained mainly from Argentina, Egypt and south-eastern Europe.

ACTION Anti-inflammatory; antispasmodic.

MEADOWSWEET Rosaceae

Spiraeae herba

Synonym: Queen-of-the-Meadow.

Meadowsweet consists of the dried aerial parts of *Filipendula ulmaria* (L). Maxim. [*Spiraea ulmaria* L.] collected when the plant is in flower.

CHARACTERISTICS

Macroscopical Description
Stems Green, cylindrical or somewhat flattened, up to 5 mm in diameter; older stems longitudinally ridged, glabrous and hollow; younger stems more finely striated and pubescent.
Leaves Petioled, pinnate, alternate and stipulate; composed of two to five pairs of ovate, serrulate leaflets up to about 7 cm long and 4 cm wide; margin doubly serrate, apex acute; upper surface dark green, lower surface greyish-white and tomentose, stipules broadly cordate and conspicuous.
Flowers Small, creamy-white, arranged in a terminal corymb on pubescent pedicels; reflexed hairy sepals, five creamy-white petals and numerous stamens, flower buds or twisted, one-seeded follicles may occasionally occur.

Microscopical Description
Stem Epidermal cells, thin-walled and axially elongated, some with very long, unicellular covering trichomes and occasional

131

anomocytic stomata; cortex with narrow outer collenchyma especially in the ridges; inner parenchyma; vascular tissue in small groups surrounding a large central pith and separated by wide medullary rays; pericyclic fibres occurring in large masses associated with each vascular group and extending laterally to form a continuous ring; individual fibres with moderately thickened, slightly lignified walls; xylem with some large, bordered-pitted vessels and smaller spirally or annularly thickened vessels; pith of thin-walled parenchyma; cluster crystals of calcium oxalate up to 40 μm in diameter in the parenchyma of cortex and pith.

Leaf Upper epidermal cells with sinuous to slightly wavy anticlinal walls; those in the lower epidermis more wavy; anomocytic stomata in the lower epidermis only, on the upper epidermis short, thick-walled, conical covering trichomes, on the lower epidermis abundant, unicellular, long, narrow covering trichomes, often forming felted masses; occasional clavate glandular trichomes with a short, one to three-celled stalk and a head of several cells with dense brown contents also occurring on the lower epidermis especially along the veins; palisade frequently two-layered; cluster crystals of calcium oxalate in the mesophyll.

Flower Outer epidermis of sepals with abundant, long, frequently tangled, covering trichomes similar to those on the lower epidermis of the leaf; scattered anomocytic stomata; cluster crystals of calcium oxalate up to 20 μm in diameter in the mesophyll; outer epidermis of petals with thin-walled, markedly sinuous anticlinal walls and anomocytic stomata; inner epidermis papillose; small cluster crystals of calcium oxalate in the mesophyll; typical fibrous layer of stamens; pollen grains spherical, 25 μm in diameter, with three pores and faintly pitted exine.

Odour and Taste
Practically no odour; very slightly bitter taste.

IDENTIFICATION

Carry out the method for Thin-layer Chromatography as described in Appendix 1, using Solvent System A.

Apply 20 μl of each of the following solutions separately to the plate: (1) extract 1 g powdered Meadowsweet with 10 ml 60% methanol on a water-bath for 10-15 minutes cool and filter; (2) 0.025% rutin in methanol.

Spray the plate with Spray Reagent A and examine in ultraviolet light 366 nm.

Major bands relative to rutin are approximately as follows: orange 2.7, blue 2.45, orange 1.85, orange 1.4, orange 1.0.

QUANTITATIVE STANDARDS

Foreign Matter

Not more than 2%	Appendix 3

Total Ash

Not more than 8%	Appendix 4

Ash Insoluble in Hydrochloric Acid

Not more than 2%	Appendix 5

Water-soluble Extractive

Not less than 12%	Appendix 7

MATERIAL OF COMMERCE Meadowsweet is supplied as the crushed or broken herb. It is obtained from European countries, including the UK, and especially from Poland, Bulgaria and former Yugoslavia.

Powdered Meadowsweet

Complies with the requirements for Identification and Quantitative Standards stated for Meadowsweet.

Characteristic Features
Green powder with practically no odour and very little taste; epidermal cells of leaf with sinuous anticlinal walls and anomocytic stomata on lower epidermis; covering trichomes of two types - unicellular, thick-walled, conical with thickened pitted base on upper epidermis only, and numerous, long, tangled, unicellular on lower epidermis; cluster crystals of calcium oxalate in mesophyll of leaf and sepals; occasional fragments of corolla showing papillose epidermis; spherical pollen grains with faintly pitted exine.

ACTION Anti-inflammatory.

MELILOT

Meliloti herba

Synonyms: Ribbed Melilot, Yellow Melilot, King's Clover, Yellow Sweet Clover.

Melilot consists of the dried flowering tops of *Melilotus officinalis* (L.) Pall.

CHARACTERISTICS

Macroscopical Description
Stems Up to 90 - 100 cm, erect, branched, cylindrical, finely ridged, glabrous.
Leaves Trifoliate, parts almost equal, petiole about as long as leaflets, stipules short, entire margined, subulate, joined to base of petiole; leaflets up to 2.5 cm, slightly elongated-ovate, apex and base acute; margin finely serrate, entire towards base; veins numerous, closely spaced, not well-marked; surfaces dark green, upper glabrous, lower with short, fine, apically directed hairs; petiolule of terminal leaflet longer than those of lateral pair.
Flowers Racemes up to 4 - 5 cm, long-stalked, numerous closely-spaced, pale yellow papilionate flowers; pedicels very short, slightly hairy; calyx hairy, deeply divided, lobes slender, tapering.
Fruit Pod with persistent calyx, brown, short, thick, almost straight, glabrous, transversely wrinkled.

Microscopical Description
Stem Section almost circular, small irregularly-spaced protuberances; epidermal cells shallow, rectangular, outer wall thick, cuticle coarsely ridged, inner wall thickened adjoining hypodermal collenchyma; cortex narrow, small-celled parenchyma; tangentially elongated groups of unlignified pericycle fibres, walls stratified, more or less collapsed, lumen large; phloem narrow; continuous ring of xylem, rows of larger, strongly lignified vessels surrounded by less strongly lignified sclerenchyma; pith, central area broken-down, large, thin-walled parenchyma; cells near xylem smaller, thicker-walled, simple-pitted, lignified. Epidermal cells in surface view straight-walled, slightly elongated, ends pointed, some with thinner transverse ends; cuticle weakly ridged, anticlinal walls occasionally beaded; stomata present.

Leaf Dorsiventral; upper epidermal cells more or less isodiametric or somewhat elongated, slightly sinuous, infrequently beaded; stomata numerous, anisocytic or anomocytic, three to six subsidiary cells; lower epidermal cells similar to upper, larger, more markedly sinuous, stomata more frequent; glandular trichomes few, short two or three-celled stalk, ovoid biseriate head, usually of four cells; numerous covering trichomes, terminal cell long, narrowed at base, straight or slightly undulate, thick-walled, cuticle with widely-spaced, often indistinct, warts, two very short, smooth basal cells; surrounding epidermal cells in rosette arrangement; trichomes over midrib larger; veinlets in mesophyll associated with well-defined prism crystal sheath.
Flower Epidermal cells of sepals larger than those of leaf, variable rectangular, walls straight or slightly wavy, thicker, more regularly beaded, cuticle finely striated, stomata less frequent, some paracytic; covering trichomes variable in length and wall thickness, many partly collapsed; small glandular trichomes on outer surface; inner epidermal cells of petal papillose near apex, cuticle striated; others shortly rectangular, variable from slightly sinuous to almost straight-walled; fibrous layer of anther cells small, polygonal, closely-spaced lignified bars of thickening; pollen grains, spherical to ovoid, about 25 µm, thin-walled, smooth, three pores.

Odour and Taste
Odour slight, reminiscent of new-mown hay; taste slight, faintly bitter.

IDENTIFICATION

Carry out the method for Thin-layer Chromatography as described in Appendix 1, using Solvent System D with non-saturated conditions.

Apply 40 µl of each of the following solutions separately to the plate: (1) extract 1 g powdered Melilot with 10 ml methanol by warming on a water-bath for 30 minutes, cool, filter and concentrate to approximately 2 ml; (2) 1% coumarin in methanol.

Examine the plate under ultraviolet light 366 nm.

The chromatogram is characterised by multiple red and white bands throughout the full Rf range. Major bands relative to the solvent front are approximately as follows: red 0.9, red 0.8, red 0.6, red 0.45, red 0.4. At this stage no coumarin band will be visible at approximately Rf 0.7.

If the plate is then sprayed with 1.8M ethanolic potassium hydroxide solution and re-examined in ultraviolet light 366 nm, the characteristic band of coumarin will become visible for both sample and standard.

Without potassium hydroxide treatment, both *Asperula odorata* and Melilot exhibit similar chromatograms, with the exception that Melilot does not exhibit an intense blue fluorescence at Rf 0. This feature may be employed to differentiate beween the two plants.

QUANTITATIVE STANDARDS

Foreign Matter
Not more than 2%   Appendix 3

Total Ash
Not more than 8%   Appendix 4

Ash insoluble in Hydrochloric acid
Not more than 2%   Appendix 5

Water-soluble Extractive
Not less than 25%   Appendix 7

MATERIAL OF COMMERCE Melilot is supplied cut or broken. It is obtained mainly from eastern European countries.

Powdered Melilot

Complies with the requirements for Identification and Quantitative Standards stated for Melilot.

Characteristic Features
Pale green to yellowish-brown powder with a leafy odour and a slightly bitter taste; fragments of the leaves, the epidermal cells in surface view with unevenly thickened, straight to sinuous walls and anomocytic or anisocytic stomata; veinlets in the mesophyll with prism crystal sheaths; characteristic uniseriate covering trichomes with the long terminal cell thick-walled and distinctly warty, glandular trichomes with ovoid, biseriate heads; groups of unlignified fibres and lignified vascular tissue from the stem; fibrous layer of the anthers and spherical to ovoid pollen grains; occasional fragments of the petals, some showing papillae.

ACTION Venotonic, vulnerary.

MILK THISTLE FRUIT   Compositae

Cardui mariae (or mariani) fructus

Synonyms: Marian Thistle, Mediterranean Milk Thistle, *Carduus marianus*.

Milk Thistle Fruit consists of the dried ripe fruits of *Silybum marianum* (L.) Gaertn.

CHARACTERISTICS

Macroscopical Description
Obovoid, strongly compressed achenes about 6-8 mm long, 3 mm broad, and 1.5 mm thick, outer surface smooth and shining, of a greyish-buff ground colour but variably streaked dark brown longitudinally to give an overall colour ranging from pale greyish-

brown to dark chocolate brown; tapering at the base and crowned at the apex with a glistening, pale yellow extension forming a collar about 1 mm high surrounding the remains of the style. Cut transversely shows a narrow, brown outer area and two large, dense, white and oily cotyledons.

Microscopical Description
Epicarp composed of a layer of colourless cells, narrow, much elongated radially and somewhat undulating, outer walls very thick, radial walls narrowing rapidly towards the base giving a flask-shaped lumen; underlying this a pigment layer with thin-walled, narrow, longitudinally elongated cells con-

taining reddish-brown colouring matter turning bright red with acid; innermost layers of the pericarp composed of collapsed parenchyma with occasional large, elongated prism crystals of calcium oxalate. Testa epidermis a conspicuous sclerenchymatous layer of large, yellow cells, 125-150 μm high, somewhat twisted and arranged as a palisade, walls thickened, pitted and striated; lumen narrow, widening at either end; subepidermal layers of small, rather indistinct cells with narrow bands of thickening appearing as beads in surface view. Cotyledons parenchymatous, showing some differentiation into palisade and mesophyll, the cells thin-walled and filled with aleurone grains and globules of fixed oil accompanied by abundant cluster crystals of calcium oxalate.

Odour and Taste
Odour slight; taste oily and somewhat bitter and unpleasant.

IDENTIFICATION

Carry out the method for Thin-layer Chromatography as described in Appendix 1, using a mixture of chloroform: acetone: formic acid (150:33:17) as the solvent system.

Apply 40 μl of the following solution to the plate: (1) 1 g powdered Milk Thistle Fruit is defatted by heating under reflux on a water-bath with 50 ml petroleum spirit 40:60 for 30 minutes, filter. The residue is extracted with 10 ml methanol by warming on a water-bath for 10-15 minutes, cool and filter.

Spray the plate with Spray Reagent A and examine in ultraviolet light 366 nm.

Major bands relative to the solvent front are approximately as follows: pale yellow 0.5, pale yellow 0.45, orange 0.3, pale yellow 0.25.

Note: If the tank is not fully saturated, bands will appear at higher Rf.

QUANTITATIVE STANDARDS

Foreign Matter
Not more than 2%   Appendix 3

Total Ash
Not more than 8%   Appendix 4

Ash Insoluble in Hydrochloric Acid
Not more than 1%   Appendix 5

Water Soluble Extractive
Not less than 10%   Appendix 7

MATERIAL OF COMMERCE Milk Thistle Fruit is supplied in the whole condition. Native to the Mediterranean area, *Silybum marianus* is naturalized in many temperate countries. Fruits from cultivated crops are obtained from Argentina, China and several European countries, particularly Romania and Hungary.

Powdered Milk Thistle Fruit
Complies with the requirements of Identification and Quantitative Standards stated for Milk Thistle Fruit.

Characteristic Features
An oily, mid-brown powder with darker specks, odour slight, taste rather bitter and unpleasant; fragments of the epicarp composed of colourless cells, polygonal in surface view, the lumen appearing fairly large or as a small slit, depending on the orientation; groups of parenchymatous cells of the pigment layer, some containing colouring matter which appears bright red in a Chloral Hydrate mount; very abundant groups of large sclereids of the testa with bright lemon-yellow, pitted walls and a narrow lumen; occasional fragments of small-celled parenchyma with beaded walls; abundant parenchyma of the cotyledons containing oil globules and cluster crystals of calcium oxalate, which also occur scattered; few larger, prism crystals.

ACTION Hepatoprotective.

MISTLETOE HERB Viscaceae

Visci albi herba

Synonyms: Viscum, European Mistletoe.

Mistletoe Herb consists of the dried, young leafy twigs, free from berries, of *Viscum album* L., collected in the spring.

CHARACTERISTICS

Macroscopical Description
Stems Yellow green, dichotomously branched, surface longitudinally striated, up to 7 mm in diameter with white central area.
Leaves Paired, yellowish-green, thick, leathery and glabrous, 2-8 cm in length; elliptical-linear obovate with parallel venation; margin entire, apex obtuse, base narrows to short petiole.

Microscopical Description
Stem Thick-walled, cube shaped, polygonal epidermal cells covered by thick, yellow cuticle forming papilla-like projections; numerous paracytic stomata; narrow cortex composed of thickened, sometimes beaded, parenchyma; ring of collateral vascular bundles with secondary growth, separated by rays widening towards the cortex; occasional arc-shaped groups of pericyclic fibres; collenchymatous phloem; large area of lignified xylem containing narrow diameter (about 10 µm), pitted tracheidal vessels and occasional vessels with spiral, annular or reticulate thickening, fibres similar to those of pericycle, average length 90 µm but up to 200 µm with thick-walled, irregular surfaces, tapering or occasionally forked apices and infrequent oblique pits; rectangular, irregular and isodiametric, thick-walled, pitted parenchyma, some sclereid-like. Some parenchymatous cells of cortex and phloem contain clusters of calcium oxalate up to 50 µm in diameter; infrequent oval or spherical starch grains about 5 µm occur throughout the stem.
Leaf Epidermal cells of both surfaces polygonal with thickened, straight, anticlinal walls, thick, yellow cuticle, smooth but forming papilla-like ridges on leaf margins; numerous paracytic stomata. Isobilateral, undifferentiated mesophyll cells, many containing clusters of calcium oxalate about 40 µm in diameter, others contain a few oval

starch grains. Parallel row of collateral vascular bundles containing yellow or yellowish-brown collenchymatous phloem and small area of lignified conducting elements, fibres and pitted parenchyna.

Odour and Taste
Sharp, characteristic odour and taste.

IDENTIFICATION

Carry out the method for Thin-layer Chromatography as described in Appendix 1, using Solvent System A.

Apply 40 µl of each of the following solutions separately to the plate: (1) extract 1 g powdered Mistletoe Herb with 20 ml methanol (50%) by warming on a water-bath for 10-15 minutes, cool, filter and concentrate to 10 ml; (2) 0.025% rutin in methanol.

Spray the plate with Spray Reagent A and examine in ultraviolet light 366 nm.

Major bands relative to rutin are approximately as follows: white 1.4, white 0.6.

There is yellow fine detail in the range 1.4-0.6.

The chromatogram for Mistletoe Herb may vary and depends to some extent upon its host. However, the two major bands above should be consistent for all samples.

QUANTITATIVE STANDARDS

Foreign Matter
Not more than 2% Appendix 3

Total Ash
Not more than 10% Appendix 4

Ash insoluble in Hydrochloric Acid
Not more than 1.5% Appendix 5

Water-soluble Extractive
Not less than 20% Appendix 7

MATERIAL OF COMMERCE Mistletoe Herb is supplied in whole or cut pieces. It is collected from the wild and obtained mainly from Bulgaria, former Yugoslavia, Albania, Turkey and the former USSR.

Powdered Mistletoe Herb

Complies with the requirements for Identification and Quantitative Standards stated for Mistletoe Herb.

Characteristic Features
Yellowish-green with distinctive odour and taste; fragments of leaf and stem epidermis with thick-walled, polygonal cells with straight anticlinal walls and frequent paracytic stomata; thick, yellow, cuticle, smooth but some areas forming papilla-like projections; abundant lignified tracheids, tracheidal vessels and parenchyma with pitted thickening, occasional small vessels with annular or reticulate thickening; frequent, thick-walled, lignified, pitted fibres; clusters of calcium oxalate free and in parenchymatous cells; occasional starch grains. Frequent, tricolpate pollen grains about 50 μm in diameter, exine with blunt spines.

ACTION Hypotensive.

MOTHERWORT   Labiatae

Leonuri cardiacae herba

Synonym: Leonurus.

Motherwort consists of the dried aerial parts of *Leonurus cardiaca* L. collected when the plant is in flower.

CHARACTERISTICS

Macroscopical Description
Stems Erect, pale green or purplish-brown, stout, square, hairy, up to 1.2 m long with stalked, opposite and decussate leaves and verticillasters of six or twelve small flowers in the axils of the upper leaves.
Leaves Lower leaves palmately three to five-lobed, upper leaves entire, oval with an irregularly serrate margin, an acute apex and the base tapering to a long petiole; upper surface green, smooth; lower surface paler and markedly pubescent.
Flowers Calyx green, bell-shaped with five, equal, pointed lobes; corolla two-lipped, pubescent, white with purplish spots on the lower lip.

Microscopical Description
Stem Ridged, four-angled with a central hollow; epidermal cells longitudinally elongated with occasional diacytic stomata and numerous covering and glandular trichomes; covering trichomes uniseriate, composed of from two to eight cells with slight swellings at the junctions and thick, warty walls; glandular trichomes of the typical Labiatae type with a short, unicellular stalk and a head composed of a single cell or, less frequently, multicellular and rounded, composed of eight cells; cortex narrow, parenchymatous with collenchyma in the ridges; phloem narrow, thin-walled; xylem lignified with small, spirally and annularly thickened vessels and groups of thick-walled fibres.
Leaf Upper epidermal cells straight-walled with a striated cuticle and scattered large, rounded, diacytic stomata; lower epidermal cells with sinuous walls and more numerous stomata; abundant covering and glandular trichomes on both surfaces, particularly on the lower surface, similar to those occurring on the stem, with both types of glandular trichomes equally numerous.
Flower Epidermal cells of the calyx with sinuous anticlinal walls; mesophyll cells containing numerous, small, cluster crystals of calcium oxalate; inner epidermis of the corolla with very numerous covering trichomes similar to those occurring on the stem and leaves; fibrous layer of the anther; pollen grains spherical, 25-30 μm in diameter, with a smooth exine, three pores and three furrows.

Odour and Taste
Strongly aromatic odour; bitter taste.

IDENTIFICATION

Carry out the method for Thin-layer Chromatography as described in Appendix 1, using Solvent System A.

Apply 20 µl of each of the following solutions separately to the plate: (1) extract 1 g powdered Motherwort with 10 ml 60% methanol on a water-bath for 10-15 minutes, cool and filter; (2) 0.025% rutin in methanol.

Spray the plate with Spray Reagent A and examine in ultraviolet light 366 nm.

Major bands relative to rutin are approximately as follows: blue 2.8, blue 2.4, blue 1.4, orange 1.0, whitish-blue 0.75.

QUANTITATIVE STANDARDS

Foreign Matter
Not more than 2%   Appendix 3

Total Ash
Not more than 12%   Appendix 4

Ash Insoluble in Hydrochloric Acid
Not more than 2%   Appendix 5

Water-soluble Extractive
Not less than 15%   Appendix 7

MATERIAL OF COMMERCE Motherwort is supplied as the crushed or chopped herb. It is obtained from many European countries.

Powdered Motherwort

Complies with the requirements for Identification and Quantitative Standards stated for Motherwort.

Characteristic Features
Greyish-green powder with a strong, aromatic odour and a bitter taste; fragments of leaf epidermis with sinuous anticlinal walls and large diacytic stomata; numerous long uniseriate, multicellular covering trichomes and typical Labiatae glandular trichomes of two types; thick-walled, lignified fibres and spirally and annularly thickened vessels from the stem; fragments of the calyx containing small cluster crystals of calcium oxalate; spherical pollen grains with a smooth exine.

ACTION Antispasmodic.

MUGWORT   Compositae

Artemisiae herba

Mugwort consists of the dried leaves and flowering tops of *Artemisia vulgaris* L.

CHARACTERISTICS

Macroscopical Description
Stems Erect, rigid, up to 120 cm, branched, angled and conspicuously grooved; reddish-brown to purple; glabrous or sparsely hairy.
Leaves Base leaves largest, up to 8 cm long, 5 cm wide, lyrate, bipinnately divided, secondary lobes small; margin entire or finely serrate near apex; very shortly petiolate; stem leaves spirally arranged, sessile-amplexicaul, progressively simpler and smaller, leaves near stem apex undivided, lanceolate; all thin and flexible; upper surface dark green, glabrous or very few hairs; lower surface pale greyish-green with thin, cobweb-like, tangled covering of fine hairs; veins not well-marked.
Flower Heads ovoid, 2-4 mm, more or less erect, pedicel short, very small linear bracteoles; grouped in dense leafy terminal panicles; involucre cup-shaped, several rows of densely hairy bracts with narrow central green rib and wide scarious margins; florets orange-brown, sometimes yellow, all tubular and fertile, project only slightly beyond involucre; tips of corolla lobes pointed, recurved.
Fruit Brown achene, up to 1 mm, smooth or finely ribbed, subcylindrical; pappus absent.

Microscopical Description

Stem Section with more or less well-marked rounded protruberances at regular, close intervals; epidermal cells small, outer wall convex, slightly thickened, cuticle slightly irregular; cortex narrow; thin-walled collenchyma in protuberances; endodermis oval to rectangular lignified cells; arcuate groups of moderately thick-walled, lignified pericycle fibres, groups merged in larger stems; narrow phloem; complete ring of lignified xylem from alternating large and small vascular bundles; predominately fibres, larger vessels bordered-pitted; pith extensive, cells large, moderately thickened, variably lignified, few pits. Epidermal cells in surface view long, straight walled, with oblique ends; cuticle smooth or faintly ridged; stomata absent; subepidermal cells with reddish-purple pigment.

Leaf Dorsiventral; palisade one or two, rarely three, layered; midrib slightly raised above, prominent below, meristele small, sclerenchymatous elements absent; epidermal cells, outer wall slightly thickened; above and below midrib cuticle ridged; stomata, in lower epidermis, slightly raised; in surface view upper epidermal cells variably polygonal, anticlinal walls thin, almost straight or slightly sinuous; stomata absent; trichomes very infrequent, T-form with erect stalk of up to four short cells, arms long, almost straight or slightly undulate, tapering gently to point, walls moderately thick; glandular trichomes few; small, stalk biseriate, head sub-spherical; lower epidermal cells much smaller, thin-walled, outline and shape irregular; anomocytic stomata; very numerous T-form trichomes, a few with straight arms, majority with thinner, much longer, coiled and convoluted arms, lumen narrow; few small glandular trichomes.

Flower Central, pigmented, rib of bracts, epidermal cells slightly elongated, straight, thin-walled, occasional stomata; colourless margins, a layer of elongated thin-walled cells; very numerous T-form trichomes, few glandular; edges ciliate. Petal epidermis, reddish-brown, elongated rectangular straight-walled cells. Fibrous layer of anther, fine, widely spaced thickening, lignified; pollen grains about 25 µm, spherical, slightly thick-walled, three well-marked pores, exine smooth. Stigma epidermal cells with short, finger-like papillae.

Odour and Taste

Odour very slightly aromatic; taste weak, faintly bitter.

IDENTIFICATION

Carry out the method for Thin-layer Chromatography as described in Appendix 1, using Solvent System A.

Apply 20 µl of each of the following solutions separately to the plate: (1) extract 1 g powdered Mugwort with 10 ml methanol by warming on a water-bath for 10-15 minutes, cool and filter; (2) 0.025% rutin in methanol.

Spray the plate with Spray Reagent A and examine in ultraviolet light 366 nm.

Major bands relative to rutin are approximately as follows: white/turquoise 2.0, white/turquoise 1.9, yellow 1.5, white/turquoise 1.4, yellow 1.0.

QUANTITATIVE STANDARDS

Foreign Matter
Not more that 3%   Appendix 3

Total Ash
Not more than 8%   Appendix 4

Ash Insoluble in Hydrochloric Acid
Not more than 2%   Appendix 5

Water-soluble Extractive
Not less that 15%   Appendix 7

MATERIAL OF COMMERCE Mugwort is supplied in the cut condition. It is mainly collected from the wild and is obtained from many European countries.

Powdered Mugwort

Complies with the requirements for Identification and Quantitative Standards stated for Mugwort.

Characteristic Features

Yellowish-green powder with an aromatic odour and a faintly aromatic and bitter taste; very abundant T-form covering trichomes occurring in felted masses and on fragments of the epidermises; epidermal cells of the leaves and bracts, in surface view, with straight to sinuous walls and anomocytic stomata; epidermal cells of the stem elongated with underlying layer containing reddish-purple pigment; few glandular

139

trichomes with biseriate stalks and subspherical heads; groups of lignified fibres and vascular tissue from the stems, the larger vessels with bordered pits; large-celled parenchyma from the pith, some with lignified walls; numerous spherical pollen grains, scattered and in dense groups, each with three distinct pores and a smooth exine; fibrous layer of the anther with characteristic, beaded walls; papillose lobes of the stigmas.

ACTION Emmenogogue.

MULLEIN LEAF   Scrophulariaceae

Verbasci folium

Synonyms: Orange Mullein (*Verbascum phlomoides*); Great Mullein, Aaron's Rod (*V. thapsus*).

Mullein Leaf consists of the dried leaves of *Verbascum densiflorum* Bertol. [*V. thapsiforme* Schrad.], *Verbascum phlomoides* L. or *Verbascum thapsus* L.

CHARACTERISTICS

Macroscopical Description
Whole leaves obovate to oblong, sometimes lanceolate, up to 45 cm long and 15 cm broad; thick, soft and felted; apex frequently rounded, occasionally acute or subacute; margin crenate or dentate and somewhat undulating; base decurrent and narrowing to form wings down the short petiole, up to 1 cm wide; upper surface dark greyish-green, lower surface paler, both surfaces and the petiole densely pubescent and woolly; venation pinnate, distinctly raised on the lower surface with the main veins anastomosing near the margin and the smaller veins forming a dense reticulum throughout the lamina.

Microscopical Description
Dorsiventral, the palisade sometimes not well differentiated, composed of one long or two shorter cells, loosely packed; spongy mesophyll with numerous strands of vascular bundles from the smaller veins; upper epidermal cells with wavy walls, those of the lower epidermis more wavy; anomocytic stomata, with three to five surrounding cells on both epidermises, but more numerous on the lower; both surfaces bearing very abundant pluricellular, branched covering trichomes of the candelabra type, composed of a central uniseriate axis of two to eight cells, from which whorls of up to seven or more branch cells arise at the position of the cross walls and from the apex; individual cells with evenly thickened walls, slightly lignified, those of the branches slender, tapering to a point and very long, measuring up to 500 μm, the narrow lumen frequently containing entrapped air; scattered glandular trichomes also occur, composed of a unicellular or bicellular uniseriate stalk and a spheroidal head with one or, occasionally, two cells; midrib with the central meristele containing radiating bands of xylem vessels and a band of collenchyma in the pericycle.

Odour and Taste
No odour; taste mucilaginous and slightly bitter.

IDENTIFICATION

Carry out the method for Thin-layer Chromatography as described in Appendix 1, using Solvent System A.

Apply 20 μl of each of the following solutions separately to the plate: (1) extract 1 g powdered Mullein Leaf with 10 ml methanol by warming on a water-bath for 10-15 minutes, cool and filter; (2) 0.025% rutin in methanol.

Spray the plate with Spray Reagent A and examine in ultraviolet light 366 nm.

Major bands relative to rutin are approximately as follows: bright yellow 2.1, turquoise 1.5, yellow 1.0, turquoise 0.9, yellow 0.75.

QUANTITATIVE STANDARDS

Foreign Matter
Not more than 5%   Appendix 3

Total Ash
Not more than 14%   Appendix 4

Acid Insoluble in Hydrochloric Acid
Not more that 4%   Appendix 5

Water-soluble Extractive
Not less than 20%   Appendix 7

MATERIAL OF COMMERCE Mullein Leaf is supplied in the whole or broken condition. It is harvested mainly from cultivated plants and obtained from European countries, particularly Bulgaria and former Czechoslovakia; also from Egypt.

Powdered Mullein Leaf

Complies with the requirements for Identification and Quantitative Standards stated for Mullein Leaf.

ACTION Expectorant.

MYRRH   Burseraceae

Myrrha

Synonym: Commiphora Resin.

Myrrh is the oleo-gum resin obtained from the stems of *Commiphora molmol* Engler and other species of *Commiphora*.

CHARACTERISTICS

Description
Masses of round or irregular tears of variable size; externally reddish-brown to yellowish-brown covered with a dry, fine powder; fracture brittle, surface oily, rich brown and translucent, frequently showing whitish patches or lines.

Odour and Taste
Aromatic odour; bitter, aromatic and acrid taste.

IDENTIFICATION

A. Triturate 0.1 g crushed Myrrh with 0.5 g sand, shake with 5 ml ether and filter; evaporate the filtrate to dryness in a porcelain dish and expose the residue to bromine vapour. A violet colour is produced.
B. Carry out the method for Thin-layer Chromatography as described in Appendix 1, using a mixture of toluene:ethyl acetate (93:7) as the solvent system.

Apply 20 µl of each of the following solutions separately to the plate: (1) extract 0.5 g finely crushed Myrrh with 5 ml ethanol (96%) on a water-bath for 5 minutes, cool and filter; (2) 0.25% d-bornyl acetate in methanol.

Spray the plate with Spray Reagent D, heat at 105°C for 5-10 minutes then examine in daylight.

Major bands relative to d-bornyl acetate are approximately as follows: red 1.4, red 0.88, red 0.8, pale pinkish red 0.25.

QUANTITATIVE STANDARDS

Foreign Matter
Not more than 4%   Appendix 3

Total Ash
Not more than 9%   Appendix 4

Ash Insoluble in Hydrochloric Acid
Not more than 5%   Appendix 5

Ethanol (90%)-insoluble Residue
Not more than 70%   Appendix 6B

Volatile Oil
Not less than 6%   Appendix 9

MATERIAL OF COMMERCE Myrrh is supplied as irregular masses of agglutinated tears or as small crushed lumps. It is obtained mainly from the Horn of Africa and Arabia.

ACTION Antiseptic.

NETTLE HERB
Urticaceae

Urticae herba

Synonym: Stinging Nettle.

Nettle Herb consists of the dried aerial parts of *Urtica dioica* L., collected during the flowering period.

CHARACTERISTICS

Macroscopical Description

Stems Erect, square, green to purplish or brown, hairy, up to 1.2 m long, bearing stalked, opposite and decussate leaves and four stipules at each node.

Leaves Ovate with an acute to acuminate apex, cordate base and a coarsely serrate margin; dark green on the upper surface with scattered whitish hairs; lower surface paler with numerous prominent hairs particularly over the mid-rib and main veins.

Flowers Small, green, dioecious, occurring as panicles in axils of upper leaves, the male flowers spreading, the female clusters pendulous.

All parts of the plant have stinging hairs, the tips of which break off when touched and cause itching and blistering of the skin.

Microscopical Description

Stem Epidermal cells longitudinally elongated, some enlarged forming cystoliths containing dense, granular masses of calcium carbonate, and occasional anomocytic stomata; covering trichomes of two types, some unicellular, slender, thick-walled, up to 700 μm long, slightly curved and tapering to a pointed apex, others which form the stinging hairs much larger, up to 2 mm long, composed of an elongated tapering cell with a slightly swollen stinging tip which readily breaks off, arising from a raised, multicellular base; occasionally more than one stinging hair arising from the same multicellular base; small glandular trichomes also occur, composed of a unicellular stalk and a rounded head formed of two cells; cortex narrow, parenchymatous with collenchyma in the ridges; vascular tissue composed of a wide phloem and a lignified xylem containing vessels with bordered pits and a few fibres; pith parenchymatous, the inner part often collapsed in older stems; the parenchyma of the phloem and pith containing numerous, small cluster crystals of calcium oxalate arranged in longitudinal rows.

Leaf Dorsiventral; upper epidermal cells with sinuous anticlinal walls, those of the lower epidermis wavy with numerous anomocytic stomata which are absent from the upper epidermis, abundant cystoliths similar to those on the stem occur on both epidermises, also covering trichomes, stinging hairs and glandular trichomes, all of which are especially numerous on the lower epidermis; small cluster crystals of calcium oxalate occur in the spongy mesophyll.

Odour and Taste

Slight odour; bitter taste.

IDENTIFICATION

Carry out the method for Thin-layer Chromatography as described in Appendix 1, using Solvent System A and allowing the solvent front to move a distance of 10 cm above the line of application.

Apply 20 μl of each of the following solutions separately to the plate: (1) extract 1 g powdered Nettle Herb with 10 ml methanol on a water-bath for 10 minutes, cool and filter, (2) 0.025% rutin in methanol.

Spray the plate with Spray Reagent A and examine in ultraviolet light 366 nm.

Major bands relative to rutin are approximately as follows: narrow deep blue 1.9, pale blue 1.8, greenish-blue 1.2.

QUANTITATIVE STANDARDS

Stems above 3 mm in Diameter
Not more than 2%

Foreign Matter
Not more than 2%   Appendix 3

Total Ash
Not more than 20%   Appendix 4

Ash Insoluble in Hydrochloric Acid
Not more than 5%   Appendix 5

Water-soluble Extractive
Not less than 18%   Appendix 7

MATERIAL OF COMMERCE Nettle Herb is usually supplied as broken or crushed material. It is obtained from European countries including the UK. It may cause skin irritation when handled.

Powdered Nettle Herb

Complies with the requirements for Identification and Quantitative Standards stated for Nettle Herb.

Characteristic Features
Green powder with a slight odour and a bitter taste; fragments of leaf epidermis with sinuous or wavy cell walls and anomocytic stomata in the lower epidermis only; cystoliths containing calcium carbonate and numerous covering trichomes; less frequent glandular trichomes; stinging hairs usually with the end cells broken off and the multicellular base still attached to portions of the epidermis; small groups of lignified, bordered-pitted vessels from the stem; parenchyma containing small cluster crystals of calcium oxalate arranged in rows.

ACTION Diuretic.

NETTLE ROOT   Urticaceae

Urticae radix

Synonym: Stinging Nettle Root.

Nettle Root consists of the dried rhizomes and roots of *Urtica dioica* L.

CHARACTERISTICS

Macroscopical Description
Rhizomes cylindrical and tapering, occasionally branched, up to about 6 mm thick at the upper end, and composed of internodes about 1 cm long, alternating with short, slightly swollen nodes, the internodes becoming longer, up to about 3 cm, in the younger part; outer surface yellowish-brown, the internodes with deep longitudinal furrows, numerous smooth, very thin and wiry roots arising from the nodes, pale yellowish-brown, and up to about 5 cm long, but frequently broken off near their origin; fracture of the rhizome fibrous and tough in the outer part, inner surface creamish-white with a central hollow.

Microscopical Description
Rhizome with a narrow cork composed of brown, thin-walled cells, a few rows of tangentially-elongated cortical parenchyma and a pericyclic region with fairly numerous fibres, occurring singly or, more usually, in small groups, individual fibres much elongated with very thick and lignified walls; some cells of the pericycle and outer part of the secondary phloem containing fairly large cluster crystals of calcium oxalate. Cambial region distinct and continuous, with narrow radial groups of vascular tissue separated by very wide medullary rays; secondary phloem mainly parenchymatous with groups of thin-walled sieve tissue; xylem groups dense and completely lignified, containing scattered vessels, isolated or in small groups, associated with moderately thickened xylem parenchymatous cells and numerous thicker-walled fibres with slit-shaped pits; individual vessels with fairly large, closely-arranged bordered pits; the adjacent parenchyma with simple or bordered pits. Medullary rays in the secondary xylem showing alternating areas of lignified and unlignified cells, appearing in transverse section as tangential bands between the groups of vascular tissue, each composed of about five or six layers of cells; the lignified cells have moderately thickened walls and numerous simple pits. Pith composed of rounded, unlignified parenchyma, collapsed in the central part to form a hollow. Root in transverse section showing a very thin cork, narrow phelloderm and secondary phloem and xylem with alternating areas of lignified and unlignified parenchyma in the wide medullary rays, as in the rhizome; in the centre, a diarch strand of primary xylem with a few small vessels.

Odour and Taste
Odourless; taste faintly aromatic and distinctly bitter.

IDENTIFICATION

Carry out the method for Thin-layer Chromatography as described in Appendix 1 using a mixture of toluene: ethyl formate: formic acid (50:40:5) as the solvent system.

Apply 20 µl of each of the following solutions separately to the plate: (1) extract 1 g powdered Nettle Root by refluxing with 10 ml chloroform for 15 minutes. Cool, filter and evaporate to approximately 1 ml; (2) 0.025% quercetin in methanol.

Spray the plate with Spray Reagent C, heat at 105°C for 10-15 minutes and examine in daylight.

Major bands relative to quercetin are approximately as follows: dark grey 3.5, light grey 2.9, light grey 2.45, purple/blue 2.0, blue/grey 0.75, dark grey 0.3.

QUANTITATIVE STANDARDS

Foreign Matter
Not more than 2%   Appendix 3

Total Ash
Not more than 12%   Appendix 4

Ash Insoluble in Hydrochloric Acid
Not more than 3.5%   Appendix 5

Water-soluble Extractive
Not less than 15%   Appendix 7

MATERIAL OF COMMERCE Nettle Root is supplied in whole or cut condition. It is obtained mainly from central and eastern European countries.

Powdered Nettle Root

Complies with the requirements for identification and quantitative standards stated for Nettle Root.

Characteristic Features
A fibrous, pale fawn powder with no odour and a slightly bitter taste; fragments of much elongated pericyclic fibres with thick and lignified walls, occurring singly or in groups; xylem vessels with bordered pits, associated with thick-walled fibres with slit-shaped pits; lignified, moderately thick-walled and pitted parenchyma from the medullary rays of the xylem; abundant thin-walled parenchymatous cells, some containing large cluster crystals of calcium oxalate, which also occur scattered; fragments of brownish cork.

ACTION Prostatic.

OAK BARK   Fagaceae

Quercus cortex

Synonyms: Common, English or Pedunculate Oak Bark (*Quercus robur*); Sessile or Durmast Oak Bark (*Quercus petraea*).

Oak Bark consists of the dried bark from younger stems and branches of *Quercus robur* L. [*Q. pedunculata* Ehrh.] or *Quercus petraea* (Matt.) Liebl. [*Q. sessiliflora* Salisb.].

CHARACTERISTICS

Macroscopical Description
Curved pieces, varying in size and up to about 3.5 mm thick, outer surface usually with a dark, greyish-brown rhytidome, uneven and deeply fissured, but sometimes, on thinner pieces, with a smooth, greyish-green cork marked with darker, transverse lenticels; inner surface pale reddish-brown, fibrous and strongly longitudinally striated; fracture granular in the outer part, fibrous and splintery in the inner part.

Microscopical Description
Cork cells polygonal in surface view, with slightly thickened tangential walls and dense brown contents; parenchyma of the

phelloderm and cortex sometimes with collenchymatous thickening; dense groups of lignified fibres and stone cells in the pericycle and outer part of the secondary phloem, some groups consisting only of fibres or stone cells, but the majority mixed with the fibres usually around the periphery; the stone cells very large, rounded to irregular, with thick, striated walls, a small lumen and numerous branching pits or smaller, more rectangular, with thinner walls and simple pits; the smaller stone cells often with brown colouring matter; some of the parenchymatous cells adjacent to the groups of stone cells containing prisms or cluster crystals of calcium oxalate; fibres thick-walled with a narrow, partially occluded lumen and few pits; the groups surrounded by a calcium oxalate prism crystal sheath with the parenchyma frequently thick-walled and lignified; remainder of the secondary phloem composed of narrow tangential bands of fibres, alternating with wider bands of sieve tissue and parenchyma and separated by narrow medullary rays; fibres similar to those of the pericycle with calcium oxalate prism crystal sheaths; sieve tubes fairly large and thin-walled, with numerous sieve areas on the oblique end walls; parenchyma frequently containing clusters, or occasionally prisms, of calcium oxalate, arranged in short, vertical rows of cells; medullary ray cells with slightly thickened walls.

Odour and Taste
No odour; taste bitter and astringent.

IDENTIFICATION

Carry out the method for Thin-layer Chromatography as described in Appendix 1, using Solvent System E.

Apply 20 µl of the following solution to the plate; extract 5 g of powdered Oak Bark in 20 ml methanol by warming on a water-bath for 20 minutes, cool and filter.

Spray the plate with Spray Reagent F, followed by a separate application of 5 ml potassium hydroxide solution; inspect in daylight.

Major bands relative to the solvent front are approximately as follows: brown 0.6, brown 0.4, brown 0.35, brown 0.3.

QUANTITATIVE STANDARDS

Foreign Matter
Not more than 2%   Appendix 3

Total Ash
Not more than 8%   Appendix 4

Ash Insoluble in Hydrochloric Acid
Not more than 1%   Appendix 5

Water-soluble Extractive
Not less than 10%   Appendix 7

MATERIAL OF COMMERCE Oak Bark is supplied as large cut pieces. It is obtained mainly from eastern and south-eastern European countries.

Powdered Oak Bark

Complies with the requirements for Identification and Quantitative Standards stated for Oak Bark.

Characteristic Features
Reddish-brown powder with no odour and a slightly bitter and astringent taste; abundant groups of sclereids, some large, irregular, thick-walled with branching pits, others smaller, thinner-walled and with simple pits; numerous fibre groups with calcium oxalate prism crystal sheaths; fragments of reddish-brown cork; cluster crystals of calcium oxalate, some contained in parenchyma; occasional fragments of thin-walled sieve tissue with sieve areas on the oblique end walls.

ACTION Astringent.

PARSLEY HERB
Umbelliferae

Petroselini herba

Parsley Herb consists of the dried aerial parts of *Petroselinum crispum* (Mill.) Nyman ex A. W. Hill, especially subsp. *crispum*, normally collected in the second year of growth before flowering.

CHARACTERISTICS

Macroscopical Description
Stems Branched, green, cylindrical and striated, up to 1 mm wide with alternate, trifoliate, stalked leaves and terminal, compound umbels.

Leaves Bright green, glabrous, petiolate, dentate and three-pinnate, segment lobes linear, up to 3 cm long.

Microscopical Description
Stem Epidermal cells polygonal and elongated, some with beaded walls and occasional anomocytic stomata; narrow cortex of collenchyma and parenchymatous cells; xylem of lignified vessels and tracheids with reticulate or bordered-pitted thickening, 30-60 µm in diameter and associated with fibres; pericycle of mature stems may exhibit pitted fibres; pith of isodiametric parenchyma, some with lignified walls; cortical and pith parenchyma containing infrequent starch granules up to 8 µm in diameter; yellow oil ducts occur in the cortex and outer phloem.

Leaf Epidermal cells wavy-walled with intermittently striated cuticle; anomocytic stomata frequent on lower epidermis but present only on margin and tip of upper epidermis; elongated papillose epidermal cells with strongly striated cuticle over veins; single layer of palisade cells frequently containing small cluster and prismatic crystals of calcium oxalate up to 5 µm; midrib with an open arc of collateral bundles with secretory ducts in the phloem of larger bundles containing yellow oil; xylem with lignified vessels having spiral or annular thickening.

Odour and Taste
Characteristic odour; strong and characteristic taste.

IDENTIFICATION

Carry out the method for Thin-layer Chromatography as described in Appendix 1, using Solvent System A.

Apply 20 µl of each of the following solutions separately to the plate: (1) extract 1 g powdered Parsley Herb with 10 ml methanol by warming on a water bath for 10-15 minutes, cool and filter; (2) 0.025% rutin in methanol.

Spray the plate with Spray Reagent A, and examine in ultraviolet light 366 nm.

The major band relative to rutin is approximately as follows: very broad green 1.15.

QUANTITATIVE STANDARDS

Foreign Matter
Not more than 2%   Appendix 3

Total Ash
Not more than 15%   Appendix 4

Ash Insoluble in Hydrochloric Acid
Not more than 4%   Appendix 5

Water-soluble Extractive
Not less than 25%   Appendix 7

MATERIAL OF COMMERCE Parsley Herb is supplied in the rubbed or powdered condition. It is cultivated worldwide in several varieties including curly-leafed and plain-leafed. For medicinal purposes the latter is commonly used, being obtained from European countries.

Powdered Parsley Herb

Complies with the requirements for Identification and Quantitative Standards stated for Parsley Herb.

Characteristic Features
Bright green powder with characteristic odour and strong, characteristic taste. Fragments of leaf with wavy-walled epidermal cells and intermittently striated cuticle, some

with anomocytic stomata; elongated epidermal cells with papillae and strongly striated cuticle; lignified vessels with spiral, annular, reticulate or bordered-pitted thickening; palisade cells containing small cluster or prismatic crystals of calcium oxalate; stem epidermal cells with beaded walls.

ACTION Diuretic.

PARSLEY ROOT Umbelliferae

Petroselini radix

Parsley Root consists of the dried roots of *Petroselinum crispum* (Mill.) Nyman ex A. W. Hill, especially subsp. *tuberosum* (Bernh. ex Rchb.) Soó.

CHARACTERISTICS

Macroscopical Description
Root unbranched, slender, napiform, up to 15 cm long, 1.5-3 cm thick at crown; yellowish-white or pale reddish-yellow; external surface uneven, coarsely wrinkled and transversely furrowed, most markedly in upper part; transversely cut surface shows a distinct brownish cambium zone; outer tissues pale yellowish-white, indistinctly radiate; xylem lemon yellow, darker and distinctly radiate near cambium; central area lighter, less obviously radiate; fracture short, uneven. Few small adventitious roots or scars.

Microscopical Description
Outer layer of three or four rows of small suberised cells; within, a narrow zone of thin-walled parenchymatous cells; phloem wide, medullary rays of varying length, straight or slightly wavy, multiseriate, closely spaced; sieve tissue not well-defined; narrow secretion canals in parenchyma, most numerous near cambium, fewer in outer phloem; xylem of small diameter reticulately-thickened vessels in narrow, irregular radial rows; fibres and secretion canals absent. Parenchyma of bark and xylem contains few, small starch granules.

Odour and Taste
Odour aromatic, characteristic; taste weakly aromatic, sweetish, somewhat sharp.

IDENTIFICATION
Carry out the method for Thin-layer Chromatography as described in Appendix 1, using Solvent System C.

Apply 60 µl of each of the following solutions separately to the plate: (1) extract 1 g powdered Parsley Root by shaking with 10 ml dichloromethane for 20 minutes. Filter, evaporate the filtrate just to dryness and dissolve the residue in 1 ml toluene; (2) 0.1% cineole in toluene.

Spray the plate with Spray Reagent D, heat at 105°C for 10-15 minutes, then examine in daylight.

Major bands relative to cineole are approximated as follows: purple 2.0, dark red 1.6, red 1.3, red 0.55.

The chromatogram exhibits an area of fine detail between 1.25-0.6.

QUANTITATIVE STANDARDS

Foreign Matter
Not more than 2%   Appendix 3

Total Ash
Not more than 8%   Appendix 4

Ash Insoluble in Hydrochloric Acid
Not more than 1%   Appendix 5

MATERIAL OF COMMERCE Parsley Root is supplied in sliced or cut condition. It is obtained mainly from northern and central Europe.

147

Powdered Parsley Root

Complies with the requirements for Identification and Quantitative Standards stated for Parsley Root.

Characteristic Features

Pale creamish-yellow; odour characteristic, aromatic; taste pleasantly aromatic, slightly sweet. Abundant thin-walled parenchyma, unpitted, small intercellular spaces; few, small starch granules; reticulately-thickened lignified vessels, up to 60-70 µm diameter, singly or in small groups, vessel segments short, ends oblique; very few, much narrower, spiral vessels; in some parenchyma, scattered, small, colourless or pale yellowish droplets of oil; ill-defined, pale yellowish secretion canals.

ACTION Carminative, diuretic.

PASSIFLORA   Passifloraceae
Passiflorae herba

Synonym: Passion Flower.

Passiflora consists of the dried aerial parts of *Passiflora incarnata* L. collected during the flowering and fruiting period.

CHARACTERISTICS

Macroscopical Description

Stems Green, greyish-green or brownish, usually less than 5 mm in diameter; rounded, longitudinally striated and often hollow.

Leaves Alternate with furrowed, often twisted petioles, possessing at the apex two extra-floral nectaries; lamina 6-15 cm long, broad, green to brownish-green, palmatifid with three lanceolate lobes covered with fine hairs on the lower surface; margin serrate; tendrils occurring in the axils of the leaves, smooth, round and terminating in cylindrical spirals.

Flowers 5-9 cm in diameter with pedicels up to 8 cm long, arising in the axils of the leaves; five white, elongated petals; calyx of five thick sepals, green on the upper surface, white on the under surface and exhibiting on the upper surface a horn-like extension; involucre of three pointed bracts with papillose margins; five large stamens; greyish-green superior ovary; hairy style with three elongated stigmatic branches.

Fruit 4-5 cm long, oval, flattened and greenish-brown containing numerous seeds 4-6 mm long, 3-4 mm wide and 2 mm thick, with a brownish-yellow, pitted surface.

Microscopical Description

Stem Transverse section of older stem showing epidermis of isodiametric cells with strongly thickened, convex, external walls; some cells containing crystals of calcium oxalate, others developing uniseriate trichomes two to four cells long, terminating in a rounded point and frequently hooked; hypodermis consisting of a layer of tangentially elongated cells, outer cortex with groups of collenchyma, both containing cells with brown, tanniferous contents; isolated yellow fibres in the pericycle with partially lignified walls; inner cortex of parenchymatous cells containing cluster crystals of calcium oxalate; xylem consisting of groups of vessels up to 300 µm in diameter with pitted, lignified walls accompanied by yellow-walled, lignified tracheids; pith of lignified parenchyma containing numerous starch granules 3-8 µm in diameter, simple or as aggregates.

Leaf Both epidermises with sinuous anticlinal walls and numerous anomocytic stomata in the lower epidermis, which also shows numerous uniseriate covering trichomes of one to three cells, terminal cells comparatively long, pointed and curved; groups of brown tannin cells occur in the marginal teeth and in the mesophyll; cluster crystals of calcium oxalate 10-20 μm isolated in the mesophyll or arranged in files associated with the veins.

Flower Upper epidermis of the sepals consisting of large, irregular, polygonal cells with some thickened walls, striated cuticle, rare stomata and numerous small crystals of calcium oxalate; the lower epidermis comprising two layers, the outer layer consisting of polygonal cells with numerous stomata and small crystals of calcium oxalate and the inner layer of smaller polygonal cells. Epidermal cells of the petals papillose, especially in the filiform appendices. Pollen grains 65-75 μm in diameter with cross-ridged surface and three acuminate germinal pores.

Fruit Pericarp composed of large cells with few stomata and groups of calcium oxalate crystals; endocarp of thickened, sclerous cells.

Odour and Taste
No distinctive odour; bitter taste.

IDENTIFICATION

Carry out the method for Thin-layer Chromatography as described in Appendix 1, using Solvent System A.

Apply 20 μl of each of the following solutions separately to the plate: (1) extract 1 g powdered Passiflora with 10 ml 60% methanol on a water-bath for 10-15 minutes cool and filter; (2) 0.025% rutin in methanol.

Spray the plate with Spray Reagent A and examine in ultraviolet light 366 nm.

Major bands relative to rutin are approximately as follows: blue 2.3, orange 1.35, green 0.7, orange 0.6.

QUANTITATIVE STANDARDS

Foreign Matter
Not more than 3%   Appendix 3

Total Ash
Not more than 11%   Appendix 4

Ash Insoluble in Hydrochloric Acid
Not more than 3%   Appendix 5

Water-soluble Extractive
Not less than 15%   Appendix 7

MATERIAL OF COMMERCE Passiflora may be supplied as the chopped or crushed herb. It is obtained chiefly from the USA and the West Indies.

Powdered Passiflora

Complies with the requirements for Identification and Quantitative Standards stated for Passiflora.

Characteristic Features
Greenish-brown powder with no odour and a bitter taste; leaf epidermis with anomocytic stomata and uniseriate trichomes with large, curved, terminal cells; tanniferous cells; cluster crystals of calcium oxalate; yellow, partially lignified fibres; brownish-yellow, pitted fragments of seed testa.

ACTION Sedative.

PEPPERMINT LEAF   Labiatae

Menthae piperitae folium

Peppermint Leaf consists of the whole or cut dried leaves of *Mentha × piperita* L.

This material complies with the requirements of the European Pharmacopoeia for Peppermint Leaf.

MATERIAL OF COMMERCE Peppermint Leaf is supplied in the whole, broken or crushed condition. It is obtained principally from northern and eastern Europe and the USA.

ACTION Carminative.

PILEWORT HERB

Ranunculaceae

Ficariae herba

Synonym: Lesser Celandine.

Pilewort Herb consists of the dried aerial parts of *Ficaria ranunculoides* Moench [*Ranunculus ficaria* L.] collected during the flowering period.

CHARACTERISTICS

Macroscopical Description

Leaves Rosette of larger leaves, petiole long, sheathed at base; smaller, shortly petiolate, stem leaves; all soft, fleshy; leaves simple, angular-cordate, up to 3 or 4 cm long, somewhat wider; margin variable from almost entire to crenate, rarely dentate; venation obscurely palmate, larger veins slightly depressed on upper surface; petiole smooth with shallow groove above; sheathing bases colourless or pale mauve.

Stems Erect, simple or infrequently branched, up to 20-25 cm, fine longitudinal ridges. Stem, leaf and petiole largely glabrous; infrequent, caducous, white, cottony trichomes on younger organs.

Flowers Solitary, terminal, up to 3 cm diameter, three sepals, ovate, light green, margin yellowish, narrow, markedly recurved; eight to twelve petals, elongated ovoid, bright yellow, glossy above, somewhat greenish-yellow below; stamens numerous, darker yellow, filaments short; carpels numerous, free, pale green.

Microscopical Description

Leaf Dorsiventral; palisade, single layer, cells short; spongy mesophyll, multilayered, intercellular spaces well-defined; upper epidermal cells rectangular to polygonal, variable, anticlinal walls thin, some very finely beaded, almost straight or slightly undulate, stomata numerous, anomocytic; lower epidermal cells similar shape and size to upper, anticlinal walls more wavy, sinuations shallow, not angular, stomata almost twice as frequent; petiole epidermal cells narrow, elongated rectangular, anticlinal walls thin, straight, cuticle finely striated, stomata infrequent; towards leaf base infrequent unicellular trichomes, long, mostly bent or twisted, smooth, moderately-thickened wall, wide lumen, apex bluntly pointed, base con-spicuously constricted.

Flower Epidermal cells of pedicel like those of petiole, stomata relatively large, axially orientated, more numerous; long unicellular trichomes, towards upper region; sepal upper epidermal cells slightly elongated-rectangular, variable, anticlinal walls almost straight or with slight angular sinuations, few stomata; lower epidermal cells similar, sinuations less angular, stomata more numerous; marginal epidermal cells longer, almost straight-walled, stomata infrequent; petal upper and lower epidermal cells similar, at tip, small, irregularly shaped, feebly sinuous, progressively longer, narrower and straight-walled towards base, faint longitudinal striations, stomata absent; anther fibrous layer, cells small, thickenings well-marked, pollen grains yellowish, about 40-45 µm, almost spherical, three indistinct pores, exine very finely pitted; carpels with bluntly-pointed or slightly bulbous papillae at apex, lower region with short, erect, unicellular lanceolate trichomes, conspicuously constricted at base, apex acutely pointed, wall smooth, only moderately thickened, lumen wide.

Odour and Taste

Little odour; taste slightly bitter and acrid.

IDENTIFICATION

Carry out the method for Thin-layer Chromatography as described in Appendix 1, using Solvent System B, allowing the solvent to ascend 13.5 cm.

Apply 40 µl of the following solutions to the plate: (1) extract 2 g powdered Pilewort Herb by heating under reflux with 10 ml ethanol (70%) for 10 minutes, cool and filter. Evaporate the clear filtrate to approximately 5 ml; (2) 0.1% aescin in methanol.

Spray the plate with Spray Reagent D, heat at 105°C for 10 minutes and examine in daylight.

Major bands relative to aescin are approximately as follows: purple 1.7, brown 0.65, grey 0.45.

The chromatogram exhibits an area of yellow and purple fine detail in the range 1.4-0.9.

QUANTITATIVE STANDARDS

Foreign Matter
Not more than 4%   Appendix 3

Total Ash
Not more than 16%   Appendix 4

Ash Insoluble in Hydrochloric Acid
Not more than 9%   Appendix 5

Water-soluble Extractive
Not less than 12%   Appendix 7

MATERIAL OF COMMERCE Pilewort Herb is supplied as cut herb. It is obtained from European countries.

Powdered Pilewort Herb

Complies with the requirements for Identification and Quantitative Standards stated for Pilewort Herb.

Characteristic Features
Dull green, slight leafy odour, faintly bitter taste; sinuous-walled epidermal cells, numerous anomocytic stomata, relatively large palisade cells; thin-walled elongated rectangular parenchyma, strands of narrow spiral and annular xylem elements, embedded in parenchyma; few short lanceolate trichomes, pollen grains, fibrous layer of anther.

ACTION Astringent.

POKE ROOT   Phytolaccaceae

Phytolaccae americanae radix

Synonym: Pokeweed Root.

Poke Root consists of the dried roots of *Phytolacca americana* L. [*Phytolacca decandra* L.] collected in autumn.

CHARACTERISTICS

Macroscopical Description
Root large and tuberous but occurring in commerce in transverse or longitudinal slices or chopped pieces; outer surface yellowish, reddish or greyish-brown, longitudinally wrinkled and sometimes with narrow, transverse annulations; inner surface hard, light brown or cream; fracture fibrous; transverse surface showing several concentric rings of fibro-vascular bundles, alternating with lighter bands of parenchyma.

Microscopical Description
Cork composed of a few layers of thin-walled cells, polygonal in surface view; phelloderm parenchymatous and thin-walled; narrow vascular bundles in concentric rings produced by successive cambia, each bundle with a small group of sieve tissue, a conspicuous cambium and a larger group of xylem composed of numerous fibres and scattered vessels associated with xylem parenchyma; the fibres and vessels show no reaction for lignin; vessels occurring singly or in small groups, fairly large with reticulately thickened walls or with transversely elongated bordered pits; parenchyma between the bundles and forming the ground tissue thin-walled and filled with starch granules or containing bundles of closely-packed needle crystals of calcium oxalate; occasional cells with brownish resin.

Odour and Taste
Odour faint, somewhat 'earthy'; taste sweetish and acrid.

IDENTIFICATION

Carry out the method for Thin-layer Chromatography as described in Appendix 1, using Solvent System B, allowing the solvent to ascend 13.5 cm.

Apply 40 µl of the following solutions to the plate: (1) extract 2 g powdered Poke Root by heating under reflux with 10 ml ethanol (70%) for 10 minutes, cool and filter. Evaporate the clear filtrate to approximately

5 ml; (2) 0.1% aescin in methanol.

Spray the plate with Spray Reagent D, heat at 105°C for 10 minutes and examine in daylight.

Major bands relative to aescin are approximately as follows: brown 1.65, brown 1.4, brown 1.15, brown 0.6, brown 0.4*.

* This is the most prominent band of the chromatogram.

QUANTITATIVE STANDARDS

Foreign Matter
Not more than 3%   Appendix 3

Total Ash
Not more than 14%   Appendix 4

Ash Insoluble in Hydrochloric Acid
Not more than 6%   Appendix 5

Water-soluble Extractive
Not less than 20%   Appendix 7

MATERIAL OF COMMERCE Poke Root is supplied in sliced form. It is obtained from the USA.

Powdered Poke Root

Complies with the requirements for Identification and Quantitative Standards stated for Poke Root.

Characteristic Features
Brownish-buff with a slightly bitter taste, strongly sternutatory. Starch granules occasionally compound but mostly simple, spherical to ovoid, up to 35 µm in diameter; abundant fibres, usually in groups, long with moderately thickened walls and few pits; groups of xylem parenchymatous cells with numerous pits and slightly thickened walls; fairly large vessels, singly or in small groups, usually associated with fibres and xylem parenchyma, reticulately thickened or with bordered pits; abundant thin-walled parenchyma, some cells containing long needle crystals of calcium oxalate which also occur broken and scattered; occasional fragments of cork.

ACTION Anti-inflammatory.

PRICKLY ASH BARK   Rutaceae

Zanthoxyli cortex

Synonym: Southern Prickly Ash Bark.

Prickly Ash Bark consists of the dried bark of *Zanthoxylum clava-herculis* L.

CHARACTERISTICS

Macroscopical Description
Transversely curved or flattened pieces, 1-4 mm thick, or single quills, 5-40 cm long; outer surface light grey to greyish-brown with prominent limpet-shaped cork projections often bearing short spines; inner surface light yellowish-brown with no obvious striations or glistening crystals; fracture short, fractured surface yellowish-white.

Microscopical Description
Stratified cork comprising several layers of cells with lignified walls alternating with several rows of tabular cells with thickened walls, both types containing cluster crystals of calcium oxalate; outer cortex of collenchymatous cells, inner cortex parenchymatous with occasional scattered groups of lignified sclereids and fibres; occasional prismatic crystals of calcium oxalate 20-25 µm long in cortex; phloem containing bands of large, yellow secretion cells, cluster crystals of calcium oxalate, 20-35 µm in diameter, and frequent simple or two to four

compound spherical starch granules in the medullary rays and phloem parenchyma.

Odour and Taste
Slight odour; bitter, acrid taste, becoming pungent.

IDENTIFICATION

Carry out the method for Thin-layer Chromatography as described in Appendix 1, using a mixture of toluene:ethyl formate:anhydrous formic acid (50:40:10) as the Solvent System.

Apply 20 μl of each of the following solutions separately to the plate: (1) extract 1 g powdered Prickly Ash Bark with 10 ml methanol by refluxing on a water-bath for 10-15 minutes, cool, filter and concentrate to about 5 ml; (2) 0.025% rutin in methanol.

Spray the plate with Spray Reagent A and examine in ultraviolet light 366 nm.

Major bands relative to rutin are approximately as follows: blue 3.0, yellow 1.5, blue 1.2, blue 0.8.

There should be no whitish bands at 2.85, 2.6 and 1.5, to confirm absence of Northern Prickly Ash Bark (*Zanthoxylum americanum* Mill.)

QUANTITATIVE STANDARDS

Foreign Matter
Not more than 2%   Appendix 3

Total Ash
Not more than 6%   Appendix 4

Ash Insoluble in Hydrochloric Acid
Not more than 1.5%   Appendix 5

Water-soluble Extractive
Not less than 10%   Appendix 7

MATERIAL OF COMMERCE Prickly Ash Bark is supplied as curved or flattened pieces, occasionally as quills and frequently in small broken pieces. It is obtained from central and southern USA.

Powdered Prickly Ash Bark

Complies with the requirements for Identification and Quantitative Standards stated for Prickly Ash Bark.

Characteristic Features
Light greyish-brown powder with a slight odour and a bitter, acrid taste; fragments of lignified cork; abundant parenchymatous cells, some with large yellow secretion cells; groups of thickened, pitted fibres, some with only the middle lamella lignified; pitted lignified sclereids; frequent cluster crystals of calcium oxalate, occasional prismatic crystals of calcium oxalate, frequent starch granules.

ACTION Circulatory stimulant.

PSYLLIUM SEED   Plantaginaceae

Psyllii semen

Synonyms: Dark, Spanish or French Psyllium, Flea Seed.

Psyllium Seed consists of the ripe, whole, dry seeds of *Plantago afra* L. *[Plantago psyllium* L.] or *Plantago indica* L. *[Plantago arenaria* Waldst. et Kit.].

This material complies with the requirements

of the European Pharmacopoeia for Psyllium Seed.

MATERIAL OF COMMERCE Psyllium is supplied as whole seeds or powder. It is obtained mainly from southern France.

ACTION Bulk-forming laxative.

PULSATILLA

Ranunculaceae

Pulsatillae herba

Synonym: Pasque Flower.

Pulsatilla consists of the dried aerial parts of *Pulsatilla vulgaris* Miller [*Anemone pulsatilla* L.] or *Pulsatilla pratensis* (L.) Miller collected during the flowering stage.

CHARACTERISTICS

Macroscopical Description

Scape Unbranched flower-bearing rigid scape, up to 20 cm long and 2-4 mm wide, arising in a rosette of basal, petiolate leaves from a more or less vertical rhizome; fracture short, solid in the lower region, hollow in the upper region; 2-3 cm below the terminal flower, at a slight swelling, three closely approximated, almost sessile, involucral bracteoles each divided almost to the base into a number of narrow, linear segments; numerous hairs on the bracteoles and at the swelling.

Leaves Slender, flexible petioles, angular or somewhat flattened, greenish-fawn and bearing numerous silky hairs; lamina light greyish-green, bi- or tri-pinnately divided, incisions quite deep; in *P. vulgaris* the ultimate lobes almost linear and the apex acute; in *P. pratensis* incisions less deep and the apex sub-acute; veins slightly sunken on upper surface, more prominent on lower surface; hairs numerous along the margins and over the veins, especially on the lower surface.

Flowers Single, terminal, campanulate; perianth of six imbricated, more or less elliptical, petaloid sepals, usually violet to purple in *P. vulgaris*, but more variable, purple, red, greenish-yellow or white in *P. pratensis*; outer surface lighter coloured with silky hairs; stamens indefinite. Flowers of *P. vulgaris* erect, sepals spreading and two to three times the length of the stamens; flowers of *P. pratensis* nodding, sepals not spreading and less than one and a half times the length of the stamens.

Fruit (if present) Dark brown, elongated ovoid-conical, slightly laterally compressed achenes, up to 5 or 6 mm long and 1-2 mm wide, with a tail up to 5 cm long and 0.5 mm thick, tapering to a point, densely covered with upwardly directed silky hairs.

Microscopical Description

Scape Epidermis of cuboid cells, finely ridged cuticle; cortex one tenth of radius, small parenchymatous cells containing chloroplasts; xylem of radially alternating large and small vascular bundles within a complete ring of sclerenchymatous cells; bundles with an outer cap of slender fibres with narrow lumen, surrounded by a sheath of two to three cells of thin-walled, non-lignified parenchymatous cells and separated by lignified parenchymatous cells, pith comprising more than half the diameter, rounded cells with moderately thickened, lignified walls; leaf stalk similar.

Leaf Upper epidermal cells almost equal sided or elongated rectangular, with almost straight to slightly sinuous, inconspicuously beaded anticlinal walls, slightly and unevenly thickened; few unicellular covering trichomes over the veins, arising from a single small cell surrounded by a rosette of five or six cells, up to 500 µm long, almost straight, of uniform diameter 15-20 µm along most of the length, tapering gradually near the apex to a point; lumen narrow or almost obliterated; stomata absent or very infrequent. Lower epidermal cells similar in shape and size to upper epidermal cells but anticlinal walls distinctly sinuous, thicker and more beaded; covering trichomes similar but more numerous; numerous anomocytic stomata.

Flower Outer epidermal cells of petaloid sepals markedly sinuous with thin anticlinal walls, numerous covering trichomes and anomocytic stomata; inner epidermal cells papillose with slightly wavy walls. Pollen grains ellipsoidal to globular, relatively thick exine finely granular, 25-35 µm in diameter, three furrows and three pores.

Odour and Taste

Very little odour; slight but acrid and pungent taste.

IDENTIFICATION

Carry out the method for Thin-layer Chromatography as described in Appendix 1, using Solvent System A.

Apply 20 µl of each of the following solutions separately to the plate: (1) extract 1 g powdered Pulsatilla with 10 ml methanol by warming on a water-bath for 10-15 minutes, cool and filter; (2) 0.025% rutin in methanol.

Spray the plate with Spray Reagent A and examine in ultraviolet light 366 nm.

Major bands relative to rutin are approximately as follow: narrow blue 1.8, whitish 1.67, reddish-orange 1.3, blue 1.05.

QUANTITATIVE STANDARDS

Foreign Matter
Not more than 3%   Appendix 3

Total Ash
Not more than 10%   Appendix 4

Ash Insoluble in Hydrochloric Acid
Not more than 2%   Appendix 5

Water-soluble Extractive
Not less than 20%   Appendix 7

MATERIAL OF COMMERCE Pulsatilla is supplied in the broken or crushed condition. It is obtained from many countries of Europe.

Powdered Pulsatilla

Complies with the requirements for Identification and Quantitative Standards stated for Pulsatilla.

Characteristic Features
Greenish-brown powder with little odour and a slight but acrid taste with a lingering pungent sensation; leaf epidermis with mainly sinuous, beaded-walled cells with numerous anomocytic stomata; scape epidermis with elongated cells, cuticular striations and few stomata; unicellular, smooth-walled covering trichomes with narrow lumen; a few more or less rectangular, moderately thick-walled, sclerenchymatous cells; pollen grains.

ACTION Sedative.

PUMPKIN SEED   Cucurbitaceae

Cucurbitae peponis semen

Pumpkin Seed consists of the dried, ripe seeds of *Cucurbita pepo* L. or its cultivars.

CHARACTERISTICS

Macroscopical Description
The seeds are ovate, constricted at one end forming a short, blunt extension; flat or weakly biconvex; up to 25 mm long and 12-14 mm wide, 3-4 mm thick; on both faces, close to edge, an encircling ridge and groove, 1-2 mm wide, absent from projection; testa creamish-white to pale beige with a satiny sheen, smooth or with irregular wrinkles; texture brittle, somewhat papery; inner surface of seed coat fawnish-white, dull, rough or scurfy. The seed is non-endospermic. Embryo easily separated from testa, more or less entirely covered in a dark olive-green pellicle, with metallic lustre; light patches of inner seed coat may be adherent. Embryo pale greenish-yellow, oily; large, almost flat cotyledons, small conical radical at constricted end of seed; inner surfaces of cotyledons with three or five rudimentary veins, palmately arranged.

Microscopical Description
Epidermal cells of testa, erect, prismatic, up to 200 µm long; walls thin, bearing slender vertical strips of thickening, usually sinuous in upper portion; in surface view polygonal, large with conspicuous beads; starch grains abundant, up to 5 µm, simple but frequently clumped; a band, about six cells deep, of small, thin-walled, isodiametric or little elongated parenchymatous cells, finely reticulately thickened and strongly lignified; a few larger, irregular simple pits; a single layer of large, sub-rectangular sclereids, lumen narrow, ovoid, walls very thick and conspicuously layered, pits few and not well-defined, only middle lamella

and primary wall strongly lignified; in surface view the sclereids are somewhat elongated and the anticlinal walls deeply sinuous. Internal to the sclereid band several layers of progressively larger lignified parenchymatous cells with very fine reticulate thickening; the cells, having short arm-like projections, form a spongy, lacunose tissue; areas of contact between branches of cells have quite large simple perforations. Innermost layers less well-defined, parenchymatous, largest cells internally; greenish chromoplasts present. Cotyledon cells variable, very thin-walled, containing oily globules and aleurone grains up to 4 µm.

Odour and Taste
The seed is odourless. The embryo has a bland, oily, slightly nut-like taste.

IDENTIFICATION

Carry out the method for Thin-layer Chromatography as described in Appendix 1, using a mixture of chloroform: absolute ethanol (95:5) as the solvent system.

Apply 20 µl of the following solution to the plate: extract 1g powdered Pumpkin Seed with 10 ml methanol by warming on a water bath for 10-15 minutes, cool and filter. Evaporate the filtrate to approximately 2 ml.

Spray the plate with Spray Reagent D, heat at 105°C for 15 minutes and examine in daylight.

Major bands relative to the solvent front are approximately as follows: red 0.85, red 0.8, red 0.75, red 0.65, red 0.5, red 0.2.

QUANTITATIVE STANDARDS

Foreign Matter
Not more than 2%   Appendix 3

Total Ash
Not more than 7%   Appendix 4

MATERIAL OF COMMERCE Pumpkin Seed is supplied as whole seed. It is obtained from many countries but the cultivars used medicinally are grown mainly in south-eastern Europe.

Powdered Pumpkin Seed

Complies with the requirements for the Identification and Quantitative Standards stated for Pumpkin Seed.

ACTION Prostatic.

QUASSIA   Simaroubaceae

Quassiae lignum

Synonyms: Bitter Wood, Jamaica Quassia.

Quassia consists of the dried stem-wood of *Picrasma excelsa* (Sw.) Planch.

CHARACTERISTICS

Macroscopical Description
Chips of varying length, yellowish-white in colour, smooth-grained and easily splitting longitudinally, transverse surface diffuse porous with distinct medullary rays and false annual rings; tangential surface rippled.

Microscopical Description
Transverse section showing vessels up to 200 µm in diameter, occurring isolated or in

groups of two to eleven, associated with thin-walled xylem parenchyma and forming tangential bands alternating with bands of thick-walled fibres; other, more continuous bands of parenchyma forming false annual rings; medullary rays composed of radially elongated cells containing scattered starch granules, mostly simple and spherical, up to 20 µm in diameter, and prism crystals of calcium oxalate, each enclosed in a lignified sheath; starch granules and calcium oxalate crystals also occurring in xylem parenchyma; longitudinal sections showing the vessels with numerous small, closely arranged bordered pits and fibres, up to 900 µm long and 18 µm wide, in storied arrangement; medullary rays mostly multiseriate. All elements lignified.

Odour and Taste
Odourless; intensely bitter taste.

IDENTIFICATION

Carry out the method for Thin-layer Chromatography as described in Appendix 1 using a mixture of chloroform: methanol (9:1) as the solvent system.

Apply 20 µl of each of the following solutions separately to the plate: (1) extract 1 g powdered Quassia with 10 ml methanol on a water-bath for 10-15 minutes, cool, filter and concentrate to about 2 ml; (2) 0.1% quercetin in methanol.

Spray the plate with Spray Reagent C, heat at 105°C for 5-10 minutes then examine in both daylight and ultraviolet light 366 nm.

Major bands relative to quercetin are approximately as follows:

In daylight - purple bands at 5.9, 4.5 and 3.0.

In ultraviolet light 366 nm - purplish-brown bands at 4.9, 4.5, 3.5 and 2.6.

QUANTITATIVE STANDARDS

Foreign Matter
Not more than 2%   Appendix 3

Total Ash
Not more than 6%   Appendix 5

Water-soluble Extractive
Not less than 4%   Appendix 7

MATERIAL OF COMMERCE Quassia is supplied as chips or rasping. It is obtained from the West Indies.

Powdered Quassia

Complies with the requirements for Identification and Quantitative Standards stated for Quassia.

Characteristic Features
Pale yellowish-buff powder with no odour and an intensely bitter taste; totally lignified; fragments of vessels with minute oval or hexagonal bordered pits; abundant thick-walled fibres; parenchymatous cells, some containing prismatic crystals of calcium oxalate; scattered starch granules.

ACTION Appetite stimulant.

QUEEN'S DELIGHT   Euphorbiaceae

Stillingiae radix

Synonyms: Queen's Root, Yaw Root.

Queen's Delight consists of the dried roots of *Stillingia sylvatica* L.

CHARACTERISTICS

Macroscopical Description
Cylindrical or fusiform pieces of varying length, 0.5-2 cm in diameter but larger pieces usually split longitudinally; outer surface dull reddish-brown and finely longitudinally striated, the thicker pieces with deep transverse cracks at intervals; bark easily removed revealing a yellowish-brown wood with deep longitudinal grooves and projecting fibres; fracture tough and fibrous. Transversely cut surface showing a narrow bark, dark reddish-brown in the outer part and paler on the inner side, and a porous, finely radiate xylem, pinkish-white to yellowish in colour.

Microscopical Description
Cork composed of several layers of brown, thin-walled lignified cells, polygonal in surface view; secondary phloem parenchymatous with scattered fibres occurring singly or, more usually, in small groups, individual fibres very long and narrow, thick-walled and slightly lignified with a small lumen; some of the parenchymatous cells with red-

dish-brown contents, the remainder containing abundant starch granules and fairly large cluster crystals of calcium oxalate; secondary xylem distinctly radiate with numerous unlignified, uniseriate or biseriate medullary rays alternating with bands of lignified vascular tissue one to three cells wide; the medullary ray cells thin-walled and containing abundant starch granules or, occasionally, reddish-brown resin or cluster crystals of calcium oxalate; the rays of vascular tissue containing scattered groups of from one to six vessels with reticulate thickening embedded in a ground tissue composed of tracheids, tracheidal-vessels, fibres and pitted xylem parenchyma. Pith, when present, composed of unlignified parenchyma containing starch granules or, occasionally, reddish-brown resinous matter.

Odour and Taste
Odour faintly aromatic; taste slightly bitter, acrid and unpleasant.

IDENTIFICATION

Carry out the method for Thin-layer Chromatography as described in Appendix 1, using Solvent System C.

Apply 60 µl of each of the following solutions separately to the plate: (1) extract 1 g powdered Queen's Delight by shaking with 10 ml of dichloromethane for 20 minutes. Filter, evaporate the filtrate just to dryness and dissolve the residue in 1 ml of toluene; (2) 0.1% cineole in toluene.

Spray the plate with Spray Reagent D, heat at 105°C for 10-15 minutes and examine in daylight.

Major bands relative to cineole are approximately as follows: purple 2.05, brown 1.25, brown 0.75, purple 0.2.

QUANTITATIVE STANDARDS

Foreign Matter
Not more than 3%   Appendix 3

Total Ash
Not more than 6%   Appendix 4

Ash Insoluble in Hydrochloric Acid
Not more than 2%   Appendix 5

Water-soluble Extractive
Not less than 5%   Appendix 7

MATERIAL OF COMMERCE Queen's Delight is supplied as tough pieces of very fibrous root. It is obtained from southeastern USA.

Powdered Queen's Delight

Complies with the requirements for Identification and Quantitative Standards stated for Queen's Delight.

Characteristic Features
Pale buff to pinkish-brown with an aromatic odour and a bitter and acrid taste; the powder is sternutatory; abundant starch granules, very variable in size, up to about 40 µm in diameter, spherical to ovoid or irregular in outline, mostly simple but occasionally compound with two or three components, central hilum distinct, circular or more usually a two or three-rayed cleft; scattered cluster crystals of calcium oxalate up to about 70 µm in diameter; long, narrow fibres, singly or in groups, with strongly thickened walls; numerous groups of vascular tissue composed of tracheids with moderately thickened walls and small bordered pits associated with fibres and pitted parenchyma; vessels with reticulate thickening; large-celled thin-walled parenchyma, some with reddish-brown contents; occasional fragments of cork.

ACTION Expectorant.

RASPBERRY LEAF

Rosaceae

Rubi idaei folium

Raspberry Leaf consists of the dried leaflets of *Rubus idaeus* L.

CHARACTERISTICS

Macroscopical Description

Leaves, three pinnate, sometimes five or seven; laterals opposite and sessile, terminal leaflet larger and petiolate. Leaflets, upper surface olive green, lower white and densely pubescent; ovate, 3-12 cm long and 1.5-9 cm wide; apex acute, base subcordate or cordate, margin irregularly serrate; venation pinnate terminating in mucronate marginal teeth; occasional prickles occur at base of midrib lower surface. Rachis 2-7 cm long, pale green, cylindrical, with small recurved prickles and longitudinal furrow on upper surface; paired, adnate, basal stipules.

Microscopical Description

Epidermal cells of upper surface polygonal with sinuous anticlinal walls, some beaded; oval hydathodes present in marginal teeth; lower surface with wavy, thin-walled cells and numerous anomocytic stomata; cuticle smooth; upper surface with frequent cicatrices or unicellular, conical, thick-walled, lignified, covering trichomes, some with spiral markings and up to 500 µm in length, base pitted; lower surface with numerous unicellular, thick-walled, non-lignified covering trichomes with blunt apices and smooth base, curled and convoluted to form a 'tomentum' which obliterates the surface cells; occasional glandular trichomes composed of multicellular, biseriate stalk and a multicellular head occur on epidermises of midrib and larger veins. Dorsiventral, a double palisade layer may occur in cultivated varieties; scattered cluster crystals of calcium oxalate, about 30 µm in diameter, in rounded palisade idioblasts, crystals up to 45 µm in the midrib mesophyll. Midrib with single, crescent-shaped collateral bundle containing narrow lignified vessels and tracheids with spiral or annular thickening; parenchyma associated with bundle often containing files of small clusters or prisms of calcium oxalate. Prickles of lower midrib composed of elongated sclereids with thickened walls and occasional pits.

Odour and Taste

Odour faint; taste slightly bitter and astringent.

IDENTIFICATION

Carry out the method for Thin-layer Chromatography as described in Appendix 1, using Solvent System A.

Apply 20 µl of each of the following solutions separately to the plate: (1) extract 1 g powdered Raspberry Leaf with 10ml methanol by warming on a water-bath for 10-15 minutes; cool, filter and concentrate to 2 ml; (2) 0.025% rutin in methanol.

Spray the plate with Spray Reagent A and examine in ultraviolet light 366 nm.

Major bands relative to rutin are approximately as follows: yellow 1.6, yellow 1.5, yellow 1.4, yellow 0.85, yellow 0.8. These yellow bands are interspersed by turquoise fine detail.

QUANTITATIVE STANDARDS

Foreign Matter
Not more than 3%   Appendix 3

Total Ash
Not more than 8%   Appendix 4

Ash Insoluble in Hydrochloric Acid
Not more than 2%   Appendix 5

Water-soluble Extractive
Not less than 12%   Appendix 7

MATERIAL OF COMMERCE Raspberry Leaf is supplied as large felted masses. It is obtained from European countries.

Powdered Raspberry Leaf

Complies with the requirements for Identification and Quantitative Standards stated for Raspberry Leaf.

Characteristic Features

Pale greyish-green powder with a faint odour

159

and slightly bitter, astringent taste; polygonal cells with thickened, sinuous, often beaded anticlinal walls; thin-walled polygonal cells with wavy anticlinal walls, accompanied by numerous anomocytic stomata; abundant, unicellular, covering trichomes, some with thick, lignified walls and pitted bases, others non-lignified, thick-walled, curled and convoluted, free or forming a 'tomentum'; abundant cluster crystals of calcium oxalate; narrow, lignified vessels and tracheids with spiral or annular thickening; occasional elongated sclereids from the prickles and fibres from the rachis.

ACTION Partus praeparator.

RED CLOVER FLOWER

Leguminosae-
Papilionoideae

Trifolii flos

Red Clover Flower consists of the dried flower-heads of *Trifolium pratense* L.

CHARACTERISTICS

Macroscopical Description
Flower-heads globose to ovoid, up to about 3 cm long, usually on a very short stalk and composed of numerous purplish-red or pinkish-brown flowers up to about 15 mm long, attached to a central receptacle; individual flowers with a calyx consisting of a more or less campanulate tube, colourless with pinkish-purple veins, surmounted by five narrow, green, strongly pubescent, unequal spreading teeth; a papillionate, pinkish-purple, glabrous corolla about three times as long as the calyx tube; diadelphous stamens and a small, ovoid ovary with a long style and capitate stigma. Some small green leaflets may be present, up to 20 mm long, oblong to obovate with an acute apex and an entire, ciliate margin, both surfaces pubescent.

Microscopical Description
Epidermis of calyx composed of polygonal cells with faintly striated cuticle and occasional anomocytic stomata on the outer epidermis only; abundant uniseriate covering trichomes with two small, thin-walled basal cells and a thick-walled, tapering end cell, up to 1 mm long with a warty cuticle; glandular trichomes also present, particularly on the lower epidermis, each with a one or two-celled stalk and a large, cylindrical head composed of several cells arranged in two rows. Epidermal cells of corolla elongated with slightly wavy walls and a strongly striated cuticle, papillose at the tip; vascular strands of corolla and calyx surrounded by a crystal sheath containing prismatic crystals of calcium oxalate. Fibrous layer of anthers; subspherical pollen grains, 25 μm in diameter with a smooth exine, three distinct pores and three furrows. Upper epidermal cells of leaflets with sinuous and slightly beaded anticlinal walls; lower epidermis with sinuous to wavy walls; anomocytic stomata on both surfaces, more frequent on the lower; abundant covering trichomes on both surfaces and on the margins; fibro-vascular strands surrounded by crystal sheath containing prismatic crystals of calcium oxalate.

Odour and Taste
Faint, fragrant odour; slightly bitter taste.

IDENTIFICATION

Carry out the method for Thin-layer Chromatography as described in Appendix 1, using Solvent System A.

Apply 20 μl of each of the following solutions separately to the plate: (1) extract 1 g powdered Red Clover Flower with 10 ml 60% methanol on a water-bath for 10-15 minutes, cool and filter; (2) 0.025% rutin in methanol.

Spray the plate with Spray Reagent A and examine in ultraviolet light 366 nm.

Major bands relative to rutin are approximately as follows: blue 1.95, yellowish-green 1.55, yellowish-orange 1.45.

QUANTITATIVE STANDARDS

Foreign Matter
Not more than 2%   Appendix 3

Total Ash
Not more than 10%   Appendix 4

Ash Insoluble in Hydrochloric Acid
Not more than 2%   Appendix 5

Water-soluble Extractive
Not less than 15%   Appendix 7

MATERIAL OF COMMERCE Red Clover Flower is supplied in the whole or crushed condition. It is obtained from many European countries.

Powdered Red Clover Flower

Complies with the requirements for Identification and Quantitative Standards stated for Red Clover Flower.

Characteristic Features
Pinkish-grey powder with a faint, fragrant odour and a slightly bitter taste. Fragments of corolla with slightly wavy walls and a striated cuticle; fragments of calyx with rectangular cells and a faintly striated cuticle; abundant uniseriate, warty-walled covering trichomes with part of the end cell frequently broken off; glandular trichomes less frequent; sub-spherical pollen grains, scattered or associated with fragments of fibrous layer of anthers; abundant strands of vascular tissue with associated crystal sheath containing prismatic crystals of calcium oxalate; occasional portions of green leaf with wavy-walled epidermis and anomocytic stomata.

ACTION Anti-inflammatory.

RHATANY ROOT   Krameriaceae

Ratanhiae radix

Synonym: Peruvian Rhatany.

Rhatany Root consists of the dried, usually fragmented, underground organs of *Krameria triandra* Ruiz and Pavon.

This material complies with the requirements of the European Pharmacopoeia for Rhatany Root and the British Pharmacopoeia for Rhatany Root or, when the material is in powder, Powdered Rhatany Root.

MATERIAL OF COMMERCE Rhatany Root is supplied as straight, tortuous pieces or in chopped or broken condition. It is obtained from Bolivia and Peru.

ACTION Astringent.

RHUBARB
Polygonaceae

Rhei radix

Rhubarb consists of the whole or cut, dried underground parts of *Rheum palmatum* L. or *of Rheum officinale* Baillon, or of hybrids of these two species, or of a mixture. The underground parts are often divided; the stem and most of the bark with the rootlets are removed.

This material complies with the requirements of the European Pharmacopoeia for Rhu-barb and the British Pharmacopoeia for Rhubarb or, when the material is in powder, Powdered Rhubarb.

MATERIAL OF COMMERCE Rhubarb is supplied as cut pieces of root, or sliced or fragmented rhizome. It is obtained mainly from China.

ACTION Laxative.

ROMAN CHAMOMILE FLOWER
Compositae

Chamomillae romanae flos

Synonyms: Chamaemelum, Anthemis.

Roman Chamomile Flower consists of the dried flower-heads of the cultivated double variety of *Chamaemelum nobile* (L.) All. [*Anthemis nobilis* L.].

This material complies with the requirements of the European Pharmacopoeia for Roman Chamomile Flower and the British Pharma-copoeia for Chamomile Flowers.

MATERIAL OF COMMERCE Roman Chamomile Flower is supplied in the whole or partially broken condition. It is obtained mainly from France, Belgium and Eastern Europe.

ACTION Antispasmodic.

ROSEMARY LEAF
Labiatae

Rosmarini folium

Rosemary Leaf consists of the dried leaves of *Rosmarinus officinalis* L.

CHARACTERISTICS

Macroscopical Description
Leaves linear to linear-lanceolate, curved, up to 3.5 cm long, 2-3 mm broad, coriaceous, greyish-green or occasionally brownish; mar-gins entire and strongly revolute, apex ob-tuse, base tapering and non-petiolate; upper surface reticulately pitted, lower surface tomentose. Occasional pieces of stems up to 4 cm long, 1-2 mm wide, dark brown to greenish, tomentose or woody with numer-ous opposite and decussate leaf scars.

Microscopical Description
Leaf dorsiventral; upper epidermal cells po-lygonal with slightly thickened walls and

occasional pits; lower epidermal cells sinuous; numerous diacytic stomata on the lower surface only; very abundant uniseriate, multicellular, much-branched covering trichomes on the lower epidermis, also glandular trichomes with a unicellular stalk and unicellular or bicellular head occurring on both epidermises; hypodermis underlying the upper epidermis composed of large, ovoid cells with thickened and beaded anticlinal walls; these cells extending across the lamina at intervals, separating the two-layered palisade into large, crescent-shaped areas, each with a group of spongy mesophyll.

Odour and Taste
Odour strongly aromatic and characteristic; taste camphoraceous and slightly bitter.

IDENTIFICATION

Carry out the method for Thin-layer Chromatography as described in Appendix 1, using Solvent System C.

Apply 60 µl of each of the following solutions separately to the plate: (1) extract 1 g of powdered Rosemary Leaf by shaking with 10 ml of dichloromethane for 20 minutes. Filter, evaporate the filtrate just to dryness and dissolve the residue in 1 ml toluene; (2) 0.1% cineole in toluene.

Spray the plate with Spray Reagent D, heat at 105°C for 10-15 minutes and examine in daylight.

Major bands relative to cineole are approximately as follows: purple 2.05, yellow 1.45, blue 1.0, pink 0.75, purple 0.5.

QUANTITATIVE STANDARDS

Woody Stems
Not more than 10%

Foreign Matter
Not more than 2%   Appendix 3

Total Ash
Not more than 8%   Appendix 4

Ash Insoluble in Hydrochloric Acid
Not more than 1.5%   Appendix 5

Water-soluble Extractive
Not less than 15%   Appendix 7

MATERIAL OF COMMERCE Rosemary Leaf is supplied as whole or cut leaves. It is obtained mainly from Mediterranean countries, especially Spain, Morocco and Tunisia.

Powdered Rosemary Leaf

Complies with the requirements for Identification and Quantitative Standards stated for Rosemary Leaf.

Characteristic Features
Greyish-green powder with a characteristic, aromatic odour and taste; dense, felted masses of covering trichomes, individual trichomes uniseriate, multicellular, much-branched with the branches arising from swollen joints and each terminating in a single, tapering cell; abundant glandular trichomes of the labiate type; fragments of leaf epidermises, those of the upper surface straight-walled with underlying hypodermis composed of large, rounded cells with thickened and beaded anticlinal walls, those of the lower surface with sinuous walls and numerous diacytic stomata; occasional cork fragments, fibres, vascular tissue and lignified parenchyma from the stems.

ACTION Carminative, spasmolytic.

SAGE LEAF   **Labiatae**

Salviae folium

Synonyms: Garden Sage, Red Sage.

Sage Leaf consists of the dried leaves of *Salvia officinalis* L.

CHARACTERISTICS

Macroscopical Description
Leaves oblong-lanceolate to ovate, up to 10 cm long and 3 cm broad, pale green on the upper surface, greyish-green on the lower surface, texture soft and velvety; margin finely crenulate, apex acute, base rounded or tapering and frequently lobed; upper surface pubescent, lower surface tomentose, both surfaces with conspicuous, reticulate venation; petiole up to about 4 cm long, grooved on the upper surface, greenish-grey to purplish, densely pubescent.

Microscopical Description
Dorsiventral with a two-layered palisade; cells of the upper epidermis polygonal with thickened and markedly beaded anticlinal walls and a faintly striated cuticle; lower epidermal cells thin-walled and sinuous; diacytic stomata on both epidermises; abundant covering and glandular trichomes on both epidermises and also on the petiole; the covering trichomes uniseriate with a short basal cell and one or two long, undulating terminal cells tapering to a blunt apex or, occasionally, unicellular with a warty wall; the glandular trichomes of the typical labiate type with a unicellular stalk and a radiate eight-celled head containing reddish-brown secretion, or smaller with a one to three-celled uniseriate stalk and a uni- or bicellular head.

Odour and Taste
Odour strongly aromatic and characteristic; taste aromatic, stringent and bitter.

IDENTIFICATION

Carry out the method for Thin-layer Chromatography as described in Appendix 1, using Solvent System C.
Apply 60 µl of each of the following solutions separately to the plate: (1) extract 1 g of powdered Sage Leaf by shaking with 10 ml of dichloromethane for 20 minutes. Filter, evaporate the filtrate just to dryness and dissolve the residue in 1 ml toluene; (2) 0.1% cineole in toluene.
Spray the plate with Spray Reagent D, heat at 105°C for 10-15 minutes and examine in daylight.
Major bands relative to cineole are approximately as follows: purple 2.0, grey 1.4, pink 1.2, blue 1.0*.
There is an area of purple and pink fine detail between 0.8 and 0.4.

* This is the major band in the chromatogram.

QUANTITATIVE STANDARDS

Foreign Matter
Not more than 3%   Appendix 3

Total Ash
Not more than 8%   Appendix 4

Ash Insoluble in Hydrochloric Acid
Not more than 2%   Appendix 5

Water-soluble Extractive
Not less than 16%   Appendix 7

MATERIAL OF COMMERCE Sage Leaf is supplied as whole or broken leaves. It is cultivated in many countries and obtained particularly from south-eastern Europe.

Powdered Sage Leaf

Complies with the requirements for Identification and Quantitative Standards stated for Sage Leaf.

Characteristic Features
Dark, greyish-green powder with a very strongly aromatic and characteristic odour and taste; abundant covering trichomes, uniseriate and whip-like with a short basal cell and one or more long, tapering, undulating terminal cells; numerous glandular trichomes of the labiate type; fragments of leaf epidermises with diacytic stomata, the cells of the upper epidermis with thickened

and distinctly beaded anticlinal walls; groups of vascular tissue from the petiole and main veins showing vessels with annular and reticulate thickening.

ACTION Antiseptic, astringent.

SARSAPARILLA

Smilacaceae

Sarsaparillae radix

Synonym: Smilax.

Sarsaparilla consists of the dried root and rhizomes of various species of *Smilax*, particularly *S. aristolochiaefolia* Mill., *S. febrifuga* Kunth, *S. ornata* Hook. f. and *S. regelii* Killip et Morton.

CHARACTERISTICS

Macroscopical Description
Roots up to 75 cm long and 1-6 mm in diameter with a greyish-brown, yellowish-brown, reddish-brown or dark brown outer surface, longitudinally ridged or furrowed; thin, wiry, flexible secondary rootlets frequently attached, fracture short in the outer part, uneven and fibrous in the inner part.

Microscopical Description
Roots Thin-walled epidermal cells with brown granular contents, root hairs often present, two to four layers of lignified, thick-walled, tangentially elongated hypodermal cells, innermost layer more strongly lignified; cortex of thin-walled, rounded parenchymatous cells, some with bundles of acicular crystals of calcium oxalate up to 150 μm long embedded in mucilage, others containing simple or sometimes two to six compound, spherical or ovoid starch granules, 3-24 μm in diameter; endodermis a single layer of tangentially elongated cells with thickened walls with middle lamella strongly lignified, passage cells absent; pericycle a single layer composed of isolated or small groups of lignified, pitted parenchymatous cells; polyarch vascular tissue comprising slightly more than half the radius of the stele consisting of thirty to forty small ovoid phloem groups immediately within the pericycle and flanked laterally by two to three layers of lignified fibrous cells; xylem with lignified vessels up to 160 μm wide, occurring singly or in small groups arranged in radial rows and surrounded by fibrous cells.

Rhizomes Similar but with an outer pith of lignified, pitted, thick-walled parenchymatous cells and a central region with thinner-walled, non-lignified cells packed with starch granules. The relative proportions of cortex, xylem and pith may vary according to the species.

Odour and Taste
Odourless; bitter and acrid taste.

IDENTIFICATION

A. Shake 1 g powdered Sarsaparilla with 10 ml water; copious frothing occurs immediately .

B. Carry out the method for Thin-layer Chromatography as described in Appendix 1, using Solvent System A.

Apply 20 μl of each of the following solutions separately to the plate: (1) extract 1 g powdered Sarsaparilla with 10 ml methanol on a water-bath for 10-15 minutes, cool, filter and concentrate the filtrate to about 2.5 ml; (2) 0.025% rutin in methanol.

Spray the plate with Spray Reagent A and examine in ultraviolet light 366 nm.

Major bands relative to rutin are approximately as follows: light green 2.6, orange 1.0.

QUANTITATIVE STANDARDS

Foreign Matter
Not more than 5%   Appendix 3

Total Ash
Not more than 10%   Appendix 4

Ash Insoluble in Hydrochloric Acid
Not more than 4%   Appendix 5

Water-soluble Extractive
Not less than 14%   Appendix 7

MATERIAL OF COMMERCE Sarsaparilla is imported in large bundles bound with root or wire, but is usually supplied in the chopped condition. It is obtained from Mexico, Central America and Ecuador.

Powdered Sarsaparilla

Complies with the requirements for Identification and Quantitative Standards stated for Sarsaparilla.

Characteristic Features
Fawn to reddish-brown powder with no odour and a bitter, acrid taste; abundant simple and compound starch granules, occurring free and in parenchymatous cells; large acicular crystals of calcium oxalate scattered and in bundles embedded in mucilage; elongated sclereid-like cells with fine pits and tapering ends often associated with cortical parenchyma; polygonal cells of epidermis; fragments of vessels with scalariform thickening or small bordered pits.

ACTION Anti-inflammatory.

SAW PALMETTO FRUIT   Palmae

Serenoae repentis fructus

Synonym: Sabal

Saw Palmetto Fruit consists of the dried, ripe fruits of *Serenoa repens* (Bartram) Small [*Serenoa serrulata* Hook.; *Sabal serrulata* (Michx.) Nutt. ex Schult.]

CHARACTERISTICS

Macroscopical Description
Sub-spherical to ovoid drupes, about 12-25 mm long and 8-15 mm wide, dark brown to black, with a smooth, dull surface, and with large, irregular depressions and ridges caused by shrinkage on drying; remains of style at the summit; base bearing a small depression with the scar of the stalk; epicarp and underlying sarcocarp forming a fragile layer, which partially peels off, revealing the hard, pale brown layer of endocarp surrounding the seed. Seed irregularly spherical to ovoid, up to about 12 mm long and 8 mm wide, hard, surface finely pitted and reddish-brown with a paler, raised and membranous area over the raphe and micropyle; cut transversely, shows a thin testa, narrow perisperm and a large area of dense, horny, greyish-white endosperm.

Microscopical Description
Epicarp composed of several layers of thin-walled, polygonal cells with brown contents; sarcocarp mostly parenchymatous, the cells large, irregularly shaped and loosely packed, filled with reddish-brown pigment and numerous globules of volatile oil; scattered stone cells occur, usually singly, but occasionally in groups of two or three, varying in size and shape and sometimes quite large, with pitted and stratified walls, which may be much thickened; endocarp sclerenchymatous, the cells polygonal in surface view with thick walls and numerous small pits; epidermis of the testa composed of small, thin-walled cells containing brown pigment; endosperm cells thick-walled with large, conspicuous, oval or rounded pits and filled with fixed oil and aleurone grains.

Odour and Taste
Odour aromatic and fruity; taste sweetish, oily, and distinctly acrid and soapy.

IDENTIFICATION

Carry out the method for Thin-layer Chromatography as described in Appendix 1, using chloroform as the solvent system.

Apply 20 µl of each of the following solutions separately to the plate: (1) extract 1 g powdered Saw Palmetto Fruit* by shaking with 5 ml methanol for 15 minutes, filter; (2) 0.1% cineole in toluene.

Spray the plate with Spray Reagent C, heat at 105° C for 10-15 minutes and examine in daylight.

Major bands relative to cineole are approximately as follows: pink/purple 1.8, purple 1.55, purple fine detail 0.65, purple fine detail 0.5.

* To powder Saw Palmetto Fruit it is helpful to freeze the whole material (ideally in liquid nitrogen for 5 minutes) prior to milling.

QUANTITATIVE STANDARDS

Foreign Matter
Not more than 1%   Appendix 3

Total Ash
Not more than 4%   Appendix 4

Ash Insoluble in Hydrochloric Acid
Not more than 1%   Appendix 5

Water-soluble Extractive
Not less than 8%   Appendix 7

MATERIAL OF COMMERCE Saw Palmetto Fruit is supplied as whole fruits. It is harvested from the wild in coastal regions of south-eastern USA and obtained mainly from Florida.

Powdered Saw Palmetto Fruit

Complies with the requirements for the Identification and Quantitative Standards stated for Saw Palmetto Fruit.

ACTION Prostatic.

SENEGA ROOT   Polygalaceae

Polygalae radix

Synonyms: Snake Root, Rattlesnake Root.

Senega Root consists of the dried and usually fragmented root and root crown of *Polygala senega* L. or of certain closely-related species of *Polygala* or of a mixture of these.

This material complies with the requirements

of the European Pharmacopoeia for Senega Root and the British Pharmacopoeia for Senega Root or, when the material is in powder, Powdered Senega Root.

MATERIAL OF COMMERCE Senega Root is supplied in the whole or broken condition. It is obtained mainly from Canada.

ACTION Expectorant.

SENNA FRUIT, ALEX.

Leguminosae-Caesalpinioideae

Sennae fructus acutifoliae

Synonyms: Cassia Fruit, Alexandrian Senna Pods.

Alexandrian Senna Fruit consists of the dried fruit of *Cassia senna* L. [*C. acutifolia* Delile].

This material complies with the requirements of the European Pharmacopoeia for Alexandrian Senna Pods and the British Pharmacopoeia for Alexandrian Senna Fruit

or, when the material is in powder, Powdered Alexandrian Senna Fruit.

MATERIAL OF COMMERCE Alexandrian Senna Fruit is supplied in the whole or broken condition. It is obtained mainly from Egypt and Sudan.

ACTION Stimulant laxative.

SENNA FRUIT, TINN.

Leguminosae-Caesalpinioideae

Sennae fructus angustifoliae

Synonyms: Cassia Fruit, Tinnevelly Senna Pods.

Tinnevelly Senna Fruit consists of the dried fruit of *Cassia angustifolia* Vahl.

This material complies with the requirements of the European Pharmacopoeia for Tinnevelly Senna Pods and the British Pharmacopoeia for Tinnevelly Senna Fruit or,

when the material is in powder, Powdered Tinnevelly Senna Fruit.

MATERIAL OF COMMERCE Tinnevelly Senna Fruit is supplied in the whole or broken condition. It is obtained mainly from India.

ACTION Stimulant laxative.

SENNA LEAF

Leguminosae-Caesalpinioideae

Sennae folium

Synonym: Cassia Leaf.

Senna Leaf consists of the dried leaflets of *Cassia senna* L. [*C. acutifolia* Delile], known as Alexandrian or Khartoum Senna, or *Cassia angustifolia* Vahl, known as Tinnevelly Senna, or a mixture of the two species.

This material complies with the requirements of the European Pharmacopoeia for Senna

Leaf and the British Pharmacopoeia for Senna Leaf or, when the material is in powder, Powdered Senna Leaf.

MATERIAL OF COMMERCE Senna Leaf is supplied in the whole or broken condition. It is obtained from Egypt, Sudan and India.

ACTION Stimulant laxative.

SHEPHERD'S PURSE Cruciferae

Bursae pastoris herba

Shepherd's Purse consists of the dried, aerial parts of *Capsella bursa-pastoris* (L.) Medik., harvested towards the end of the flowering period when seed pods are present.

CHARACTERISTICS

Macroscopical Description

Stems Up to 40 cm, 2-3 mm thick, sparsely branched, more or less cylindrical or roundly angled, unevenly grooved, shiny, almost glabrous.

Leaves Basal leaves up to 7 cm, in a rosette, petiolate, elongated lanceolate; margin with hairs on minute projections, variable from entire to serrate to deeply pinnatifid; stem leaves few, smaller, sessile, amplexicaul, with two small auricles, margin variable; surfaces with few scattered hairs, most numerous above.

Flowers 2-3 mm in diameter, in a compact raceme, petals white, about twice as long as sepals, glabrous; sepals pale green, glabrous or with few long hairs.

Fruit Obcordate to almost triangular, flattened, 6-9 mm, pedicels long; widely-spaced, in progressive state of development, along upper part of stem; pale green to yellowish-green, smooth, shiny, glabrous; small remains of style at apex; numerous small, reddish-brown seeds.

Microscopical Description

Stem Section almost circular, epidermal cells more or less rectangular, outer wall thickened, cuticle smooth, occasional stomata; cortex a few layers of small parenchymatous cells; well-defined endodermis; lignified pericycle fibres in irregular tangential groups of up to about ten, lumen large; vascular tissue with alternating larger and smaller bundles linked by sclerenchyma; larger bundles projecting into pith, have groups of sclerenchymatous cells at inner radial end; pith of thin-walled, unlignified parenchymatous cells; xylem vessels bordered-pitted and spirally thickened; epidermal cells in surface view elongated, straight-walled, cuticle smooth, frequent stomata with small subsidiary cells.

Leaf Dorsiventral, palisade one or two layers of short cells; upper epidermal cells isodiametric or slightly elongated; shorter sides almost straight, the longer gently sinuous; numerous anisocytic stomata, three or four subsidiary cells, guard cells comparatively small; lower epidermal cells slightly larger, shape similar, walls more sinuous, stomata more abundant; unlignified, covering trichomes of two forms on both epidermises; unicellular, conical, more or less erect, smooth-walled, lumen wide and continuous almost to tip; unicellular, stellately-branched, very closely appressed to the epidermis, surface coarsely warted, lumen, wide at base, narrows close to point of branching, almost occluded in terminal part of pointed branches; most with three, four or five arms, very infrequently two or six; erect trichomes on lower surface somewhat larger.

Flower Epidermal cells of sepal elongated, walls angularly sinuous, beaded, cuticle finely striated, anisocytic stomata; infrequent, long unicellular trichomes; epidermal cells of petal, near apex, small, shortly papillose, towards base cells progressively elongated, almost straight-walled, cuticular striations throughout; pollen grains spherical about 25 µm, three pores, exine very finely granular.

Fruit Epicarp cells thin-walled, quite large, elongated. markedly sinuous, anisocytic stomata, cuticle longitudinally striated; endocarp, single layer of thick-walled, finely pitted, weakly lignified, slightly sinuous fusiform cells, elongated parallel to long axis of fruit.

Seed Epidermal cells colourless, thin-walled; underlying is a brown layer of shallow beaker cells, rectangular in surface view with almost straight anticlinal walls.

Odour and Taste

Weak, rather unpleasant odour; taste slightly saline and astringent.

IDENTIFICATION

Carry out the method for Thin-layer Chromatography as described in Appendix 1, using Solvent System A.

Apply 20 µl of each of the following solutions separately to the plate: (1) extract 1 g powdered Shepherd's Purse with 10 ml methanol by warming on a water-bath for 10-15 minutes, cool and filter; (2) 0.025% rutin in methanol.

Spray the plate with Spray Reagent A and examine in ultraviolet light 366 nm.

Major bands relative to rutin are approximately as follows: yellow 1.6, yellow 1.25, yellow 1.0, yellow 0.65.

Fine detail is exhibited below the band corresponding to rutin.

QUANTITATIVE STANDARDS

Foreign Matter
Not more than 3%   Appendix 3

Total Ash
Not more than 10%   Appendix 4

Ash Insoluble in Hydrochloric Acid
Not more than 2.5%   Appendix 5

Water-soluble Extractive
Not less than 12%   Appendix 7

MATERIAL OF COMMERCE Shepherd's Purse is supplied in cut condition. It is collected from the wild and obtained mainly from south-eastern Europe.

Powdered Shepherd's Purse

Complies with the requirements for Identification and Quantitative Standards stated for Shepherd's Purse.

Characteristic Features
Green to greenish-yellow with a faint, unpleasant odour and a slightly bitter, astringent taste; stellately-branched, thick-walled, coarsely-warted trichomes, frequently whole; smooth, thin-walled, conical trichomes, mostly fragmented; single-layered groups of pigmented, narrow fusiform cells of endocarp; wavy-walled leaf epidermal cells with anisocytic stomata; narrow vessels with small bordered pits; fragments of sparsely-pitted, wide-lumened, pericycle fibres; spherical pollen grains with three pores, often clumped in small masses; fibrous layer of anther with small cluster crystals; thin-walled pith parenchyma.

ACTION Anti-haemorrhagic.

SKULLCAP   Labiatae

Scutellariae herba

Synonyms: Scullcap, Hoodwort, Quaker Bonnet, Helmet Flower.

Skullcap consists of the dried aerial parts of *Scutellaria lateriflora* L. collected during the flowering period.

CHARACTERISTICS

Macroscopical Description
Stems Quadrangular, hollow, up to about 4 mm wide, frequently branched, with longitudinal ridges and bearing pairs of opposite and decussate leaves at the nodes; pale yellowish-green and glabrous in the lower part, darker green or purplish in the upper part with scattered long white hairs, particularly along the ridges.

Leaves Ovate, ovate-oblong or ovate-lanceolate, up to about 5 cm long and 2.5 cm broad, apex acute or acuminate, base rounded or subcordate, margin coarsely dentate to serrate; upper surface dark green, glabrous, lower surface paler with scattered hairs along the veins; petiole slender and up to about 1 cm long.

Flowers Axillary, solitary or in one-sided racemes; calyx campanulate, two-lipped, hairy, the upper lip bearing a small scale on the back; corolla 4-6 mm long, blue, or occasionally white, two-lipped, the upper lip helmet-shaped with small lateral lobes; stamens four, didynamous; carpels two, joined, with a two-cleft style, ovary four-lobed; nutlets about 1 mm long, ovoid, enclosed in the persistent calyx.

Microscopical Description

Stem Epidermal cells polygonal or longitudinally elongated with occasional diacytic stomata and, on young stems, scattered covering trichomes similar to those on the leaf; cortex narrow, parenchymatous, with collenchyma in the ridges; endodermis distinct; pericyclic fibres in dense groups in the ridges and continuing laterally to form a complete cylinder of two or three layers, individual fibres with moderately thickened and pitted walls; vascular tissue with small vessels showing bordered pits or with spiral or annular thickening; pith broken down forming a central hollow.

Leaf Dorsiventral, the cells of the palisade layer relatively large and closely packed; epidermal cells wavy-walled in surface view with numerous diacytic stomata on the lower epidermis; covering trichomes infrequent, mainly on the lower surface along the veins, uniseriate, conical, composed of from one to three cells, wide at the base and tapering towards the apex, with thin, warty walls; multicellular glandular trichomes scattered on both surfaces, each with a small, rounded uni- or bicellular stalk and a large globular head composed of four radiating cells containing brown secretion and with the common cuticle raised to form a bladder.

Flower Calyx outer epidermis with diacytic stomata and densely covered with short, conical covering trichomes, composed of one or two cells with conspicuously warty walls, interspersed with longer, glandular trichomes with a uniseriate one or two-celled stalk and a spherical unicellular or occasionally bicellular head. Corolla purple-violet, the inner epidermis papillose, the outer epidermis with abundant long glandular trichomes similar to those on the calyx and also numerous covering trichomes similar to those on the leaf; other multicellular glandular trichomes with a four-celled head, as occurring on the leaf, also found scattered on the outer surfaces of the calyx and the corolla. Pollen grains spherical to ovoid,

25-30 µm in diameter, with three pores and a smooth exine.

Odour and Taste
Odour slight; taste bitter.

IDENTIFICATION

Carry out the method for Thin-layer Chromatography as described in Appendix 1, using Solvent System A.

Apply 20 µl of each of the following solutions separately to the plate: (1) extract 1 g powdered Skullcap with 10 ml methanol by warming on a water-bath for 10-15 minutes, cool and filter; (2) 0.025% rutin in methanol.

Spray the plate with Spray Reagent A and examine in ultraviolet light 366 nm.

Major bands relative to rutin are approximately as follows: yellow 2.3, turquoise 1.5, yellow 1.3.

QUANTITATIVE STANDARDS

Foreign Matter
Not more than 2%   Appendix 3

Total Ash
Not more than 12%   Appendix 4

Ash Insoluble in Hydrochloric Acid
Not more than 4%   Appendix 5

Water-soluble Extractive
Not less than 15%   Appendix 7

MATERIAL OF COMMERCE Skullcap is supplied in cut or broken condition. It is obtained from the USA.

Powdered Skullcap

Complies with the requirements for Identification and Quantative Standards stated for Skullcap.

Characteristic Features
A greyish to greenish-yellow powder with a slight odour and a bitter taste; fragments of the leaf epidermis, cells wavy-walled with numerous diacytic, occasionally anisocytic, stomata on the lower surface; conical covering trichomes, uniseriate, one to three cells with distinctly warty walls; glandular trichomes with a small, uni- or bicellular

stalk and a spherical head composed of four radiating cells with brown contents; others with a uniseriate, one or two-celled stalk and a globular, unicellular head; dense groups of pericyclic fibres and small vessels, with bordered pits or spiral, or annular, thickening from the stem; occasional pinkish-purple fragments of the corolla, some showing papillae; characteristic fibrous layer of the anther and smooth, spherical to ovoid pollen grains.

ACTION Mild sedative.

SLIPPERY ELM BARK Ulmaceae

Ulmi rubrae cortex

Synonym: Red Elm.

Slippery Elm Bark consists of the dried inner bark of *Ulmus rubra* Muhl. [*Ulmus fulva* Michaux].

CHARACTERISTICS

Macroscopical Description
Large flat pieces, outer surface light brown to reddish-brown, longitudinally wrinkled and furrowed with occasional pieces of rhytidome; inner surface yellowish-white to yellowish-brown, finely striated longitudinally and often cracked transversely; fracture fibrous, fractured surface porous.

Microscopical Description
Secondary phloem completely traversed by medullary rays between which are tangential groups of 6-30 sclerenchymatous fibres, each up to 20 μm wide, with thick, slightly lignified walls; bundles of fibres surrounded by a crystal sheath containing prismatic crystals of calcium oxalate 10-60 μm long; very large mucilage cells about 200 μm in diameter, the mucilage staining red with Ruthenium Red Solution; parenchymatous cells packed with spheroidal starch granules 10-25 μm in diameter.

Odour and Taste
Slight, fenugreek-like odour; bland and mucilaginous taste.

IDENTIFICATION

A. Mix 1 g powdered Slippery Elm Bark with 40 ml cold water and allow to stand for 1 hour; a thick, light brown jelly is formed.
B. Carry out the method for Thin-layer Chromatography as described in Appendix 1, using Solvent System A.

Apply 20 μl of each of the following solutions separately to the plate: (1) extract 1 g powdered Slippery Elm Bark with 10 ml 60% methanol on a water-bath for 10-15 minutes, cool, filter and concentrate the filtrate to about 2.5 ml; (2) 0.025% rutin in methanol.

Spray the plate with Spray Reagent A and examine in ultraviolet light 366 nm.

Major bands relative to rutin are approximately as follows: blue 1.05, orange 0.8.

QUANTITATIVE STANDARDS

Loss on Drying
Not more than 12% when dried in an oven at 100-105°C. Use 2-3 g   Appendix 2

Foreign Matter
Not more than 2%   Appendix 3

Total Ash
Not more than 14% calculated with reference to the oven-dried material Appendix 4

Ash Insoluble in Hydrochloric Acid
Not more than 1.5% calculated with reference to the oven-dried material Appendix 5

MATERIAL OF COMMERCE Slippery Elm Bark is supplied in small pieces. It is obtained from eastern North America.

Powdered Slippery Elm Bark

Complies with the requirements for Identification and Quantitative Standards stated for Slippery Elm Bark.

Characteristic Features
Pale buff powder with a slight, fenugreek-like odour and a bland, mucilaginous taste; numerous fibres, thick-walled, slightly lignified and occurring in groups; abundant mucilage staining red with Ruthenium Red Solution; prismatic crystals of calcium oxalate, fairly abundant starch granules; only very occasional fragments of brown cork cells.

STORAGE Store in a cool, dry place in well closed containers.

ACTION Demulcent.

SQUILL   Hyacinthaceae

Scillae bulbus

Synonym: White Squill.

Squill consists of the bulb of *Drimia maritima* (L.) Stearn, collected soon after the plant has flowered, divested of its dry, outer, membranous coats, cut into transverse slices and dried.

This material complies with the requirements

of the British Pharmacopoeia for Squill or, when the material is in powder, Powdered Squill.

MATERIAL OF COMMERCE Squill is supplied as slices of bulb. It is obtained from the Mediterranean region.

ACTION Expectorant.

SQUILL, INDIAN   Hyacinthaceae

Scillae indicae bulbus

Synonym: Urginea.

Indian Squill consists of the bulb of *Drimia indica* (Roxb.) J. P. Jessop, collected soon after the plant has flowered, divested of dry, outer membranous coats and usually cut longitudinally into slices and dried.

This material complies with the requirements

of the British Pharmacopoeia for Indian Squill or, when the material is in powder, Powdered Indian Squill.

MATERIAL OF COMMERCE Indian Squill is supplied as slices of bulb. It is obtained from India.

ACTION Expectorant.

173

ST. JOHN'S WORT Guttiferae

Hyperici herba

Synonym: Hypericum.

St. John's Wort consists of the dried flowering tops or aerial parts of *Hypericum perforatum* L., harvested shortly before or during the flowering period.

CHARACTERISTICS

Macroscopical Description
Stems Major portion of herb. Cylindrical with two equidistant longitudinal ridges, base brown and woody with hollow centre, upper portion green and branched to form terminal cyme.

Leaves Opposite, sessile pairs; grey-green, linear-oblong, 8-30 mm in length, entire margin, revolute when dried, obtuse apex, base even. Surface glabrous but exhibiting brown 'dots', on heating with chloral hydrate solution those in central areas become translucent but in marginal positions reveal red pigment.

Flowers 2 cm in diameter; five green, lanceolate sepals, acuminate apex, joined at base, surface with brown 'dots'; five yellow, linear-ovate petals, longer than sepals, dark 'dots' on terminal margins only; numerous stamens with long filaments and anthers with single, terminal pigment 'dot'; ovary, elongated and conical with parietal placentation, containing numerous brown, triangular seeds with one rounded surface.

Microscopical Description
Stem Elongated epidermal cells with straight, beaded, anticlinal walls; cuticle smooth; frequent parallel orientated stomata with two small, adjacent epidermal cells; cortex of five to six rows of collenchyma; stele with secondary growth consisting of compacted ring of phloem, wide area of lignified xylem and small areas of intraxylary phloem; parenchymatous pith, lignified and pitted in older stems; oil cells may occur in the cortex and phloem.

Leaf Upper surface, polygonal cells with sinuous, slightly beaded, anticlinal walls; cells of lower surface smaller, anticlinal walls more wavy with frequent paracytic, sometimes anomocytic stomata; smooth cuticle, thicker on upper surface; straight-walled, elongated epidermal cells of veins occasionally beaded. Dorsiventral, single palisade layer; large oil cells equal to depth of spongy mesophyll. Midrib containing single, collateral bundle with small area of lignified xylem.

Flower Characteristics of sepal resemble those of the leaf. Petal, narrow, elongated, thin-walled, epidermal cells with straight anticlinal walls on outer surface and wavy on the inner surface. Stamen, lignified fibrous layer of anther wall; elongated, thin-walled cells of filament with striated cuticle; subprolate pollen grains, about 20 μm in diameter with three pores and a smooth exine. Ovary, small polygonal cells with underlying oil cells; seed testa, brown, thick-walled hexagonal cells.

Odour and Taste
Aromatic and balsamic odour; taste bitter and acrid.

IDENTIFICATION

Carry out the method for Thin-layer Chromatography as described in Appendix 1, using Solvent System A.

Apply 20 μl of each of the following solutions separately to the plate: (1) extract 1g powdered St. John's Wort with 10 ml methanol by warming on a water-bath for 10-15 minutes, cool and filter; (2) 0.025% rutin in methanol.

Spray the plate with Spray Reagent A and examine in ultraviolet light 366 nm.

Major bands relative to rutin are approximately as follows: red 2.0, yellow 1.9, yellow 1.7, yellow 1.5, turquoise 1.3, yellow 1.0.

QUANTITATIVE STANDARDS

Foreign Matter
Not more than 2%   Appendix 3

Total Ash
Not more than 8%   Appendix 4

Ash Insoluble in Hydrochloric Acid
Not more than 2.5%   Appendix 5

Water-soluble Extractive

Not less than 12%   Appendix 7

MATERIAL OF COMMERCE St. John's Wort is supplied in the cut condition. It is harvested from the wild in July-August and obtained mainly from eastern Europe.

Powdered St. John's Wort

Complies with the requirements for Identification and Quantitative Standards stated for St. John's Wort.

Characteristic Features

Buff to greenish-brown, with an aromatic and balsamic odour and bitter, acrid taste; elongated and polygonal epidermal cells with thickened and beaded anticlinal walls, some accompanied by paracytic (occasionally anomocytic) stomata; fragments of leaf and sepal with schizogenous oil and pigment cells; narrow, thin-walled, elongated epidermal cells with straight and wavy anticlinal walls from petal; narrow, lignified vessels with annular or reticulate thickening; tracheids and tracheidal vessels with lignified, pitted thickening; thick-walled, lignified fibres with tapering apices and occasional oblique pits; rectangular, lignified, pitted parenchyma; fibrous layer of anther wall; pollen grains with smooth exine.

ACTION Antidepressant.

STRAMONIUM LEAF   Solanaceae

Stramonii folium

Synonym: Datura.

Stramonium Leaf consists of the dried leaf or the dried leaf, the flowering tops and, occasionally, the fruit-bearing tops of *Datura stramonium* L. and its varieties.

This material complies with the requirements of the European Pharmacopoeia for Stramonium Leaf and the British Pharmacopoeia for Stramonium Leaf or, when the material is in powder, Powdered Stramonium Leaf.

MATERIAL OF COMMERCE Stramonium Leaf is supplied in the whole, broken or crushed condition. It is obtained from eastern and southern Europe.

ACTION Antispasmodic.

THYME   Labiatae

Thymi herba

Synonyms: Common Thyme, Garden Thyme (*Thymus vulgaris*); Spanish Thyme (*T. zygis*).

Thyme consists of the whole leaves and flowers separated from the previously dried stems of *Thymus vulgaris* L. or *Thymus zygis* L. or a mixture of both species.

This material complies with the requirements of the European Pharmacopoeia for Thyme.

MATERIAL OF COMMERCE Thyme is usually supplied as whole, dried leaves and flowers. It is obtained mainly from the Iberian peninsula, Morocco, France, Turkey and eastern Europe.

ACTION Expectorant.

VALERIAN ROOT

Valerianaceae

Valerianae radix

Synonym: Valeriana.

Valerian Root consists of the subterranean organs of *Valeriana officinalis* L.s.l., including the rhizome, roots and stolons, carefully dried at a temperature below 40°C.

This material complies with the requirements of the European Pharmacopoeia for Valerian Root and the British Pharmacopoeia for

Valerian or, when the material is in powder, Powdered Valerian.

MATERIAL OF COMMERCE Valerian Root is supplied in the whole or broken condition. It is cultivated in northern and eastern European countries, Japan and the USA and is obtained mainly from Europe.

ACTION Sedative.

VERVAIN

Verbenaceae

Verbenae herba

Synonym: Verbena.

Vervain consists of the dried aerial parts of *Verbena officinalis* L. harvested during the flowering period.

CHARACTERISTICS

Macroscopical Description

Stems Axis up to 1 m, four-sided, finely-striated, smooth to roughly hairy, dark green, terminal pubescent spike, compact in bud, elongating in flower; up to eight pairs of shorter, decussate branches in leaf axils, with terminal inflorescences.

Leaves Simple, base tapering, sessile or very shortly pedicellate, narrowly oblanceolate to rhomboidal; up to 10 cm long, 4.5 cm wide; largest deeply, often widely, pinnately-lobed, margin bluntly dentate; smaller not lobed, margin irregular, crenate-dentate; surfaces rough, hairy, dark green, lower somewhat lighter; venation pinnate, veins light coloured, prominent below, with bristly hairs.

Flowers Numerous, almost sessile, in axil of small, slender, leaf-like bract; calyx ribbed, hairy, sepals united forming narrow tube having four or five short, acute pointed lobes; corolla petals joined forming tube about twice calyx in length, white to pale lilac, with five-part, two-lipped margin at top, 3-4 mm diameter, lilac to pink; entrance

of tube pubescent within; stamens four, not exerted; ovary superior, becoming four-celled; dehiscent fruit with four small, reddish-brown nutlets, surfaces reticulated, striated.

Microscopical Description

Stem Section square, corners rounded; epidermal cells subrectangular, outer wall considerably thickened; long-stalked glandular trichomes; single-layered hypodermis; small, round-celled collenchyma groups at angles; multilayered zones of photosynthetic tissue, outer layers short, columnar, palisade-like; distinct, large-celled endodermis; band of thin-walled, weakly lignified, pericycle fibres; narrow, continuous ring of lignified xylem with inconspicuous medullary rays; extensive pith, large, round, thin-walled cells; epidermal cells in surface view, narrow, elongated, at intervals areas of thicker-walled, finely beaded, variable cells containing numerous anomocytic, rarely anisocytic, stomata with three or four subsidiary cells; xylem, bordered-pitted and spiral vessels; rectangular, square-ended pitted parenchymatous cells.

Leaf Dorsiventral; upper epidermal cells thin-walled, isodiametric, or shortly rectangular, straight or slightly sinuous, anomocytic or anisocytic stomata, short, wide-based, unicellular covering trichomes, upper part of lumen very narrow; glandular trichomes with long-celled stalk, very short cell just below a flattened four to eight-celled head; fewer, almost sessile or very shortly stalked multicellular glands; glandular heads pale brown; lower epidermal cells a little smaller, walls markedly sinuous, stomata numerous, covering and glandular trichomes; longer covering trichomes on veins.

Bract Margins with unicellular, wide-based conical, covering trichomes and fewer, shorter, stalked glands; epidermal cells elongated, rectangular, sinuous.

Flower Calyx, trichomes very numerous, especially on ribs of tube and lobes, frequent stomata; corolla, upper lobes glabrous, epidermal cells small, polygonal, papillose; lower outer region of lobes and upper part of tube with short, covering trichomes, thin, warty-walled; lower corolla tube with few glandular trichomes, short unicellular stalk and almost spherical head, epidermal cells elongated, cuticle wrinkled; inner corolla at throat with numerous long, granular or warty-surfaced trichomes with closely-spaced, balloon-like swellings; a few short, with very granular surface, one to three-celled, terminal cell enlarged, bulbous; stamens; fibrous layer cells small, polygonal, well-marked thickenings; pollen 30 µm, triangular, sides slightly curved, three pores, exine thin, smooth.

Odour and Taste
Odour faint, becoming aromatic, reminiscent of citrus, when rubbed; taste strongly and unpleasantly bitter.

IDENTIFICATION

Carry out the method for Thin-layer Chromatography as described in Appendix 1, using Solvent System A.

Apply 20 µl of each of the following solutions separately to the plate: (1) extract 1 g powdered Vervain with 10 ml methanol by warming on a water-bath for 10-15 minutes, cool and filter; (2) 0.025% rutin in methanol.

Spray the plate with Spray Reagent A and examine in ultraviolet light 366 nm.

Major bands relative to rutin are approximately as follows: turquoise 1.45, yellow 1.3, yellow 0.65.

QUANTITATIVE STANDARDS

Foreign Matter
Not more than 2%   Appendix 3

Total Ash
Not more than 10%   Appendix 4

Ash Insoluble in Hydrochloric Acid
Not more than 2%   Appendix 5

Water-soluble Extractive
Not less than 14%   Appendix 7

MATERIAL OF COMMERCE Vervain is supplied in the cut or broken condition. It is cultivated in eastern Europe and harvested from the wild in south-eastern Europe.

Powdered Vervain

Complies with the requirements for Identification and Quantitative Standards stated for Vervain.

Characteristic Features
A greenish-brown powder with a faintly aromatic odour and a rather bitter taste; leaf epidermis with straight or sinuous walls and anomocytic stomata; covering and glandular trichomes scattered or attached to fragments of the stems, leaves, calyx or corolla; covering type short, unicellular, glandular, with long-celled stalk and a flattened head of four to eight cells, or, less frequently, shortly-stalked with multicellular heads; abundant groups of thin-walled fibres, vessels with bordered pits or spiral thickening and large, rounded parenchyma, from the stem; fibrous layer of the anther with well-marked thickenings; triangular pollen grains with three pores and a smooth exine.

ACTION Tonic.

VIOLET LEAF
Violaceae

Violae odoratae folium

Synonym: Sweet Violet Leaf.

Violet Leaf consists of the dried leaves of *Viola odorata* L., harvested in late Spring.

CHARACTERISTICS

Macroscopical Description
Leaf stipulate, dark grey-green; lamina, 1.5-6 cm long, subglabrous, ovate to orbiculate, margin crenate-serrate, apex obtuse but acute in summer leaves, base deeply cordate; petiole long, downy; stipules ovate or ovate-lanceolate.

Microscopical Description
Epidermal cells with wavy, slightly beaded anticlinal walls, more angular on lower surface; cuticle faintly striated; anisocytic stomata, more numerous on the lower surface; unicellular, thick-walled, covering trichomes mainly on veins of upper surface, generally more frequent on lamina of lower surface, up to 400 µm long, walls distinctly warty; cuticle strongly striated over beaded, elongated epidermal cells of veins and epidermal cells surrounding trichome bases. Dorsiventral, single palisade, sometimes continuous over midrib; calcium oxalate cluster crystals 25-40 µm in diameter occurring as an intermittent crystal layer in the mesophyll. Midrib with a collateral bundle containing narrow, lignified xylem vessels with spiral, annular or reticulate thickening.

Odour and Taste
Pleasant, sweet-scented odour; taste not distinctive.

IDENTIFICATION

Carry out the method for Thin-layer Chromatography as described in Appendix 1, using Solvent System A.

Apply 20 µl of each of the following solutions separately to the plate; (1) extract 1 g powdered Violet Leaf with 10 ml methanol by warming on a water-bath for 10-15 minutes, cool and filter; (2) 0.025% rutin in methanol.

Spray the plate with Spray Reagent A and examine in ultraviolet light 366 nm.

Major bands relative to rutin are approximately as follows: turquoise 2.1, blue 1.1, yellow 0.85, yellow 0.75.

There is an area of fine detail from 1.0-0.

QUANTITATIVE STANDARDS

Foreign Matter
Not more than 2%   Appendix 3

Total Ash
Not more than 14%   Appendix 4

Ash Insoluble in Hydrochloric Acid
Not more than 3%   Appendix 5

Water-soluble Extractive
Not less than 20%   Appendix 7

MATERIAL OF COMMERCE Violet Leaf is supplied in the cut or broken condition. It is obtained from several European countries, particularly France and Italy.

Powdered Violet Leaf

Complies with the requirements for Identification and Quantitative Standards stated for Violet Leaf.

Characteristic Features
Greyish-green powder with a sweet-scented odour; fragments of leaf lamina with beaded, wavy-walled epidermal cells, some with anisocytic stomata; frequent, thick-walled, unicellular trichomes, some with distinctly warty walls; cuticle strongly striated over elongated epidermal cells and those surrounding trichome bases; frequent clusters of calcium oxalate free and in spongy mesophyll; narrow, lignified vessels with annular or reticulate thickening; elongated epidermal cells of petiole, some extended into unicellular, deflexed, thick-walled covering trichomes, others accompanied by parallel orientated stomata.

ACTION Expectorant.

WHITE DEADNETTLE
Labiatae

Lamii albi herba

Synonym: Archangel.

White Deadnettle consists of the dried flowering tops of *Lamium album* L.

CHARACTERISTICS

Macroscopical Description
Stems Quadrangular, hollow, up to about 4 mm wide, longitudinally ridged; light green or dark brownish-purple, surface covered with long white hairs, particularly abundant on the younger stems; pairs of opposite and decussate leaves at the nodes.

Leaves Ovate, acuminate at the apex, base cordate, petiolate, up to about 7 cm long and 4 cm wide; margin coarsely serrate or crenate-serrate; upper surface bright green with long white hairs, particularly along the veins and the margins, lower surface paler with prominent venation and more numerous hairs; petiole grooved on the upper surface and densely hairy along the margins.

Bracts Similar to the leaves.

Flowers In dense axillary whorls on the upper part of the stems. Calyx pale green, about 8mm long, tubular-campanulate with five more or less equal teeth slightly longer than the tube, mucronate at the apex; outer surface covered with long white hairs. Corolla white, about 2 cm long with an oblique ring of hairs near the base of the tube; two-lipped, the upper lip long, densely ciliate and laterally compressed forming a hood, the lower lip three-lobed, the lateral lobes small and each with two or three small teeth, the middle lobe larger and deeply cleft. Stamens four, epipetalous; carpels two, joined, with a long style and bifid stigma.

Microscopical Description
Stem Epidermal cells polygonal to longitudinally elongated in surface view and sometimes containing purple pigment; raised covering trichomes similar to those on the leaf, with the longer type fairly abundant; scattered glandular trichomes and occasional diacytic stomata; cortex with dense areas of collenchyma in the ridges, otherwise narrow and parenchymatous; central vascular cylinder with larger vessels showing reticulate thickening.

Leaf Dorsiventral, the cells of the palisade layer small and sometimes not clearly differentiated; cells of the upper epidermis sinuous in surface view, those of the lower epidermis slightly more wavy; diacytic stomata very abundant on the lower epidermis, infrequent on the upper; covering trichomes characteristic and abundant, each arising from a group of four or more rounded epidermal cells raised up from the surface, uniseriate, conical, composed of a fairly short basal cell and a long, tapering apical cell, swollen at the joint, the walls somewhat thickened and marked with distinct longitudinal striations; some longer covering trichomes with up to five cells along the margins; small glandular trichomes also numerous, especially along the veins, each composed of a short unicellular stalk and a four-celled, spherical head.

Flower Calyx outer epidermis composed of thin-walled polygonal cells, sometimes with a purplish pigment; raised two-celled uniseriate covering trichomes, similar to those on the leaf, with the apical-cell frequently much elongated, occurring abundantly, particularly along the margins of the teeth; glandular trichomes also fairly numerous. Corolla white, the outer epidermis papillose on the lobes; raised covering trichomes, similar to those on the calyx but more filamentous, with thinner walls and frequently composed of three or more cells, forming a dense covering, especially along the margins of the lobes and near the base of the tube; glandular trichomes also numerous; inner epidermal cells irregularly polygonal to elongated in surface view. Anthers with very long filamentous covering hairs similar to those of the corolla; pollen grains spherical, about 30 μm in diameter with three pores and three rather indistinct furrows, and a finely warted exine.

Odour and Taste
Odour faint; taste slightly mucilaginous and bitter.

IDENTIFICATION

Carry out the method for Thin-layer Chromatography as described in Appendix 1, using Solvent System A.

Apply 20 µl of each of the following solutions separately to the plate; (1) extract 1 g powdered White Deadnettle with 10 ml methanol by warming on a water-bath for 10-15 minutes, cool and filter; (2) 0.025% rutin in methanol.

Spray the plate with Spray Reagent A and examine in ultraviolet light 366 nm.

Major bands relative to rutin are approximately as follows: turquoise 2.3, turquoise 2.1, turquoise 1.5, yellow 1.0, turquoise 0.8, yellow 0.65.

There is an area of fine detail from 1.0-0.4.

QUANTITATIVE STANDARDS

Foreign Matter
Not more than 3%   Appendix 3

Total Ash
Not more than 10%   Appendix 4

MATERIAL OF COMMERCE White Deadnettle is supplied in cut or broken form. It is obtained from eastern European countries.

Powdered White Deadnettle

Complies with the requirements for Identification and Quantitative Standards stated for White Deadnettle.

ACTION Astringent.

WHITE HOREHOUND   Labiatae

Marrubii herba

Synonyms: Marrubium, Hoarhound.

White Horehound consists of the dried leaves and flowering tops of *Marrubium vulgare* L.

CHARACTERISTICS

Macroscopical Description
Stems Up to 30 cm long, quadrangular, 3-5 mm wide, young stems whitish, densely covered with downy hairs, older stems less hairy, greenish-grey.

Leaves Opposite and decussate, exstipulate; lower leaves broadly ovate to almost orbicular, upper leaves less broadly ovate, both petiolate; lamina 1.5-6 cm long, 1-3.5 cm wide, petiole up to 3 cm long; apex sub-acute, base tapering on to petiole or may be cordate, margin dentate to dentate-crenate, venation pinnate, prominent on the lower surface, distinctly depressed on upper surface giving a rugose appearance; both leaf surfaces densely covered with fine white, woolly hairs, older leaves having fewer hairs on the dark greyish-green upper surface.

Flowers Small sessile, in dense axillary clusters arising in the angles of the leaves; calyx 5 mm long, persistent, with five long and five short, alternating, hooked, recurved fringing spines; throat of calyx with an internal ring of long silky hairs; corolla, 7 mm long, dull white, four-lobed, upper lobe two-lipped, lower lobe three-lipped; four short stamens; style with bifid stigma.

Microscopical Description
Stem Transverse section quadrangular with curved, enlarged corners; outer layer of young stem, green epidermis; outer layer of older stem brown, cork-like, with outer walls thickened; numerous covering trichomes, 100-200 µm long, mainly unicellular but some of two to six cells; stellate trichomes, occasionally with fifteen to twenty branches; thick-walled collenchymatous cortex, one to two layers in the younger stems and four to six layers in the older stems, increasing to eight to ten layers at the corners; pericycle, discontinuous band of tangentially elongated, moderately thick-walled, lignified fibres usually single or in small groups; dense xylem with uniseriate medullary rays, vessels up to 25 µm in diam-

eter, numerous thick-walled fibres; pith of thin-walled parenchymatous cells slightly lignified.

Leaf Upper epidermis of polygonal, thin-walled cells with sinuous anticlinal walls; anticlinal walls in lower epidermis more sinuous; numerous diacytic stomata on lower epidermis, occasional on upper surface; covering trichomes as on the stem very numerous, twisted or coiled, walls slightly lignified, smooth but occasionally inconspicuously warty, junctions of multi cellular trichomes enlarged; stellate trichomes of two types, one with fifteen to twenty branches arising from a short unicellular stalk and the other with fewer branches arising from a sessile base; sessile Labiate glandular trichomes with eight-celled head and some smaller glandular trichomes with one or two-celled stalk and a one to four-celled head.

Flower Calyx and corolla bear trichomes similar to those on the leaves, stellate trichomes somewhat smaller and the covering trichomes on the inner surface of the calyx up to 1000 µm long with two to three cells, strongly thickened at the swollen joint and with the upper cell elongated; typical fibrous layer of anthers; pollen grains spherical, smooth exine, three germinal pores and three furrows.

Odour and Taste

Faint, pleasant odour; aromatic and bitter taste.

IDENTIFICATION

Carry out the method for Thin-layer Chromatography as described in Appendix 1, using Solvent System A.

Apply 20 µl of each of the following solutions separately to the plate: (1) extract 1 g powdered White Horehound with 20 ml methanol on a water-bath for 10-15 minutes, cool, filter and concentrate to about 5 ml; (2) 0.025% rutin in methanol.

Spray the plate with Spray Reagent A and examine in ultraviolet light 366 nm.

Major bands relative to rutin are approximately as follows: blue 2.6, yellow 1.7, yellow 1.4, whitish-blue 1.0.

QUANTITATIVE STANDARDS

Foreign Matter
Not more than 2%   Appendix 3

Total Ash
Not more than 12%   Appendix 4

Ash Insoluble in Hydrochloric Acid
Not more than 3%   Appendix 5

Water-soluble Extractive
Not less than 15%   Appendix 7

MATERIAL OF COMMERCE White Horehound is usually supplied in the cut or crushed condition. It is obtained mainly from south-eastern European countries, especially Hungary, and also from France, Italy and Morocco.

Powdered White Horehound

Complies with the requirements for Identification and Quantitative Standards stated for White Horehound.

Characteristic Features
Bright greyish-green powder with a pleasant odour and a bitter, aromatic taste. Abundant stellate and unicellular covering trichomes, both lignified near the basal region; Labiate and simple glandular trichomes, slightly lignified parenchymatous cells, thin-walled epidermal cells with sinuous anticlinal walls and diacytic stomata; fibrous layer from anther; spherical, smooth pollen grains with three pores and furrows.

ACTION Expectorant.

WILD CARROT

Umbelliferae

Dauci herba

Synonym: Queen Anne's Lace.

Wild Carrot consists of the dried aerial parts of *Daucus carota* L. subsp. *carota*, collected during the flowering period.

CHARACTERISTICS

Macroscopical Description
Stems Up to 100 cm long, 2-5 mm wide, seven to ten longitudinal ridges, yellowish-brown to green with purple patches along the ridges, pubescent.
Leaves Alternate, bi- or tri-pinnate, finely divided with fairly long flattened petiole, midrib prominent on under-surface, pubescent.
Flowers Terminal compound umbel of small white flowers.

Microscopical Description
Stem Epidermis of elongated cells with straight or slightly wavy anticlinal walls, anomocytic stomata, unicellular covering trichomes 700-750 µm long; fibrovascular bundles with lignified, reticulately thickened vessels and narrow fibres; pith with abundant, large polygonal parenchymatous cells, occasionally with slightly lignified walls.
Leaf Epidermal cells with wavy anticlinal walls and anomocytic stomata; abundant unicellular, conical, covering trichomes often more than 1 mm long, with smooth or occasionally wrinkled surface and acute or acuminate apex.
Flower Petals and sepals with markedly papillose inner epidermis, wavy-walled outer epidermal cells, occasional covering trichomes on the margins; typical fibrous layer of anthers; numerous pollen grains, prolate, about 10-15 µm long with three pores and three furrows.

Odour and Taste
Faintly aromatic odour; slightly bitter taste.

IDENTIFICATION

Carry out the method for Thin-layer Chromatography as described in Appendix 1, using Solvent System A.

Apply 20 µl of each of the following solutions separately to the plate: (1) extract 1 g powdered Wild Carrot with 10 ml methanol by refluxing on a water-bath for 10-15 minutes, cool, filter and concentrate to about 5 ml; (2) 0.025% rutin in methanol.

Spray the plate with Spray Reagent A and examine in ultraviolet light 366 nm.

Major bands relative to rutin are approximately as follows: green 2.0, orange 1.75, white 1.4, pale yellowish-orange 1.0.

QUANTITATIVE STANDARDS

Foreign Matter
Not more than 2%   Appendix 3

Total Ash
Not more than 12%   Appendix 4

Ash Insoluble in Hydrochloric Acid
Not more than 2%   Appendix 5

Water-soluble Extractive
Not less than 15%   Appendix 7

MATERIAL OF COMMERCE Wild Carrot is usually supplied in the cut or crushed condition. It is obtained mainly from Europe and North America.

Powdered Wild Carrot

Complies with the requirements for Identification and Quantitative Standards stated for Wild Carrot.

Characteristic Features
Yellowish-green powder with a faint aromatic odour and a slightly bitter taste. Fragments of leaf and stem epidermis with wavy anticlinal walls and anomocytic stomata; long unicellular covering trichomes; fragments of petals and sepals with outer epidermal cells of wavy anticlinal walls and papillose inner epidermis; ovoid pollen grains, equatorially constricted.

ACTION Diuretic.

WILD CHERRY BARK
Rosaceae

Pruni serotinae cortex

Synonym: Virginian Prune Bark, Wild Black Cherry Bark.

Wild Cherry Bark consists of the dried bark of *Prunus serotina* Ehrh.

CHARACTERISTICS

Macroscopical Description
Irregular pieces, flat or slightly transversely curved. Young bark 2-5 mm thick, up to 12 cm long and 5 cm wide; surface smooth, somewhat glossy, reddish-brown to brownish-black, numerous small, almost round lenticels; cork thin, papery, variably covered with light grey to greyish-black crustaceous or, less frequently, thalloid lichen; cortex, exposed by exfoliated cork, greenish-brown, finely granular, bearing lenticel scars. Older bark up to 12-15 mm thick, pieces smaller and irregular, surface dark brown to almost black, extremely rough and uneven, randomly fissured. Inner surface of both young and older bark cinnamon-brown, lustreless, fine, slightly undulating longitudinal striations, many pieces with conspicuous open network of longitudinally elongated fissures, infrequent small, thin, patches of off-white wood, especially on younger bark; fracture short, granular, uneven, with very short projections; transverse surface of younger bark predominantly phloem and cortex, cork very thin; older bark, paler phloem rather less than half total thickness, sharply demarcated from extensive dense, nearly black outer layers.
Bark from which variable amounts of outer tissues have been mechanically removed sometimes occurs; known as 'rossed' bark.

Microscopical Description
Several layers of thin-walled cork cells, sometimes with associated fungal hyphae, in older bark extensive, variable rhytidome; two or three layers of small-celled, rounded collenchyma with chloroplasts; narrow cortex, small thin-walled parenchyma; few cluster crystals up to about 25 μm and more numerous cuboid prisms of variable size, up to about 70 μm, of calcium oxalate; thick-walled sclereids with branched pits, lumen often very narrow, singly or usually in dense groups, individual sclereids irregularly shaped, most with short projections or more-obviously branched; infrequent, only moderately thickened, sparsely pitted, lignified fibres; few small, rounded starch granules; phloem with sinuous medullary rays, three to four, or occasionally up to eight, cells wide, starch granules present; random radially elongated lacunae; sieve tissue small-celled with numerous sclereid groups, cuboid prisms and, in smaller number, cluster crystals; inner zone of small-celled sieve tissue traversed by somewhat narrower medullary rays; occasional fragments of narrow, very small-celled cambiform tissue. Xylem, if present, small thick-walled fibres and scattered bordered-pitted vessels, singly or in groups of two or three.

Odour and Taste
Odour slight, stronger when moistened, reminiscent of bitter almonds; taste bitter, astringent, aromatic.

IDENTIFICATION

Carry out the method for Thin-layer Chromatography as described in Appendix 1, using Solvent System E.

Apply 20 μl of the following solution to the plate; extract 5 g powdered Wild Cherry Bark with 20 ml methanol by warming on a water-bath for 20 minutes, cool and filter.

Spray the plate with Spray Reagent F, followed by a separate application of 5 ml potassium hydroxide solution and examine in daylight.

Major bands relative to the solvent front are approximately as follows: brown 0.8, brown 0.6, brown 0.4.

QUANTITATIVE STANDARDS

Foreign Matter
Not more than 2%   Appendix 3

Total Ash
Not more than 4%   Appendix 4

Ash Insoluble in Hydrochloric Acid
Not more than 1%   Appendix 5

Water-soluble Extractive
Not less than 6%   Appendix 7

MATERIAL OF COMMERCE Wild Cherry Bark is supplied in large pieces. It is harvested in early autumn and obtained from the USA.

Powdered Wild Cherry Bark

Complies with the requirements for Identification and Quantitative Standards stated for Wild Cherry Bark.

Characteristic Features
Fawnish-brown, somewhat gritty powder with the odour and taste of bitter almonds; abundant irregularly-shaped thick-walled sclereids with numerous branched pits; large prisms and smaller cluster crystals of calcium oxalate; cork fragments, some with associated fungal hyphae; rounded, simple starch granules; occasional fibres with moderately thickened walls; infrequent groups of fibres, vessels and lignified parenchyma from the adherent wood.

ACTION Antitussive.

WILD LETTUCE   Compositae

Lactucae folium

Synonym: Lactuca.

Wild Lettuce consists of the dried leaves of *Lactuca virosa* L.

CHARACTERISTICS

Macroscopical Description
Leaves ovate-oblong, thin and brittle; radical leaves up to 30 cm long, margin dentate, apex obtuse and base decurrent forming a stalk-like portion; stem leaves smaller, sessile, more or less deeply pinnatifid with a markedly serrate to dentate margin, obtuse apex and cordate base. Upper surface yellowish-green, lower surface greyish-green, both surfaces glabrous but on the lower surface prominent bristles occur along the mid-rib and the main veins.

Microscopical Description
Cells of upper epidermis with wavy to sinuous anticlinal walls, those on the lower epidermis more wavy; anomocytic stomata on both surfaces; brown, glandular trichomes along veins of lower surface showing considerable variation in size, each having a

multicellular, multiseriate stalk tapering to a small globular head of two to four cells; the larger trichomes which form the conspicuous bristles have a central core of lignified cells in the stalk, narrow latex vessels occur associated with the vascular tissue.

Odour and Taste
Slight odour; bitter and acrid taste.

IDENTIFICATION

Carry out the method for Thin-layer Chromatography as described in Appendix 1, using Solvent System A.

Apply 20 µl of each of the following solutions separately to the plate: (1) extract 1 g powdered Wild Lettuce with 10 ml methanol on a water-bath for 10-15 minutes cool and filter; (2) 0.025% rutin in methanol.

Spray the plate with Spray Reagent A and examine in ultraviolet light 366 nm.

Major bands relative to rutin are approximately as follows: blue 1.85, white 1.75, reddish-orange 1.4, orange 1.25.

QUANTITATIVE STANDARDS

Foreign Matter
Not more than 2%   Appendix 3

Total Ash
Not more than 10%   Appendix 4

Ash Insoluble in Hydrochloric Acid
Not more than 3%   Appendix 5

Water-soluble Extractive
Not less than 25%   Appendix 7

MATERIAL OF COMMERCE Wild Lettuce is supplied in the cut or crushed condition. It is obtained from European countries including the UK.

Powdered Wild Lettuce

Complies with the requirements for Identification and Quantitative Standards stated for Wild Lettuce.

Characteristic Features
Mid to dark green powder with a faint odour and a bitter, acrid taste; fragments of lamina showing wavy-walled epidermal cells and anomocytic stomata; small glandular trichomes attached to veins on lower surface groups of lignified parenchymatous cells from larger trichomes; fragments of vessels with annularly thickened walls and often associated with dark-brown, narrow strands of latex tissue.

ACTION Sedative.

WILD THYME   Labiatae

Serpylli herba

Synonyms: Mother of Thyme, Creeping Thyme, Serpyllum, Serpolet.

Wild Thyme consists of the dried aerial parts of *Thymus serpyllum* L. sensu latiore, harvested when the plant is in flower.

CHARACTERISTICS

Macroscopical Description
   Stems Very slender, much branched, obscurely quadrangular; green, reddish-brown or purplish, occasionally dark brown, hard and woody; markedly hairy, sometimes more so on two opposite sides.
   Leaves Opposite, 4-6 mm long by 2-4 mm broad, elliptical to ovate; somewhat thick and leathery with an obtuse apex and cuneate base, shortly petiolate; margin entire and prominently ciliate, particularly near the base; upper surface dark green, lower surface paler, both surfaces more or less glabrous but markedly punctate; midrib and two lateral veins prominent on the lower surfaces.
   Inflorescence Flowers usually six to

twelve, in rounded or ovoid, terminal heads. Calyx tubular, 3.5-4 mm long, two-lipped with the upper lip divided forming three more or less equal teeth, the lower lip with two narrow, elongated teeth edged with long cilia; green at the base with purple ribs, teeth purple; inner surface strongly pubescent. Corolla purple-violet, about 3 mm broad, tubular at the base, two-lipped, the lower lip with three lobes, upper lip slightly notched; inner surface of tube strongly pubescent. Stamens four, epipetalous; carpels two, joined, with a long style and bifid stigma.

Microscopical Description
   Stem Epidermal cells usually containing purple pigment, polygonal or longitudinally elongated in surface view with slightly thickened and beaded walls and a striated cuticle; occasional diacytic stomata and abundant uniseriate covering trichomes composed of one or two cells, wide at the base and tapering rapidly to the apex, walls thickened and somewhat warty; cortex parenchymatous; pericyclic fibres with moderately thickened and pitted walls; central vascular cylinder with small vessels show-

ing annular or spiral thickening or, occasionally, with bordered pits.

Leaf Dorsiventral, the palisade composed of two layers with the cells of the inner layer smaller and more loosely packed; cells of the upper epidermis sinuous to wavy in surface view with slightly thickened and beaded walls, those of the lower epidermis more wavy and with evenly thickened walls; diacytic stomata on both surfaces but more numerous on the lower; covering trichomes on both epidermises and along the margins, the majority short, unicellular, conical with thickened and warty walls but those on the underside of the midrib and along the margins at the base of the leaf very long, uniseriate, composed of up to eight cells, slightly swollen at the joints, with moderately thickened walls and frequently with groups of fine needle crystals in the lumen; glandular trichomes very abundant on both epidermises, of two types, multicellular and capitate; multicellular type with a small, rounded, unicellular stalk embedded in the epidermis and a large globular head composed of a number of indistinct, radiating cells containing brown secretion and with the common cuticle raised to form a bladder, the epidermal cells surrounding the stalk arranged to form a rosette; capitate glands much smaller with a unicellular stalk and a unicellular, spherical or ovoid head.

Flower Calyx outer epidermis composed of slightly sinuous cells with thin walls and a striated cuticle; occasional stomata, numerous multicellular and capitate glandular trichomes and abundant uniseriate covering trichomes with two to four cells, which also occur on the inner epidermis at the base of the teeth; teeth with purple pigment and fringed with long covering trichomes similar to those on the leaf margins; corolla purple-violet, the outer epidermis with covering and glandular trichomes similar to those on the calyx, inner surface papillose; pollen grains spherical, about 35-40 μm in diameter, with six pores, indistinct furrows and a slightly warty exine.

Odour and Taste
Odour strong, characteristic, aromatic; taste aromatic, camphoraceous and slightly bitter.

IDENTIFICATION

Carry out the method for Thin-layer Chromatography as described in Appendix 1, using Solvent System C.

Apply 60 μl of each of the following solutions to the plate: (1) extract 1 g powdered Wild Thyme by shaking with 10 ml dichloromethane for 20 minutes. Filter, evaporate the filtrate just to dryness and dissolve the residue in 1 ml toluene; (2) 0.1% cineole in toluene.

Spray the plate with Spray Reagent D, heat at 105°C for 10-15 minutes and examine in daylight.

Major bands relative to cineole are approximately as follows: purple 2.15, purple 2.0, blue 1.4, pink 1.15, grey 0.7, grey 0.45.

QUANTITATIVE STANDARDS

Foreign Matter
Not more than 2%   Appendix 3

Total Ash
Not more than 10%   Appendix 4

Ash Insoluble in Hydrochloric Acid
Not more than 4%   Appendix 5

Water-soluble Extractive
Not less than 10%   Appendix 7

MATERIAL OF COMMERCE Wild Thyme is supplied in cut or broken condition. It is obtained from European countries including the UK, and particularly from Balkan countries.

Powdered Wild Thyme

Complies with the requirements for Identification and Quantitative Standards stated for Wild Thyme.

ACTION Expectorant.

WILD YAM

Dioscoreaceae

Dioscoreae villosae rhizoma

Synonyms: Colic Root, Rheumatism Root.

Wild Yam root consists of the dried rhizome and roots of *Dioscorea villosa* L. [*D. paniculata* Michx.].

CHARACTERISTICS

Macroscopical Description
Rhizome Curved, compressed, cylindrical tuber with lateral branching. Pale brown, scaly outer surface; stem scars on upper surface, slender fibrous roots or root scars on lower; pale cream inner surface with small scattered yellow areas.

Microscopical Description
Rhizome Thin-walled, exfoliating epidermal cells of yellowish cork; outer ground tissue parenchymatous, remainder lignified, pitted parenchyma; numerous scattered collateral vascular bundles containing lignified, pitted tracheids and tracheidal vessels, some associated with thin-walled fibres with acute apices, all 10-15 µm in diameter. Cells of ground tissue packed with oval and spherical starch granules, up to 25 µm in length.
Root Thin-walled, yellowish epidermal cells; lignified, pitted cortical parenchyma; sclereid-like endodermal cells with inner and radial walls heavily thickened and lightly lignified, contain brown cell contents; stele, outer ring of thick-walled, striated, lignified, pitted fibres; alternating groups of phloem and narrow xylem conducting elements; inner ring of single tracheids/tracheidal vessels, about 30 µm diameter; lignified, pitted pith parenchyma. Starch granules infrequent.

Odour and Taste
No distinctive odour; taste initially starchy, later bitter and acrid.

IDENTIFICATION

Carry out the method for Thin-layer Chromatography as described in Appendix 1, using Solvent System B, allowing the solvent to ascend 13.5 cm.
Apply 40 µl of each of the following solutions separately to the plate: (1) extract 2 g powdered Wild Yam by heating under reflux with 10 ml ethanol (70%) for 10 minutes, cool and filter. The clear filtrate is evaporated to approximately 5 ml; (2) 0.1% aescin in methanol.
Spray the plate with Spray Reagent D, heat at 105°C for 10 minutes and examine in daylight.
Major bands relative to aescin are approximately as follows: grey 0.6, grey 0.45.
There is a characteristic series of approximately eight light brown bands in the range 1.5-0.85.

QUANTITATIVE STANDARDS

Foreign Matter
Not more than 2%   Appendix 3

Total Ash
Not more than 8%   Appendix 4

Ash Insoluble in Hydrochloric Acid
Not more than 3%   Appendix 5

Water-soluble Extractive
Not less than 15%   Appendix 7

MATERIAL OF COMMERCE Wild Yam is supplied in cut or broken condition. It is obtained from eastern and central USA.

Powdered Wild Yam

Complies with the requirements for Identification and Quantitative Standards stated for Wild Yam.

Characteristic Features
Greyish-fawn powder with bitter and acrid taste; majority of cells lignified; abundant rectangular and hexagonal pitted parenchyma; narrow tracheids and tracheidal vessels with pitted thickening; thin and thick-walled pitted fibres; thin-walled yellow cork cells; occasional groups of non-lignified parenchyma; numerous free and embedded spherical and oval starch granules; needles of calcium oxalate very rare.

ACTION Spasmolytic, anti-inflammatory.

WILLOW BARK Salicaceae

Salicis cortex

Willow Bark consists of the dried bark from young branches of *Salix alba* L., or other suitable *Salix* species, such as *S. purpurea* L., *S. daphoides* Vill., *S. fragilis* L., *S. pentandra* L. collected in early spring.

CHARACTERISTICS

Macroscopical Description
Channelled pieces of varying length, 1-2 cm wide and 1-2 mm thick; younger bark outer surface greenish-brown, smooth, slightly wrinkled longitudinally; older bark yellowish-brown to dark brown, rugged surface, irregularly wrinkled; inner surface fawn to dull cinnamon brown to pale reddish-brown, very finely longitudinally striated; fracture short and inconspicuously fibrous in the inner part; easily split longitudinally.

Microscopical Description
Two or three rows of poorly developed cork cells with thickened outer walls; cortex of collenchymatous and parenchymatous cells, the latter containing cluster crystals of calcium oxalate, 20-25 µm in diameter, and occasionally tannin; phloem characterized by tangential groups of lignified fibres associated with a crystal sheath containing prismatic crystals of calcium oxalate; simple, rounded starch granules 6-8 µm in diameter in the parenchymatous cells of the phloem and medullary rays.

Odour and Taste
Slight aromatic odour; astringent and slightly bitter taste.

IDENTIFICATION

Carry out the method for Thin-layer Chromatography as described in Appendix 1, using Solvent System B.

Apply 20 µl of each of the following solutions separately to the plate: (1) extract 1 g powdered Willow Bark with 10 ml methanol on a water-bath for 10-15 minutes, cool and filter; (2) 0.05% aescin in methanol.

Spray the plate with Spray Reagent C, heat at 105°C for 5-10 minutes then examine in daylight.

Major bands relative to aescin are approximately as follows: purple 2.0, purple 1.1, greenish-brown 0.7.

QUANTITATIVE STANDARDS

Foreign Matter
Not more than 3%   Appendix 3

Total Ash
Not more than 10%   Appendix 4

Ash Insoluble in Hydrochloric Acid
Not more than 3%   Appendix 5

Water-soluble Extractive
Not less than 10%   Appendix 7

MATERIAL OF COMMERCE Willow Bark is supplied as channelled pieces or broken pieces. It is obtained from European countries, including the UK, and particularly from south-eastern Europe.

Powdered Willow Bark

Complies with the requirements for Identification and Quantitative Standards stated for Willow Bark.

Characteristic Features
Light brown powder with a slight aromatic odour and an astringent, slightly bitter taste; numerous groups of lignified fibres accompanied by a crystal sheath containing prismatic crystals of calcium oxalate; abundant cluster crystals of calcium oxalate; fragments of pale yellowish-brown thick-walled cork cells; slightly thickened yellowish brown parenchymatous cells.

ACTION Anti-inflammatory.

WORMWOOD Compositae

Absinthii herba

Synonym: Absinthium.

Wormwood consists of the dried leaves and flowering tops of *Artemisia absinthium* L.

CHARACTERISTICS

Macroscopical Description

Stems Grooved and angled, brownish-green, the younger ones covered with a silky, grey pubescence, creamy white internally.

Leaves 2.5-10 cm long, those of the rosettes and the lower and middle parts of the stem two or three pinnate and shortly petiolate, uppermost leaves undivided and sessile; segments up to about 6 mm wide, linear to oblong, apex obtuse, margin entire or toothed; greyish-green, both surfaces densely pubescent.

Flower-heads Drooping, greenish-yellow, numerous, subspherical, 3-5 mm in diameter, arranged in much-branched racemose panicles; involucre covered with grey, silky hairs, the outer bracts linear, inner layer ovate, blunt at the apex with scarious margins; receptacle with very long, white hairs; marginal florets few, ligulate and female; central florets numerous, tubular and hermaphrodite.

Microscopical Description

Stem Epidermal cells longitudinally elongated with occasional stomata and numerous covering and glandular trichomes similar to those on the leaf; cortex narrow, with several outer layers of collenchyma and inner parenchyma; endodermis clearly defined; numerous vascular bundles arranged in a ring, separated by narrow bands of lignified and pitted parenchyma, each bundle with a dense cap of lignified pericyclic fibres, a small group of thin-walled phloem and a lignified xylem with narrow medullary rays and composed mainly of fibres with vessels and parenchyma in radial rows towards the inside; larger vessels with very numerous, closely-arranged bordered pits, with slit-shaped openings, smaller vessels spirally and annularly thickened; fibres long, thick-walled, with numerous pits; pith parenchymatous, with moderately thickened and pitted walls.

Leaf Dorsiventral, the palisade cells fairly large and loosely packed; upper epidermal cells sinuous to wavy in surface view, lower epidermal cells more wavy; large, slightly raised anomocytic stomata rare on the upper surface, very numerous on the lower; covering trichomes abundant on both epidermises and frequently forming felted masses, individual trichomes T-form with a short uniseriate stalk of one to three small cells and a very long, undulating head cell, tapering at the ends; large glandular trichomes also abundant, each with a short, biseriate two-celled stalk and a biseriate head with two or, occasionally, four cells, with the common cuticle raised to form a bladder.

Flower Epidermis of the bracts composed of longitudinally elongated cells with scattered stomata and densely covered with T-form trichomes as on the leaf, glandular trichomes also abundant; elongated stone cells in the central region, particularly near the base; epidermis of the corolla of the tubular florets with glandular trichomes, mesophyll containing numerous small cluster crystals of calcium oxalate; pollen grains spheroidal, about 30 μm in diameter, with three distinct pores and a finely warty exine; receptacle hairs, each with a small cell forming a stalk and a very long, cylindrical and thin-walled terminal cell, up to 1.5 mm long.

Odour and Taste

Odour strongly aromatic and characteristic; taste aromatic and intensely bitter.

IDENTIFICATION

Carry out the method for Thin-layer Chromatography as described in Appendix 1, using Solvent System A.

Apply 20 μl of each of the following solutions separately to the plate: (1) extract 1 g powdered Wormwood with 10 ml methanol by warming on a water-bath for 10-15 minutes, cool and filter; (2) 0.025% rutin in methanol.

Spray the plate with Spray Reagent A and examine in ultraviolet light 366 nm.

Major bands relative to rutin are approximately as follows: turquoise 2.1, turquoise

1.8, turquoise 1.3, yellow 1.0. There is an area of yellow fine detail below 1.0.

QUANTITATIVE STANDARDS

Foreign Matter
Not more than 2%   Appendix 3

Total Ash
Not more than 10%   Appendix 4

Ash Insoluble in Hydrochloric Acid
Not more than 1.5%   Appendix 5

Water-soluble Extractive
Not less than 15%   Appendix 7

MATERIAL OF COMMERCE Wormwood is supplied in the cut or broken condition. It is obtained mainly from eastern European countries.

Powdered Wormwood

Complies with the requirements for Identification and Quantitative Standards stated for Wormwood.

Characteristic Features
Greenish-yellow with an aromatic odour and a very bitter and lingering taste; abundant T-shaped covering trichomes, scattered, and in felted masses or attached to fragments of the epidermis of the leaves, stems and bracts; leaf epidermis with sinuous to wavy walls, anomocytic stomata and large, biseriate glandular trichomes; groups of fibres, some associated with pitted parenchyma; larger vessels with small, bordered pits, smaller vessels with spiral or annular thickening, pith parenchyma with moderately thickened and pitted walls; corolla fragments containing small cluster crystals of calcium oxalate; numerous spheroidal pollen grains, often forming dense groups; occasional, long, cylindrical covering trichomes of the receptacle.

ACTION Bitter.

YARROW   Compositae

Millefolii herba

Synonyms: Millefolium, Milfoil.

Yarrow consists of the dried aerial parts of *Achillea millefolium* L. sensu latiore, collected during the flowering season.

CHARACTERISTICS

Macroscopical Description
   Stems Furrowed, usually unbranched, 40 cm or more long, distinctly woolly, pale green, sometimes purplish.
   Leaves Lanceolate, up to about 15 cm long, two to three pinnate with the ultimate segments linear and subulate, pale greyish-green and covered with long white hairs; lower leaves with a short petiole, upper leaves sessile and often with two or three small axillary leaves at the base.
   Flowers Numerous, in dense terminal corymbs about 3-4 cm in diameter, each

capitulum about 0.5 cm in diameter with an ovoid involucre composed of two rows of oblong, hairy bracts, each with a dark brown to black scarious margin; five white, pink or reddish ray florets and several white or cream disc florets; achenes 2 mm long, shiny, greyish-brown, slightly curved.

Microscopical Description
   Stem Epidermal cells axially elongated with occasional anomocytic stomata and a faintly striated cuticle; abundant covering and scattered glandular trichomes, the covering trichomes uniseriate, composed of four or five small, more or less isodiametric cells at the base and a much elongated, thick-walled end cell tapering to a point; glandular trichomes of the Compositae type with a short stalk and a head formed of two rows of cells enclosed in a bladder-like membrane; cortex narrow, parenchymatous with several layers of collenchyma in the ridges;

numerous vascular bundles, arranged in a ring in transverse section, each with a small group of phloem and a wide cap of thick-walled, lignified pericyclic fibres which, in older stems, join to form a continuous band; xylem groups lignified and composed of small vessels with spiral and annular thickening and numerous fibres; parenchymatous cells of outer pith lignified and pitted, those of the central region unlignified and sometimes collapsed in older stems forming a hollow.

Leaf Isobilateral, with the palisades composed of one to three layers; upper and lower epidermal cells with sinuous anticlinal walls and numerous anomocytic stomata; abundant covering trichomes and scattered glandular trichomes, similar to those on the stem, occur on both epidermises.

Flower Epidermal cells of bracts, longitudinally elongated, thin-walled, filled with dark brown striated pigment, scattered covering trichomes and occasional stomata; the inner central region composed of elongated cells with lignified and finely pitted walls. Corolla of the ray floret with the epidermis of the ligule composed of wavy-walled cells with rounded papillae; the epidermis of the tubular florets with rectangular cells and a small group of pitted stone cells at the base; cells of the ovary wall longitudinally elongated with a finely striated cuticle; corolla of the disc floret composed of rectangular cells with moderately thickened walls; numerous small cluster crystals of calcium oxalate occur in the corolla tube of both ray and disc florets. Pollen grains spherical, 30-35 μm in diameter, with a spiny exine and three distinct pores.

Odour and Taste
Slight fragrant odour; bitter, faintly aromatic taste.

IDENTIFICATION

Carry out the method for Thin-layer Chromatography as described in Appendix 1, using Solvent System A.

Apply 20 μl of each of the following solutions separately to the plate: (1) extract 1 g powdered Yarrow with 10 ml methanol on a water-bath for 5 minutes, cool and filter; (2) 0.025% rutin in methanol.

Spray the plate with Spray Reagent A and examine in ultraviolet light 366 nm.

Major bands relative to rutin are approximately as follows: pale blue 1.75, orange 1.33, blue 1.2, orange 1.1, orange 0.9.

QUANTITATIVE STANDARDS

Foreign Matter
Not more than 2%   Appendix 3

Total Ash
Not more than 10%   Appendix 4

Ash Insoluble in Hydrochloric Acid
Not more than 2.5%   Appendix 5

Water-soluble Extractive
Not less than 15%   Appendix 7

MATERIAL OF COMMERCE Yarrow is supplied in the broken, crushed or chopped condition. It is obtained from European countries, including the UK, and especially from eastern and south-eastern Europe.

Powdered Yarrow

Complies with the requirements for Identification and Quantitative Standards stated for Yarrow.

Characteristic Features
Greyish-green powder with a slight fragrant odour and a bitter, faintly aromatic taste; epidermal fragments of stem and leaf with abundant covering trichomes and less numerous glandular trichomes, the covering trichomes frequently broken off and occurring scattered; groups of thick-walled, lignified fibres from the pericycle and xylem, those of the xylem sometimes associated with small vessels with spiral and annular thickening; lignified, pitted parenchyma from the pith; dark brown fragments of the membranous margins of the bracts and groups of lignified and pitted elongated cells from the central region; occasional fragments of the papillose epidermis of the ligulate florets; small-celled parenchyma containing cluster crystals of calcium oxalate; pollen grains with a spiny exine .

ACTION Diaphoretic.

APPENDICES

Where indicated by corresponding references, the Methods of Analysis and Reagents described are those of the European Pharmacopoeia Second Edition (Ph.Eur.2) or of the British Pharmacopoeia 1993 (BP 1993).

The kind permission of the European Pharmacopoeia Commission and the Controller of Her Majesty's Stationery Office (with respect to the British Pharmacopoeia) to reproduce the relevant texts is gratefully acknowledged.

METHODS OF ANALYSIS

Appendix 1
THIN-LAYER
CHROMATOGRAPHY

Apparatus

Plates of glass or other suitable material, 20 cm long and of suitable width for the application of test solutions and reference solutions prescribed in the monographs, commercially coated with suitable Silica Gel. Alternatively, similar chromatoplates may be prepared in the laboratory, following the supplier's instructions for the coating substance and using a suitable spreading device, provided that consistent results can be achieved.

A transparent chromatographic tank, of sufficient size for the plates to be used, preferably of glass with a ground glass fitting lid.

Method

Prepare the Solvent System prescribed in the monograph and pour into the tank to a depth not exceeding 15 mm. Line the walls of the tank with filter paper, moistening the paper with the solvent, then close the lid and allow to stand for about one hour at room temperature to achieve saturated conditions. If the monograph specifies that non-saturated conditions should be used, then the method should be followed with the exception that the tank should not be lined with filter paper and the Solvent System should be added immediately prior to placing the plate in the tank.

Apply the prescribed solutions to the adsorbent with a suitable applicator, as bands 2 cm long and 1-3 mm wide, on a line parallel to, and 20 mm from, the lower edge of the plate. No band should be nearer than 20 mm to the sides of the plate and bands should be separated by at least 15 mm. Mark the sides of the plate at 15 cm, or the distance prescribed in the monograph, above the line of application.

Allow the solvent to evaporate then place the plate in the tank, as nearly vertical as possible, ensuring that the line of applied bands is above the level of the solvent. Replace the lid tightly and allow the tank to stand at a stable temperature, about 20° C, preferably in subdued light, until the solvent has ascended the plate to the marks.

After removal of the plate from the tank, allow the solvent to evaporate completely, in a current of warm air if necessary.

Visualisation

Examine the plate in daylight and then proceed as prescribed in the monograph. When a spraying technique is prescribed, the reagent should be evenly applied as a fine spray.

Record the colour of the bands and their position relative to the marker or markers.

Solvent Systems

Solvent System A A mixture of ethyl acetate: anhydrous formic acid: glacial acetic acid: water (100:11:11:27).

Solvent System B A mixture of chloroform: methanol: water (64:50:10).

Solvent System C: a mixture of toluene: ethylacetate (93:7).

Solvent System D: a mixture of toluene: ether: 1.75M acetic acid (1:1:1) is shaken in a separating funnel for 5 minutes. The upper phase is retained as the solvent system. This system should be freshly prepared.

Solvent System E: a mixture of ethyl acetate: methanol: water (100:10:10).

Other solvent systems, where prescribed, are specified in individual monographs.

Spray Reagents

Spray Reagent A A 1% w/v solution of diphenylboric acid 2-aminoethyl ester in methanol, followed by separate application of a 5% w/v solution of polyethylene glycol 4000 in ethanol (96%).

Spray Reagent B A solution of 1% w/v iodine and 1% w/v potassium iodide in ethanol (96%), followed by separate application of a mixture of equal volumes of ethanol (96%) and 8M hydrochloric acid.

Spray Reagent C Mix 0.5 ml of anisaldehyde with 10 ml of glacial acetic acid, 85 ml of methanol and 5 ml of sulphuric acid, in that order.

The reagent should be freshly prepared.

Spray Reagent D Either a 5% v/v solution of sulphuric acid in ethanol (96%), followed immediately by separate application of a 1% w/v solution of vanillin in ethanol (96%).
or Dissolve 0. 3 g of vanillin in 85 ml of methanol and add 3 ml of sulphuric acid.
The reagent should be freshly prepared.

Spray Reagent E A 1% w/v solution of vanillin in 50% v/v aqueous orthophosphoric acid.
The reagent should be freshly prepared.

Spray Reagent F A 0.5% w/v solution of fast blue BB salt in water.

Dragendorff's Reagent and Ninhydrin Reagent are listed under Reagents.

Appendix 2
LOSS ON DRYING
Ph.Eur.2 V.6.22.

Loss on drying is the loss of mass expressed as per cent *m/m*.
Method - Place the prescribed quantity of the substance to be examined in a weighing bottle previously dried under the conditions prescribed for the substance to be examined. Dry the substance to constant mass or for the prescribed time by one of the following procedures.
a) "in a desiccator": the drying is carried out over diphosphorus pentoxide R at atmospheric pressure and at room temperature;
b) *"in vacuo"*: the drying is carried out over diphosphorus pentoxide R, at a pressure of 1.5 kPa to 2.5 kPa* at room temperature;
c) *"in vacuo"* within a specified temperature range: the drying is carried out over diphosphorus pentoxide R, at a pressure of 1.5 kPa to 2.5 kPa* within the temperature range specified in the monograph. If the drying is carried out at a temperature above 100°C the temperature range within which the desiccant is to be maintained is also specified;
d) "in an oven" within a specified temperature range: the drying is carried out in an oven within the temperature range specified in the monograph.
If other conditions are prescribed, the procedure to be used is described in full in the individual monograph.

* 1.5 kPa to 2.5 kPa is equivalent to 11 Torr to 19 Torr.

Appendix 3
FOREIGN MATTER
Ph.Eur.2 V.4.2.

Vegetable drugs should be free from moulds, insects and other animal contamination.
Unless otherwise prescribed, the amount of foreign matter is not more than 2 per cent *m/m*.
Foreign matter is material consisting of any or all of the following:
1) *Foreign organs*: matter coming from the source plant but not defined as the drug,
2) *Foreign elements*: matter not coming from the source plant and either of vegetable or mineral origin.

DETERMINATION OF FOREIGN MATTER
Weigh 100 g to 500 g of the substance to be examined or the minimum quantity prescribed in the monograph, and spread it out in a thin layer. The foreign matter should be detected by inspection with the unaided eye or by use of a lens (6 x). Separate and weigh it, and calculate the percentage present.

Appendix 4
TOTAL ASH
Ph.Eur.2 V.3.2.16.

Heat a silica or platinum crucible to redness for 30 min, allow to cool in a desiccator and weigh. Unless otherwise prescribed, evenly distribute 1.00 g of the substance or the powdered vegetable drug to be examined in the crucible. Dry at 100°C - 105°C for 1 h and ignite to constant mass in a muffle furnace at 600 ± 25 °C, allowing the crucible to cool in a desiccator after each ignition. Flames should not be produced at any time during the procedure. If after prolonged ignition, the ash still contains black particles, take up with hot water, filter through an ashless filter paper and ignite the residue and the filter paper. Combine the filtrate with the ash, carefully evaporate to dryness and ignite to constant mass.

Appendix 5

ASH INSOLUBLE IN HYDROCHLORIC ACID

Ph.Eur.2 V.4.1.

Ash insoluble in hydrochloric acid is the residue obtained after extracting the sulphated or total ash with hydrochloric acid R, calculated with reference to 100 g of drug.

To the crucible containing the residue from the determination of sulphated or total ash, add 15 ml of water and 10 ml of hydrochloric acid R, cover with a watch glass, boil the mixture gently for 10 min and allow to cool. Filter through an ashless filter, wash the residue with hot water until the filtrate is neutral, dry, ignite to dull redness, allow to cool in a desiccator and weigh. Reheat until the difference between two consecutive weighings is not more than 1 mg.

Appendix 6A

ETHANOL-SOLUBLE EXTRACTIVE

BP 1993 Appendix XI B

Macerate 5 g of the air-dried drug, coarsely powdered, with 100 ml of ethanol of the specified strength in a closed flask for 24 hours, shaking frequently during the first 6 hours and then allowing to stand for 18 hours. Filter rapidly, taking precautions against loss of ethanol, evaporate 20 ml of the filtrate to dryness in a tared, flat-bottomed, shallow dish and dry at 105° to constant weight. Calculate the percentage of ethanol-soluble extractive with reference to the air-dried drug.

BHP Note: 'Coarsely powdered' means that all particles pass through a sieve of nominal mesh aperture 1700 μm and not more than 40% by weight pass through a sieve of nominal mesh aperture 355 μm.

Appendix 6B

ETHANOL-INSOLUBLE RESIDUE

Macerate 5 g of powdered, air-dried drug with 100 ml of ethanol of the specified strength in a closed flask for 24 hours, shaking frequently during the first 6 hours and then allowing to stand for 18 hours. Filter and wash the residue with 5 ml of ethanol of the same strength. Dry the residue at 105°C to constant weight. Calculate the percentage of ethanol-insoluble residue with reference to the air-dried drug.

Appendix 7

WATER-SOLUBLE EXTRACTIVE

BP 1993 Appendix XI C

Proceed as directed for *ethanol-soluble extractive*, but using *chloroform water* in place of ethanol.

Appendix 8

SWELLING INDEX

Ph.Eur.2 V.4.4.

The swelling index is the volume in millilitres occupied by 1 gram of a drug, including any adhering mucilage, after it has swollen in an aqueous liquid for 4 h.

In a 25 ml ground-glass-stoppered cylinder graduated over a height of about 125 ± 5 mm in 0.5 ml divisions, place 1.0 g of the drug, whole or of the degree of comminution prescribed in the monograph. Unless otherwise perscribed, moisten the drug with 1.0 ml of alcohol R, add 25 ml of water and close the cylinder. Shake vigorously every 10 min for 1 h. Allow to stand for 3 h. At 1 h 30 min after the beginning of the test, release any large volumes of liquid retained in the layer of the drug and any particles of the drug floating at the surface of the liquid by rotating the cylinder about a vertical axis. Measure the volume occupied by the drug, including any adhering mucilage. Carry out three tests at the same time.

The swelling index is given by the mean of the three tests.

Appendix 9

VOLATILE OIL

Determination of Essential Oils in Vegetable Drugs
Ph.Eur.2 V.4.5.8.

The determination of essential oils in vegetable drugs is carried out by steam distillation in a special apparatus in the conditions described below. The distillate is collected in the graduated tube, using xylene to take up the essential oil; the aqueous phase is automatically returned to the distillation flask.

Apparatus. – The apparatus comprises the following parts:

(a) a suitable round-bottomed flask with a short, ground-glass neck having an internal diameter of about 29 mm at the wide end,
(b) a condenser assembly (see Figure 2) that closely fits the flask, the different parts being fused into one piece; the glass used has a low coefficient of expansion; the stopper K' is vented and the tube K has an orifice of diameter about 1 mm that coincides with the vent; the wide end of the tube K is of ground-glass and has an internal diameter of 10 mm; a pear-shaped swelling, J, of 3 ml capacity; the tube JL is graduated in 0.01 ml; above the graduation there are two circular marks H and J; the bulb-shaped swelling L has a capacity of about 2 ml; M is a three-way tap; the junction B is at a level 20 mm higher than the uppermost graduation,
(c) a suitable heating device, allowing a fine control,
(d) a vertical support with a horizontal ring covered with insulating material.

Method. – Use a thoroughly cleaned apparatus. Carry out the assay according to the nature of the drug to be examined. Place the prescribed volume of distillation liquid in the flask, add a few pieces of porous porcelain and attach the condenser assembly. Introduce water through the filling funnel N until it is at the level B. Remove the stopper K' and introduce the prescribed quantity of xylene R, using a pipette with its tip at the bottom of the tube K. Replace the stopper K' and ensure that the orifice coincides with the vent. Heat the liquid in the flask to boiling and adjust the distillation rate to 2 ml to 3 ml per minute, unless otherwise prescribed.

To determine the rate of distillation, during distillation lower the level of the water by means of the three-way tap until the meniscus is at the level of the lower mark (a) (see Figure 1). Close the tap and measure the time taken for the liquid to reach the upper mark (b). Open the tap and continue the distillation, modifying the heat to regulate the distillation rate. Distil for 30 min. Stop the heating and after at least 10 min read off the volume of xylene in the graduated tube.

Introduce into the flask the prescribed quantity of the drug and continue the distillation as described above for the time and at the rate prescribed. Stop the heating and after 10 min read the volume of liquid collected in the graduated tube and subtract the volume of xylene previously noted. The difference represents the quantity of essential oil in the mass of the drug taken. Calculate the result as millilitres per 100 g of drug.

When the essential oil is to be used for other analytical purposes, the water-free mixture of xylene and essential oil may be recovered as follows: remove the stopper K' and introduce 0.1 ml of a 0.1 per cent m/V solution of sodium fluoresceinate R and 0.5 ml of water. Lower the mixture of xylene and essential oil into the bulb-shaped swelling L by means of the three-way tap, allow to stand for 5 min and lower the mixture slowly until it just reaches the level of the tap M. Open the tap clockwise so that the water flows out of the connecting tube BM. Wash the tube with acetone R and with a little toluene R introduced through the filling funnel N. Turn the tap clockwise in order to recover the mixture of xylene and essential oil in an appropriate flask.

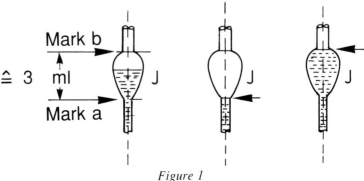

Figure 1

198

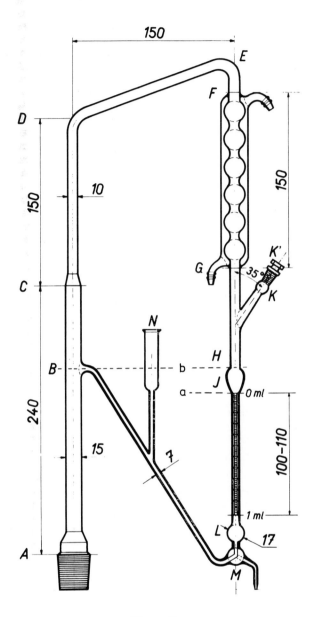

Figure 2
Apparatus for the Determination of Essential Oils
in Vegetable Drugs
Dimensions in millimetres

Appendix 10

STOMATA AND STOMATAL INDEX

Ph.Eur.2 V.4.3.

STOMATA

There are several types of stomata (see Figure), distinguished by the form and arrangement of the surrounding cells:

(1) The *anomocytic* (irregular-celled) type: the stoma is surrounded by a varying number of cells in no way differing from those of the epidermis generally,

(2) The *anisocytic* (unequal-celled) type: the stoma is usually surrounded by three subsidiary cells, of which one is markedly smaller than the others,

(3) The *diacytic* (cross-celled) type: the stoma is accompanied by two subsidiary cells, whose common wall is at right angles to the guard cells,

(4) The *paracytic* (parallel-celled) type: the stoma has on each side one or more subsidiary cells parallel to the long axis of the pore and guard cells.

STOMATAL INDEX

$$\text{Stomatal Index} = \frac{100 \times S}{E + S}$$

S = the number of stomata in a given area of leaf

E = the number of epidermal cells (including trichomes) in the same area of leaf.

For each sample of leaf make not fewer than ten determinations and calculate the mean.

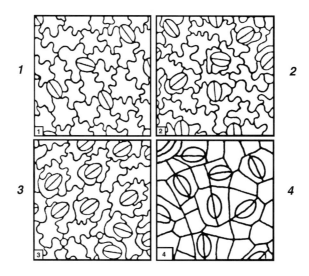

REAGENTS

Acetic Acid Solutions of molarity xM should be prepared by diluting $57x$ ml ($60x$ g) of *glacial acetic acid* to 1000 ml with *water*. †

Acetic Acid, Glacial
Analytical reagent grade of commerce. A colourless liquid with a pungent odour, about 17.5M in strength; freezing point, about 16°; weight per ml, about 1.05 g.   †

Acetone Propan-2-one; C_3H_6O = 58.08
Analytical reagent grade of commerce.
A volatile, flammable liquid; boiling point, about 56°; weight per ml, about 0.79 g.

Aescin Escin; $C_{54}H_{84}O_{23},2H_2O$ = 1138
General reagent grade of commerce.

Alcohol *See ethanol (96%).*

Ammonia NH_3 = 17.03
For 18M and 13.5M *ammonia* use analytical reagent grade solutions of commerce containing 35% and 25% w/w of NH_3 and weighing 0.88 g and 0.91 g per ml, respectively. Solutions of molarity xM should be prepared by diluting $75x$ ml of 13.5M *ammonia* or $56x$ ml of 18M *ammonia* to 1000 ml with *water*.
                                                          †

Anisaldehyde 4-Methoxybenzaldehyde;
$C_8H_8O_2$ = 136.2
General reagent grade of commerce.
A colourless to pale yellow, oily liquid with an aromatic odour; boiling point, about 248°; weight per ml, about 1.125 g.   †

Berberine Chloride $C_{20}H_{18}NO_4 \cdot Cl$ = 371.82
General reagent grade of commerce.
A bright yellow, crystalline powder.

Bismuth Subnitrate
[$4BiNO_3(OH)_2,BiO(OH)$] = 1462
A white powder, practically insoluble in *water*.

d-Bornyl Acetate $C_{12}H_{20}O_2$ = 196.3
Melting point, about 28°; $[\alpha]_D^{20}$, about +44° (10% w/v in *ethanol*).

Butan-1-ol *n*-Butyl alcohol;

$C_4H_{10}O$ = 74.12
Analytical reagent grade of commerce.
A colourless liquid; boiling point, about 117°; weight per ml, about 0.81 g.   †

Caffeine $C_8H_{10}N_4O_2$ = 194.19
General reagent grade of commerce.
White crystals or a white, crystalline powder; sublimes readily; sublimation point, 235° to 238°.

Chloroform Trichloromethane; $CHCl_3$ = 119.4
Analytical reagent grade of commerce containing 0.4 to 1.0% w/w of ethanol. A colourless liquid with a sweet, penetrating odour; boiling point, about 61°; weight per ml, about 1.48 g.   †

Chloroform Water Shake 2.5 ml of *chloroform* with 900 ml of *water* until dissolved and dilute to 1000 ml with *water*.   †

Cineole Eucalyptol; 1,8-epoxy-*p*-menthane; $C_{10}H_{18}O$ = 154.3
Use a grade of commerce specially supplied for *o*-cresol determinations.
A colourless liquid with a camphoraceous odour; boiling point, about 176°; weight per ml, about 0.92 g.   †

Copper(II) Acetate Cupric acetate;
$C_2H_6CuO_4,H_2O$ = 199.7
Analytical reagent grade of commerce.   †

Copper Acetate Solution Dissolve 50 mg of *copper(II) acetate* in sufficient *water* to produce 100 ml.

Diphenylboric Acid 2-Aminoethyl Ester
2-aminoethyl diphenyl borate;
diphenylboric acid, ethanolamine complex;
$(C_6H_5)_2BOCH_2CH_2NH_2$ = 225.10
General reagent grade of commerce.
A white, crystalline powder; melting point 192° to 194°.

Dragendorff's Reagent Dissolve 0.85 g of *bismuth subnitrate* in 40 ml of *water* and 10 ml of *glacial acetic acid*; to this add a solution of 8 g of *potassium iodide* in 20 ml of *water*.

Diphosphorus pentoxide Phosphorus pentoxide; phosphoric anhydride P_2O_5 = 142.0.

A white powder, amorphous, deliquescent. It is hydrated by *water* with the evolution of heat.

Ethanol, Absolute C_2H_6O = 46.07

Analytical reagent grade of commerce containing not less than 99.5% v/v of C_2H_6O.

A colourless, hygroscopic liquid with a characteristic odour; boiling point, about 78°; weight per ml, about 0.79 g.

Store protected from light at a temperature not exceeding 30°. †

Ethanol (96%) Analytical reagent grade ethanol of commerce containing not less than 95.1% v/v and not more than 96.9% v/v of C_2H_6O.

A colourless liquid; weight per ml, about 0.81 g.

Diluted ethanols may be prepared by diluting the volumes of *ethanol (96%)* indicated in the following table to 1000 ml with *water*. †

Strength	Volume of *ethanol (96%)* (approx)	Weight per ml
%v/v	ml	g
90	934	0.83
85	885	0.85
80	831	0.86
70	727	0.89
65	676	0.90
60	623	0.91
50	519	0.93
45	468	0.94
25	259	0.97
20	207	0.975
10	104	0.986

Ether Diethyl ether; $C_4H_{10}O$ = 74.12

Analytical reagent grade of commerce. A volatile, highly flammable, colourless liquid; boiling point, about 34°; weight per ml, about 0.71 g.

Warning It is dangerous to distil or evaporate ether to dryness unless precautions have been taken to remove peroxides.

Ethyl Acetate $C_4H_8O_2$ = 88.1

Analytical reagent grade of commerce. A colourless liquid with a fruity odour; boiling point, about 77°; weight per ml, about 0.90 g. †

Ethyl Formate $C_3H_6O_2$ = 74.08

General reagent grade of commerce.

A colourless liquid; boiling point, 52° to 54°; weight per ml, about 0.917 g.

Fast Blue BB Salt

CI 37175; 4-benzoylamino-2, 5-diethoxybenzenediazonium chloride hemi [zinc chloride] salt; $C_{17}H_{18}ClN_3O_3, \frac{1}{2}ZnCl_2$ = 415.

General reagent grade of commerce. †

Ferric Chloride $FeCl_3, 6H_2O$ = 270.3

Analytical reagent grade of commerce.

Yellowish-orange or brownish crystalline masses, deliquescent, very soluble in *water*, soluble in *alcohol* and in *ether*. On exposure to light, ferric chloride and its solutions are partly reduced.

Ferric Chloride Solution Dissolve 10 g of *ferric chloride* in sufficient *water* to produce 100 ml. The solution contains about 6.0% w/v of $FeCl_3$.

Ferric Chloride Solution, Dilute Dissolve 1.7 g of *ferric chloride* in sufficient *water* to produce 100 ml. The solution contains about 1.0% w/v of $FeCl_3$.

Formic Acid, Anhydrous CH_2O_2 = 46.03

Analytical reagent grade formic acid of commerce containing not less than 98.0% w/w of CH_2O_2.

A colourless, corrosive liquid with a pungent odour; weight per ml, about 1.22 g.

Hydrastine Hydrochloride

$C_{21}H_{21}NO_6 \cdot HCl$ = 419.9

General reagent grade of commerce.

A white, crystalline powder; melting point, about 116°.

Hygroscopic: keep well closed.

Hydrochloric Acid HCl = 36.46

Where no molarity is indicated use analytical reagent grade of commerce with a relative density of about 1.18, containing not less than 35% w/w and not more than 38% w/w of HCl and about 11.5M in strength.

A colourless, fuming liquid.

Solutions of molarity xM should be prepared by diluting $85x$ ml of *hydrochloric acid* to 1000 ml with *water*. Store in a container of polyethylene or other non-reacting material at a temperature not exceeding 30°. †

Iodine I_2 = 253.8

Analytical reagent grade of commerce.
To prepare 0.05M iodine dissolve 20 g of *potassium iodide* in the minimum amount of *water*, add 13 g of *iodine*, allow to dissolve and add sufficient *water* to produce 1000 ml. Weaker solutions should be prepared using proportionately lesser amounts of reagents or by appropriate dilution.   †

Iodine Solution Dissolve 2 g of *iodine* and 3 g of *potassium iodide* in sufficient *water* to produce 100 ml.

Lead(II) Acetate $C_4H_6O_4Pb,3H_2O = 379.3$
Analytical reagent grade of commerce.   †

Lead Acetate Solution A 9.5% w/v solution of *lead(II) acetate* in *carbon dioxide-free water*.   †

Methanol Methyl alcohol; $CH_4O = 32.04$
Analytical reagent grade of commerce.
A colourless liquid; boiling point, about 65°; weight per ml, about 0.79 g.
When '*methanol*' is followed by a percentage figure, an instruction to use *methanol* diluted with *water* to produce the specified percentage v/v of methanol is implied.   †

L-Methionine $C_5H_{11}NO_2S = 149.2$
General reagent grade of commerce.
A white, crystalline solid; $[\alpha]_D^{20}$, about + 23° (5% w/v in 1M hydrochloric acid).   †

Methyl red CI 13020;
2-(4-dimethylaminophenylazo)-benzoic acid;
$C_{15}H_{15}N_3O_2 = 269.3$
A dark-red powder or violet crystals.   †

Ninhydrin Indane-1,2,3-trione;
$C_9H_4O_3,H_2O = 178.21$
Analytical reagent grade of commerce.
A very pale yellow, crystalline powder; melting point, about 255°.
Store protected from light.   †

Ninhydrin Reagent Dissolve 30 mg of *ninhydrin* in 10 ml of *butan-1-ol* and add 0.3 ml of *glacial acetic acid*.

Orthophosphoric Acid Phosphoric acid;
$H_3PO_4 = 98.00$
Analytical reagent grade of commerce containing not less than 84% w/w of H_3PO_4 and about 15.7M in strength. A corrosive liquid; weight per ml, about 1.75 g.   †

Petroleum Spirit Petroleum ether; light petroleum
Analytical reagent grades of commerce.
Colourless, volatile, highly flammable liquids obtained from petroleum, consisting of a mixture of the lower members of the paraffin series of hydrocarbons supplied in the following fractions:
    †

boiling range,	30° to 40°;	weight per ml, about	0.63 g
boiling range,	40° to 60°;	weight per ml, about	0.64 g
boiling range,	50° to 70°;	weight per ml, about	0.66 g
boiling range,	60° to 80°;	weight per ml, about	0.67 g
boiling range,	80° to 100°;	weight per ml, about	0.70 g
boiling range,	100° to 120°;	weight per ml, about	0.72 g
boiling range,	120° to 160°;	weight per ml, about	0.75 g

Phloroglucinol Benzene-1,3,5-triol;
$C_6H_6O_3,2H_2O = 162.1$
Analytical reagent grade of commerce.
White or pale cream crystals; melting point, about 220°.

Phloroglucinol Solution Dissolve 1 g of *phloroglucinol* in sufficient *ethanol (90%)* to produce 100 ml.

Polyethylene Glycol 4000 Macrogol 4000
General reagent grade of commerce.
A white, waxy mass.
Note Polyethylene Glycol within the M_r range 3000 to 4000 will also be suitable for use as a spray reagent in thin-layer chromatography identifications

Potassium Hydroxide KOH = 56.11
Analytical reagent grade of commerce containing not less than 85.0% of total alkali calculated as KOH and not more than 2.0% of K_2CO_3.
Deliquescent pellets, sticks or slabs.
Store in an airtight container.   †

Potassium Hydroxide Solution Dissolve 5 g of *potassium hydroxide* in sufficient *water* to produce 100 ml.

Potassium Hydroxide, Ethanolic Solutions of the requisite molarity may be obtained by dissolving the appropriate amount of *potassium hydroxide* in sufficient *ethanol (96%)* to produce 1000 ml.   †

Potassium Iodide KI = 166.0
Analytical reagent grade of commerce.
A white, crystalline powder.   †

203

Propan-1-ol *n*-Propyl alcohol; $C_3H_8O = 60.10$
Analytical reagent grade of commerce.
A colourless liquid; boiling point, about 97°; weight per ml, 0.802 to 0.806 g. Not less than 95% distils between 96° and 99°. †

Quercetin 3,3', 4', 5, 7-Pentahydroxyflavone; $C_{15}H_{10}O_7 \cdot 2H_2O = 338.27$
General reagent grade of commerce.
A yellow-green, amorphous powder; melting point, above 300°.

Ruthenium Red Ammoniated ruthenium oxychloride; $H_{42}C1_6N_{14}O_2Ru_3, 4H_2O = 858$
Microscopical staining grade of commerce.
A brownish red powder. †

Ruthenium Red Solution A 0.08% w/v solution of *ruthenium red* in *lead acetate solution*. †

Rutin Vitamin P; rutoside;
3,3',4',5,7-pentahydroxy-flavone
3-rutinoside; $C_{27}H_{30}O_{16}, 3H_2O = 664.6$
General reagent grade of commerce.
A yellow, crystalline powder, darkening on exposure to light. Solutions of *rutin* used as markers in thin-layer chromatography should always be freshly prepared.

Sodium Fluoresceinate CI 45350
$C_{20}H_{10}Na_2O_5 = 376.3$
An orange-red powder, freely soluble in water. Aqueous solutions display an intense yellowish-green fluorescence.

Sodium Hydroxide NaOH = 40.00
Analytical reagent grade of commerce containing not less than 97% of total alkali calculated as NaOH and not more than 2.0% of Na_2CO_3. White, deliquescent pellets, sticks or slabs.
Store in an airtight container.

Sodium Hydroxide Solution Dissolve 10 g of *sodium hydroxide* in sufficient *water* to produce 100 ml.

Sodium Nitrite $NaNO_2 = 69.00$
Analytical reagent grade of commerce con-

taining not less than 97.0% of $NaNO_2$. †

Sodium Nitrite Solution A 10% w/v solution of *sodium nitrite*.
Prepare immediately before use. †

Sulphuric Acid $H_2SO_4 = 98.08$
When no molarity is indicated use analytical reagent grade of commerce containing about 98% w/w of sulphuric acid and about 18M in strength; an oily, corrosive liquid; weight per ml, about 1.84 g.
When solutions of molarity xM are required, they should be prepared by carefully adding $54x$ ml of *sulphuric acid* to an equal volume of *water* and diluting to 1000 ml with *water*. When '*sulphuric acid*' is followed by a percentage figure, an instruction to add, carefully, *sulphuric acid* to *water* to produce the specified percentage v/v proportion of *sulphuric acid* is implied. †

Toluene Methylbenzene; $C_7H_8 = 92.14$
Analytical reagent grade of commerce.
A colourless liquid with a characteristic odour; weight per ml, 0.865 to 0.870 g; boiling point, about 110°. †

Vanillin 4-Hydroxy-3-methoxybenzaldehyde; $C_8H_8O_3 = 152.2$
Analytical reagent grade of commerce.
White to yellowish white, needles or crystalline powder, with an odour of vanilla.
Melting point, about 81°, determined without previous drying. †

Water Purified water, prepared by distillation, ion exchange or any other appropriate method, from suitable potable water.

Water, Carbon Dioxide-free *Water* that has been boiled vigorously for a few minutes and protected from the atmosphere during cooling and storage. †

Xylene A mixture of *o*-, *m*- and *p*-isomers; $C_8H_{10} = 106.2$
Analytical reagent grade of commerce.
A colourless, clear, flammable liquid; boiling point, about 140°. †

INDEX